Contribution of FDG to Modern Medicine, Part I

Editors

SØREN HESS
POUL FLEMMING HØILUND-CARLSEN

PET CLINICS

www.pet.theclinics.com

Consulting Editor
ABASS ALAVI

October 2014 • Volume 9 • Number 4

ELSEVIER

1600 John F. Kennedy Boulevard • Suite 1800 • Philadelphia, Pennsylvania, 19103-2899

http://www.pet.theclinics.com

PET CLINICS Volume 9, Number 4
October 2014 ISSN 1556-8598, ISBN-13: 978-0-323-32626-1

Editor: John Vassallo (j.vassallo@elsevier.com)
Developmental Editor: Susan Showalter

PET Clinics (ISSN 1556-8598) is published quarterly by Elsevier Inc., 360 Park Avenue South, New York, NY 10010-1710. Months of issue are January, April, July, and October. Periodicals postage paid at New York, NY, and additional mailing offices. Subscription prices per year are $225.00 (US individuals), $327.00 (US institutions), $115.00 (US students), $255.00 (Canadian individuals), $369.00 (Canadian institutions), $140.00 (Canadian students), $275.00 (foreign individuals), $369.00 (foreign institutions), and $140.00 (foreign students). To receive student and resident rate, orders must be accompanied by name of affiliated institution, date of term, and the signature of program/residency coordinator on institution letterhead. Orders will be billed at individual rate until proof of status is received. Foreign air speed delivery is included in all Clinics subscription prices. All prices are subject to change without notice. POSTMASTER: Send address changes to PET Clinics, Elsevier Health Sciences Division, Subscription Customer Service, 3251 Riverport Lane, Maryland Heights, MO 63043. **Customer Service: 1-800-654-2452 (U.S. and Canada); 314-447-8871 (outside U.S. and Canada). Fax: 314-447-8029. E-mail: journalscustomerservice-usa@elsevier.com (for print support); journalsonlinesupport-usa@elsevier.com (for online support).**

Reprints. For copies of 100 or more of articles in this publication, please contact the Commercial Reprints Department, Elsevier Inc., 360 Park Avenue South, New York, NY 10010-1710. Tel.: 212-633-3874; Fax: 212-633-3820; E-mail: reprints@elsevier.com.

PET Clinics is covered in MEDLINE/PubMed (Index Medicus).

Contributors

CONSULTING EDITOR

ABASS ALAVI, MD, PhD (Hon), Dsc (Hon)
Professor of Radiology, Division of Nuclear
Medicine, Department of Radiology, University
of Pennsylvania School of Medicine, Hospital
of the University of Pennsylvania, Philadelphia,
Pennsylvania

EDITORS

SØREN HESS, MD
Consultant/Attending Physician, Department
of Nuclear Medicine, Odense University
Hospital, Odense, Denmark

**POUL FLEMMING HØILUND-CARLSEN,
MD, DMSc**
Professor, Department of Nuclear Medicine,
Odense University Hospital and Institute of
Clinical Research, University of Southern
Denmark, Odense, Denmark

AUTHORS

ABASS ALAVI, MD, PhD (Hon), Dsc (Hon)
Professor of Radiology, Division of Nuclear
Medicine, Department of Radiology, University
of Pennsylvania School of Medicine, Hospital
of the University of Pennsylvania, Philadelphia,
Pennsylvania

SANDIP BASU, MD
Professor, Radiation Medicine Center, Bhabha
Atomic Research Centre, Tata Memorial
Hospital Annexe, Mumbai, India

POUL-ERIK NIELSEN BRAAD, MSc
Department of Nuclear Medicine, Odense
University Hospital, Odense, Denmark

ANDRÉS DAMIÁN, MD
Uruguayan Centre of Molecular Imaging
(CUDIM), Montevideo, Uruguay

MAARTEN L. DONSWIJK, MD
Departments of Radiology and Nuclear
Medicine, University Medical Center Utrecht,
Utrecht, The Netherlands

GHASSAN E. EL-HADDAD, MD, PhD
Department of Interventional Radiology, Moffitt
Cancer Center, Tampa, Florida

HENRY ENGLER, MD, PhD
Uruguayan Centre of Molecular Imaging
(CUDIM), Montevideo, Uruguay; Department of
Medical Sciences, Uppsala University, Sweden

**POUL FLEMMING HØILUND-CARLSEN,
MD, DMSc**
Professor, Department of Nuclear Medicine,
Odense University Hospital and Institute of
Clinical Research, University of Southern
Denmark, Odense, Denmark

SUSANNE H. HANSSON, MD
Department of Nuclear Medicine, Næstved
Hospital, Næstved, Denmark

SØREN HESS, MD
Consultant/Attending Physician, Department
of Nuclear Medicine, Odense University
Hospital, Odense, Denmark

MARTIN HUTCHINGS, MD, PhD
Staff Specialist, Department of Hematology,
Rigshospitalet, Copenhagen University
Hospital, Copenhagen, Denmark

SIGNE INGLEV, MSc, PhD
Department of Nuclear Medicine, Odense
University Hospital, Odense, Denmark

MARNIX G.E.H. LAM, MD, PhD
Senior Staff, Department of Radiology and
Nuclear Medicine, University Medical Center
Utrecht, Utrecht, The Netherlands

LARS LUND, MD, DMSci
Institute of Clinical Research, University of
Southern Denmark; Department of Urology L,
Odense University Hospital, Odense,
Denmark

IZAAK QUINTES MOLENAAR, MD, PhD
Senior Staff, Department of Surgery,
University Medical Center Utrecht, Utrecht,
The Netherlands

TIES MULDERS, MD, PhD
Departments of Radiology and Nuclear
Medicine, University Medical Center Utrecht,
Utrecht, The Netherlands

KAREN JUUL MYLAM, MD
Department of Hematology, Odense University
Hospital, Odense, Denmark

ANNE LERBERG NIELSEN, MD
Department of Nuclear Medicine, Odense
University Hospital, Odense, Denmark

BIRGITTE BRINKMANN OLSEN, MSc, PhD
Department of Nuclear Medicine, Odense
University Hospital, Odense, Denmark

KASPER T. PEDERSEN, MD
Department of Nuclear Medicine, Odense
University Hospital, Odense, Denmark

LARS MØLLER PEDERSEN, MD
Department of Hematology, Roskilde Hospital,
Denmark

HENRIK PETERSEN, MD
Department of Nuclear Medicine, Odense
University Hospital, Odense, Denmark

MADS HVID POULSEN, MD, PhD
Institute of Clinical Research, University of
Southern Denmark; Department of Urology,
Odense University Hospital, Odense,
Denmark

WARNER PREVOO, MD
Senior Staff, Department of Interventional
Radiology, Antoni van Leeuwenhoek Hospital,
Amsterdam, The Netherlands

MORSAL SAMIM, MD
PhD Student, Department of Surgery,
University Medical Center Utrecht, Utrecht,
The Netherlands

MICHAEL SCHÖLL, PhD
MedTech West and the Department of
Clinical Neuroscience and Rehabilitation,
University of Gothenburg, Gothenburg,
Sweden; Department NVS, Center for
Alzheimer Research, Translational Alzheimer
Neurobiology, Karolinska Institute, Stockholm,
Sweden

DREW A. TORIGIAN, MD, MA, FSAR
Associate Professor, Department of Radiology,
Hospital of the University of Pennsylvania,
Philadelphia, Pennsylvania

MAURICE A.A.J. VAN DEN BOSCH, MD, PhD
Professor, Department of Radiology and
Nuclear Medicine, University Medical Center
Utrecht, Utrecht, The Netherlands

MIE HOLM VILSTRUP, MD
Department of Nuclear Medicine, Odense
University Hospital, Odense, Denmark

Contents

> Positron emission tomography (PET) imaging with 2-[^{18}F]fluoro-2-deoxy-D-glucose (FDG) forms the basis of molecular imaging. FDG-PET imaging is a multidisciplinary undertaking that requires close interdisciplinary collaboration in a broad team comprising physicians, technologists, secretaries, radio-chemists, hospital physicists, molecular biologists, engineers, and cyclotron technicians. The aim of this review is to provide a brief overview of important basic issues and considerations pivotal to successful patient examinations, including basic physics, instrumentation, radiochemistry, molecular and cell biology, patient preparation, normal distribution of tracer, and potential interpretive pitfalls.

> PET imaging with the most widely available PET tracer, 2-deoxy-2-[^{18}F]fluoro-D-glucose (FDG), is a powerful tool in the differential diagnosis of numerous neurologic and psychiatric disorders, particularly in early disease stages. It also plays an important role in the longitudinal evaluation of treatment effects and the depiction of disease courses. A selection of established and eligible application areas of FDG PET in neurology and psychiatry, such as different types of dementia, epilepsy, schizophrenia, and bipolar disorder, are reviewed in this article. A general methodology for clinical FDG PET examinations and typical diagnostic criteria and pitfalls are addressed.

> [^{18}F]Fluorodeoxyglucose (FDG) PET is a robust quantitative molecular imaging technique that complements available structural imaging techniques for the detection and characterization of malignancy. This article provides an overview of the utility and applications of FDG-PET for the evaluation of patients with thoracic malignancy.

> This article discusses the current state-of-the-art application of 2-deoxy-2-[^{18}F]fluoro-D-glucose (FDG)-PET and FDG-PET/computed tomography (CT) in the management of patients with gastrointestinal malignancies. Gastrointestinal malignancies include many different cell types, several common malignancies of which may be imaged by FDG-PET/CT. This review focuses on gastric carcinoma, pancreatic carcinoma, hepatocellular carcinoma, cholangiocarcinoma, colorectal carcinoma, and stroma cell tumors. The role of FDG-PET/CT in staging these malignancies is

discussed, in addition to (re)staging, detection of recurrent disease, patient selection/ prognostication, and response assessment, using the currently available literature.

Diffuse large B-cell lymphoma (DLBCL) is an aggressive and potentially curable type of lymphoma. Fluorine-18-fluorodeoxyglucose positron emission tomography (FDG-PET) is part of the clinical routine for DLBCL in most hospitals and also recommended for staging and end-of-therapy evaluation. FDG-PET/computed tomography (CT) is able to identify nodal and extranodal sites with greater accuracy than CT alone. Little evidence supports the use of surveillance FDG-PET imaging in the follow-up setting because of high rates of false-positive scans and because most studies are retrospective. This article discusses FDG-PET assessment methods and the clinical application of FDG-PET for management of DLBCL.

Kidney, bladder, and prostate cancer account for more than one-eighth of new cancer cases worldwide. Imaging in kidney cancer is dominated by computed tomography (CT). Positron emission tomography (PET) imaging of bladder cancer is hampered by the urinary excretion of the most common PET tracer, 18F-fluoro-deoxy-glucose (FDG). PET imaging has been applied more often in prostate cancer. FDG-PET/CT is claimed to have a high frequency of false-negative results in urologic cancers; however, this finding may instead reflect correctly the state of disease being due to slow-growing cancers with a good prognosis and without a need of therapy.

[^{18}F]Fluorodeoxyglucose (FDG) PET is a functional imaging tool that provides metabolic information, which has the potential to detect a lesion before it becomes anatomically apparent. This ability constitutes a strong argument for using FDG-PET/computed tomography (CT) in the management of oncology patients. Many studies have investigated the accuracy of FDG-PET or FDG-PET/CT for these purposes, but with small sample sizes based on retrospective cohorts. This article provides an overview of the role of FDG-PET or FDG-PET/CT in patients with liver malignancies treated by means of surgical resection, ablative therapy, chemoembolization, radioembolization, and brachytherapy, all being liver-directed oncologic interventions.

Nuclear medicine techniques have been an integral part of infection and inflammation imaging for decades; in recent years, fluorodeoxyglucose–positron emission tomography/computed tomography (FDG-PET/CT) has taken over many indications.

This review provides a comprehensive overview of the current and potential applications for FDG-PET/CT in infectious and inflammatory diseases (ie, systemic infections, bone infections, vascular infection and inflammation, thoracic and abdominal inflammation) and potential novel applications in both infection and inflammation.

PET CLINICS

PROGRAM OBJECTIVE

The goal of the PET Clinics is to keep practicing radiologists and radiology residents up to date with current clinical practice in positron emission tomography by providing timely articles reviewing the state of the art in patient care.

TARGET AUDIENCE

Practicing radiologists, radiology residents, and other health care professionals who provide patient care utilizing radiologic findings.

LEARNING OBJECTIVES

Upon completion of this activity, participants will be able to:
1. Review the basic principles of FDG-PET/CT imaging.
2. Discuss the use of FDG in urological, liver, gastrointestinal, and thoracic malignancies
3. Recognize the use of FDG-PET in neurology and psychiatry.

ACCREDITATION

The Elsevier Office of Continuing Medical Education (EOCME) is accredited by the Accreditation Council for Continuing Medical Education (ACCME) to provide continuing medical education for physicians.

The EOCME designates this enduring material for a maximum of 15 *AMA PRA Category 1 Credit*(s) ™. Physicians should claim only the credit commensurate with the extent of their participation in the activity.

All other health care professionals requesting continuing education credit for this enduring material will be issued a certificate of participation.

DISCLOSURE OF CONFLICTS OF INTEREST

The EOCME assesses conflict of interest with its instructors, faculty, planners, and other individuals who are in a position to control the content of CME activities. All relevant conflicts of interest that are identified are thoroughly vetted by EOCME for fair balance, scientific objectivity, and patient care recommendations. EOCME is committed to providing its learners with CME activities that promote improvements or quality in healthcare and not a specific proprietary business or a commercial interest.

The planning committee, staff, authors and editors listed below have identified no financial relationships or relationships to products or devices they or their spouse/life partner have with commercial interest related to the content of this CME activity:

Abass Alavi, MD, PhD, DSc; Sandip Basu, MD; Poul-Erik Nielson Braad, MSc; Andrés Damián, MD; Maarten L. Donswijk, MD; Ghassan E. El-Haddad, MD, PhD; Henry Engler, MD, PhD; Susanne H. Hansson, MD; Kristen Helm; Søren Hess, MD; Poul Flemming Høilund-Carlsen, MD, DMSc; Brynne Hunter; Signe Inglev, MSc, PhD; Marnix G.E.H. Lam, MD, PhD; Sandy Lavery; Lars Lund, MD, DMSci; Jill McNair; Izaak Quintus Molenaar, MD, PhD; Ties Mulders, MD, PhD; Karen Juul Mylam, MD; Mahalakshmi Narayanan; Anne Lerberg Nielsen, MD; Birgitte Brinkmann Olsen, MSc, PhD; Lars Møller Pedersen, MD; Kasper T. Pedersen, MD; Henrik Petersen, MD; Mads Hvid Poulsen, MD, PhD; Warner Prevoo, MD; Morsal Samim, MD; Michael Schöll, PhD; Drew A. Torigian, MD, FSAR, MA; John Vassallo; Maurice AAJ van den Bosch, MD, PhD; Mie Holm Vilstrup, MD.

The planning committee, staff, authors and editors listed below have identified financial relationships or relationships to products or devices they or their spouse/life partner have with commercial interest related to the content of this CME activity:

Martin Hutchings, MD, PhD is a consultant/advisor for Millenium, Inc.- a wholly-owned subsidiary of Takeda Pharmaceutical Company Limited.

UNAPPROVED/OFF-LABEL USE DISCLOSURE

The EOCME requires CME faculty to disclose to the participants:
1. When products or procedures being discussed are off-label, unlabelled, experimental, and/or investigational (not US Food and Drug Administration (FDA) approved); and
2. Any limitations on the information presented, such as data that are preliminary or that represent ongoing research, interim analyses, and/or unsupported opinions. Faculty may discuss information about pharmaceutical agents that is outside of FDA-approved labelling. This information is intended solely for CME and is not intended to promote off-label use of these medications. If you have any questions, contact the medical affairs department of the manufacturer for the most recent prescribing information.

TO ENROLL

To enroll in the PET Clinics Continuing Medical Education program, call customer service at 1-800-654-2452 or sign up online at http://www.theclinics.com/home/cme. The CME program is available to subscribers for an additional annual fee of USD $235.

METHOD OF PARTICIPATION

In order to claim credit, participants must complete the following:
1. Complete enrolment as indicated above.
2. Read the activity.
3. Complete the CME Test and Evaluation. Participants must achieve a score of 70% on the test. All CME Tests and Evaluations must be completed online.

CME INQUIRIES/SPECIAL NEEDS

For all CME inquiries or special needs, please contact elsevierCME@elsevier.com.

Preface
FDG-PET/CT: Quo vadis?

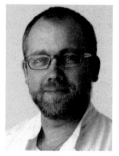 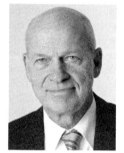

Søren Hess, MD   Poul Flemming Høilund-Carlsen, MD, DMSc

Editors

"Further studies addressing the usefulness of FDG-PET/CT are desirable." "The role of FDG-PET/CT has yet to be formally established in the diagnostic work-up and for monitoring of this disease." These and similar quotes are frequent reading in articles on the use of PET/CT applying the most common of all tracers, F-18 fluorodeoxyglucose (FDG). These quotes are often accompanied by additions such as "by the appearance and implementation of novel and more specific PET tracers, it is likely that PET/CT will have even greater influence on patient care" or "the development continues and with new and better radiopharmaceuticals, PET/CT will profoundly change management of this disease and provide a basis for updating the existing guidelines."

One could continue adding examples of a similar kind. They illustrate at least three things: (1) a peculiar defensive or apologetic attitude among those familiar with PET/CT and with FDG-PET/CT in particular, (2) a belief that it can be made even better with other, more specific tracers than FDG, and (3) that molecular clinical imaging with PET/CT has not yet found its place in modern health care, despite the fact that PET was unveiled approximately 40 years ago.[1]

All three statements call for an explanation. First, for those who have witnessed the development of nuclear medicine from its childhood or from the advent of SPECT and later PET, it remains a mystery why these modalities have not penetrated more rapidly and deeply into general clinical use, because in their (ie, our) view, the excellence and potential of these methods are almost self-evident. This contrasts, however, against a striking absence or sporadic presence in clinical guidelines, where many of us think that PET should instead be listed as first choice or a very early procedure in the workup and management of major disease entities like, for instance, atherosclerosis, inflammation, and neuropsychiatric disorders.

Second, in trying to demonstrate the benefits of FDG-PET/CT, it is commonly compared with conventional structural imaging in the form of conventional radiography, CT, or MRI, requiring that PET should provide a yes or no to a specific clinical question. However, dichotomous results are rare products also of structural imaging and, in addition, FDG imaging represents a completely different principle supplying with unsurpassed sensitivity quantitative information on the disease process that cannot be furnished by any other modality. These processes are dynamic and comprise from one patient to another an entire spectrum from negligible to aggressive disease. It is, therefore, not surprising that FDG imaging depicts a continuum of findings from invisible and barely visible to pronounced uptake in various disease processes. Consequently, to use it properly, our medical colleagues will have to understand FDG imaging better and look on it for what it is: an imaging probe system, which reflects the type of disease and gauges its extent, severity, and level of activity for use in diagnosis, staging, and response evaluation.

Third, it is surprising that after 3 or 4 decades, PET and PET/CT are still not occupying the outstanding positions in clinical guidelines they deserve. New and more specific tracers will appear. However, the time course for them to be

PET Clin 9 (2014) xi–xiii
http://dx.doi.org/10.1016/j.cpet.2014.07.007

found and emerge from bench to bed has turned out to be much longer and more costly than often anticipated. In the meantime, there is good reason to take a fresh new look on FDG imaging, to see what it can and cannot do, and where there are still white spots on the map to be filled out. There is noticeable lack of scientific evidence for the clinical usefulness of PET. In fact, by mid-2012, there were in the literature only 14 published and 15 ongoing randomized clinical studies, of which 5 and 12, respectively, did not even use a patient-important outcome.[2]

No wonder, therefore, that it has been a walk uphill to get PET introduced, let alone accepted and accredited by the medical society and its various guideline boards. It is a recurring problem for the study of the accuracy of PET that there are no ideal reference methods. On the contrary, as a rule, one is forced to compare with structural imaging, which basically shows something different with much lower sensitivity and without the possibility of quantification. The data and various diagnostic values reported in the series of articles that we have planned for two successive issues of *PET Clinics* should consequently be taken with a large grain of salt. It is all the more necessary that in the future we are planning our studies in a way that makes it possible to collect the data needed to demonstrate the excellence of FDG-PET/CT and PET in general. However, there is considerable uncertainty about how to assess the comparative effectiveness of diagnostic procedures. For PET/CT, not only diagnostic accuracy but also clinical benefit must be demonstrated, and there is a lack of consensus about how to approach this task, which is not a trivial one. In particular, it should be clarified whether there is a direct benefit of the use of PET/CT or an indirect one because of improved diagnostic accuracy, as various scenarios require different approaches.[3] Finally, in times of rising health care costs, there is an increasing need of adding economic analyses as an adjunct to studies of accuracy and the benefit that an increased accuracy may bring to patients, because the additional cost of applying a new method must be justified by the benefits provided to patient and community.[4]

Almost none of the review articles presented in this and the succeeding issue of *PET Clinics* can meet these stringent requirements. Nonetheless, they are a beginning, because they illustrate what we know and where there are gaps and holes that should be filled, recognizing that the assessment of FDG-PET/CT, its opportunities and benefits, is after all, still in its infancy.

The first article by Sandip Basu and colleagues gives a comprehensive overview of the basic technical and practical issues associated with the performance of FDG-PET/CT scans in a simple and straightforward manner that, in particular, nuclear medicine fellows and medical colleagues without specific knowledge of these methods may benefit from and have as foundation for successive reading. Subsequent articles cover the use of FDG-PET/CT in various clinical settings, malignant and nonmalignant, well-established as well as upcoming. Thus, a review by Michael Schöll and colleagues describes FDG in neurology and psychiatry, the first clinical applications of this modality. Mie Vilstrup and colleagues cover FDG in thoracic malignancies, and Karen Mylam and colleagues review FDG in hematologic malignancies, ie, two rather well-established oncologic indications with widespread clinical use. In contrast, Maarten Donswijk and colleagues describe the use of FDG-PET in gastrointestinal malignancies, and Morsal Samim and colleagues present PET-based interventional radiology, both much less investigated areas, where FDG-PET is currently utilized to a lesser extent, but has great potential. Høilund-Carlsen and colleagues review FDG in urologic malignancies covering several diseases with very different utilization of FDG, partly due to inherent differences in pathophysiology. Finally, Hess and colleagues give an overview of FDG in infectious/inflammatory diseases, a very diverse field that is increasingly explored and probably will continue to expand in years to come.

Thus, it is hoped that the various articles presented in this and the subsequent issue of *PET Clinics* provide the readers with a plethora of relevant information on the use of FDG, a truly amazing molecule, the full potential of which still remains to be uncovered and thoroughly documented to ensure the eminent position in the clinic that it deserves, and which no other, new and promising, PET tracer has so far been able to claim.

Søren Hess, MD
Department of Nuclear Medicine
Odense University Hospital
Sønder Boulevard 29
5000 Odense, Denmark

Poul Flemming Høilund-Carlsen, MD, DMSc
Department of Nuclear Medicine
Odense University Hospital and Institute of
Clinical Research
University of Southern Denmark
Sønder Boulevard 29
5000 Odense, Denmark

E-mail addresses:
soeren.hess@rsyd.dk (S. Hess)
pfhc@rsyd.dk (P.F. Høilund-Carlsen)

REFERENCES

1. Hess S, Blomberg BA, Zhu HJ, et al. The pivotal role of FDG-PET/CT in modern medicine. Acad Radiol 2014;21:232–49.
2. Siepe B, Hoilund-Carlsen PF, Gerke O, et al. The move from accuracy studies to randomized trials in PET: current status and future directions. J Nucl Med 2014; 55(8):1228–34.
3. Vach W, Høilund-Carlsen PF, Gerke O, et al. Generating evidence for clinical benefit of PET/CT in diagnosing cancer patients. J Nucl Med 2011;52(Suppl 2): 77S–85S.
4. Høilund-Carlsen PF, Gerke O, Vach W. Demonstrating benefits of clinical nuclear imaging: time for adding economic analyses. Eur J Nucl Med Mol Imaging 2014;41(9):1720–2.

The Basic Principles of FDG-PET/CT Imaging

Sandip Basu, MD[a], Søren Hess, MD[b],*, Poul-Erik Nielsen Braad, MSc[b],
Birgitte Brinkmann Olsen, MSc, PhD[b], Signe Inglev, MSc, PhD[b],
Poul Flemming Høilund-Carlsen, MD, DMSc[b]

KEYWORDS

- Positron emission tomography/computed tomography • PET/CT • Fluorodeoxyglucose • FDG
- History • Physics • Instrumentation • Radiochemistry

KEY POINTS

- The positron (β+ decay) combines with an electron, and the 2 opposite charges annihilate each other and produce 2 gamma rays (annihilation photons) of each 511 keV emitted in opposite directions at approximately 180° from each other.
- If properly corrected, positron emission tomography (PET) images are truly quantitative (ie, the reconstructed value in each image voxel can be calibrated to the in vivo absolute radioactivity concentration).
- Fluorine 18 (^{18}F) is produced in a cyclotron by bombarding oxygen 18–enriched water with protons, and ^{18}F is still the backbone of PET radiochemistry.
- Tumors consume more glucose than most other tissues because of increased glycolysis (known as the Warburg effect), and this feature is exploited in PET using the glucose analogue 2-[^{18}F]fluoro-2-deoxy-D-glucose (FDG) as the tracer.
- The spectrum of potential pitfalls with FDG is highly variable; a thorough knowledge of technical and patient-related factors, normal distribution, physiologic uptake, and common normal variants is pivotal.

INTRODUCTION

The Society of Nuclear Medicine and Molecular Imaging has defined molecular imaging as "the visualization, characterization, and measurement of biological processes at the molecular and cellular levels in humans and other living systems. Molecular imaging typically consists of 2-dimensional (2D) or 3-dimensional (3D) imaging as well as quantification over time."[1] Positron emission tomography (PET) imaging with 2-[^{18}F]fluoro-2-deoxy-D-glucose (FDG) forms the basis of this evolution in modern medicine with aims toward the mantra of contemporary health care: personalized medicine.

The commercially availability of hybrid PET/computed tomography (PET/CT) has led to widespread clinical use, and all major domains of human health are represented in current clinical applications as well as research applications (ie, neurology, oncology, cardiology, and infection/inflammation).[2] And no matter what the indication is, FDG-PET/CT imaging is a multidisciplinary undertaking that requires close collaboration that is not only between the classic constituents of the health care industry (ie, physicians, nurses, technologists, and secretaries); there is an increasing recognition of the importance of a much broader team behind the scenes (ie, radio-chemists,

[a] Radiation Medicine Center, Bhabha Atomic Research Centre, Tata Memorial Hospital Annexe, Jerbai Wadia Road, Parel, Mumbai 400012, India; [b] Department of Nuclear Medicine, Odense University Hospital, Soender Boulevard 29, Odense 5000, Denmark
* Corresponding author.
E-mail address: soeren.hess@rsyd.dk

PET Clin 9 (2014) 355–370
http://dx.doi.org/10.1016/j.cpet.2014.07.006
1556-8598/14/$ – see front matter © 2014 Elsevier Inc. All rights reserved.

hospital physicists, molecular biologists, engineers, and cyclotron technicians).

The aim of this review is to provide a brief overview of basic, but nonetheless important, issues and considerations from the physicist's, the chemist's, and the molecular biologist's point of view, as well as patient factors (ie, prescan preparation, normal distribution of tracer, normal variants, and potential pitfalls).

SHORT HISTORICAL OVERVIEW OF THE EARLY PET EVOLUTION

When Irene and Frederic Joliot-Curie in 1934 reported that alpha particle irradiation of aluminum, boron, and magnesium led to the formation of radioactive substances that decayed with relatively short half-lives by emitting positrons, it was the first demonstration that artificial radiation could be produced.[3] The Joliot-Curies first artificially produced radionuclide was nitrogen 13 (^{13}N), now a promising PET isotope for myocardial studies. Ernest O. Lawrence's cyclotron group at Berkeley immediately began producing a multitude of new, biologically significant radionuclides on a larger scale, including ^{13}N, carbon 11 (^{11}C), oxygen 15 (^{15}O), and fluorine 18 (^{18}F). Lawrence established the first "medical cyclotron" in 1938; but with the postwar abundance of reactor-produced isotopes, interest in short-lived isotopes dwindled somewhat until the pioneering work by Ter-Pogossian and coworkers in St Louis in the 1950s.[4–6] Initially, they studied oxygen tension in malignant tumors by using ^{15}O and autoradiography but went on to study cerebral metabolism using ^{15}O-labeled oxygen and other gases. The recognized potential led to further cyclotrons dedicated to medical research with short-lived positron-emitting radionuclides both nationally and abroad.[7]

Alongside these advances, several groups worked independently on improving the detection of annihilation radiation. In 1951, Wren and coworkers[8] were the first to report the use of opposing thallium-activated sodium iodide detectors to localize copper 64–phthalocyanine in brain tumors; they introduced the concept of coincidence detection compared with single-photon imaging. Independently, Brownell and Sweet[9] reported similar works on brain tumors with a positron scanner comprising 2 colinear sodium iodide detectors moving rectilinearly and attached to a writing mechanism recording the count rate on carbonized paper. During the 1960s and early 1970s, several groups developed novel designs of positron-detecting devices to improve the sensitivity and resolution; the prevailing concept

became ring detection of coincidence first introduced by Rankowitz and coworkers[10] in 1962.[4–6] Kuhl's and Edwards' tomographic scanner for single-photon imaging from 1963, although not intended for positron imaging, demonstrated the great potential of tomographic imaging; their designs still form the basis of modern PET scanners.[11] The evolution culminated in the prototype device positron-emission transaxial tomograph (PETT) II constructed in 1972 to 1973 by the Washington University group headed by Ter-Pogossian.[5] This prototype became the foundation for the further evolution of PET scanners, including the group's own clinically functional whole-body camera, the PETT III, with 48 detectors presented in 1975.[12,13] The coincidental evolution in computers provided the essential cost-effective computational power for image reconstruction and helped pave the way for the future developments of PET, including multiple ring detection systems and more efficient crystals like bismuth germinate oxide (BGO) and later cesium fluoride enabling time-of-flight detection developed by Ter-Pogossian and coworkers in the 1980s.[14–16]

The evolution in PET instrumentation coincided with similar developments in radiochemistry; by the turn of the 1970s, Ter-Pogossian and colleagues[17] published an article in Scientific American listing 30 new compounds labeled with either ^{15}O, ^{13}N, ^{11}C, or ^{18}F. One of these compounds was FDG, which was coined and developed during the first half of the 1970s in close collaboration between researchers at the Hospital of the University of Pennsylvania (PENN) (including Martin Reivich, David Kuhl, and Abass Alavi), and Brookhaven National Laboratory (BNL) (Alfred Wolf's team including Joanna Fowler and Tatsuo Ito).[18] A PET center was established at PENN; by August 1976, the first human subjects in history were injected with FDG. Initially, Kuhl's Mark IV tomographic scanner for low-energy gamma photons was modified with high-energy collimators to detect positron emission photons; they performed the first whole-body image with a dual-head rectilinear scanner with high-energy collimators. The original PETT III scanner was later transferred from Washington University to BNL to be used by the team from Pennsylvania.[5,19–21]

From the 1970s onward, the evolution of cyclotron design from large, high-energy types to smaller, low-energy types also became an important additional catalyst for radiochemical developments. It became obvious that smaller, and less costly, dedicated cyclotrons could be installed and maintained in medical centers; in the mid-1980s, the first cyclotrons dedicated to PET isotopes were introduced commercially.[5] Since then, both instrumentation and radiochemical diversity has continued to evolve with increasingly sensitive scanners, now mostly multimodality with coregistered CT, introduced at the turn of the century, or with coregistered magnetic resonance (MR) imaging introduced a decade later. Nonetheless, FDG-PET/CT remains the backbone of molecular imaging and probably will for decades to come.

BASIC PHYSICS: POSITRON EMISSION AND ANNIHILATION

Medical imaging with PET primarily encompasses short-lived positron-emitting isotopes, such as cyclotron-produced ^{11}C, ^{13}N, ^{15}O, and ^{18}F as well as generator-produced gallium 68 (^{68}Ga) and rubidium 82 (^{82}Rb). The isotopes are usually produced by proton irradiation of natural or enriched targets. **Table 1** enumerates the production equation, half-lives, and other salient characteristics of important positron-emitting radionuclides.

Positron emission, also known as beta plus decay (β^+ decay), is an isobaric decay process whereby a proton inside a radionuclide nucleus is converted into a neutron while releasing a positron and a neutrino (ν_e). The decay process is characteristic of proton-rich radionuclides. Positron decay results in an element with an atomic number that is less by one unit. Thus, this could be termed as *nuclear transmutation* (ie, the conversion of one chemical element or isotope into another). The isobaric decay process denotes that the mass number of the daughter nuclei remains the same in the parent; however, the atomic number changes.

The protons and neutrons are composed of elementary particles known as quarks. The 2 stable and common subtypes of quarks are (1) up quarks having a charge of +2/3 and (2) down quarks, with a −1/3 charge. A proton (charge +1) is composed of 2 up quarks and one down quark, whereas the neutrons (zero charge) have one up quark and 2 down quarks. The positron emission is explained by the conversion of an up quark into a down quark.

The proton-rich radionuclides have 2 options for conversion to stable nuclei: positron emission or electron capture, both of which are *isobaric decay* processes. Electron capture (whereby the proton-rich nuclide absorbs an inner shell electron, thus, converting a proton to a neutron) primarily occurs for isotopes with insufficient energy difference between it and its prospective daughter. If the energy difference between them is less than 1.022 MeV, positron emission is not possible and electron capture is the usual decay mode. For instance, positron emission is more prevalent in lower-atomic-weight nuclei like ^{11}C, ^{13}N, ^{15}O, and ^{18}F, whereas electron capture is the predominant mode of decay in iodine 123.

A positron is the electron's antiparticle. A typical positron decay equation is written as follows:

$$^A_ZX \rightarrow (^{\ A}_{Z-1}Y + e^+ + \nu_e)$$

X and Y denote the element; A is the mass number; Z is the atomic number; e^+ symbolizes the positron; and ν_e symbolizes an electron neutrino. In the positron decay, a transmutation of elements occurs; the resulting daughter nucleus possesses the same mass number but an atomic number reduced by 1.

The resulting neutrino from positron decay, more specifically an electron neutrino, is an

Table 1
Salient features of common positron emitters

Positron Emitter	Production	Half-Life (min)	Daughter	β (%)	Maximum Energy (MeV)
^{11}C	$^{14}N(p,\alpha)^{11}C$	20.4	^{11}B	99	0.96
^{13}N	$^{16}O(p,\alpha)^{15}N$	10.0	^{13}C	100	1.19
^{15}O	$^{14}N(d,n)^{15}O$ $^{15}N(p,n)^{15}O$	2.1	^{15}N	100	1.72
^{18}F	$^{18}O(p,n)^{18}F$ $^{20}Ne(d,\alpha)^{18}F$	110.0	^{18}O	97	0.64
^{68}Ga	^{68}Ga-generator ($t_{1/2}$ = 271 d)	68.0	^{68}Zn	88	1.89
^{82}Rb	^{82}Sr-generator ($t_{1/2}$ = 25 d)	1.3	^{82}Kr	96	3.35

Abbreviations: ^{11}B, boron 11; ^{82}Kr, krypton 82; ^{20}Ne, neon 20; ^{82}Sr, strontium 82; $t_{1/2}$, half-life; ^{68}Zn, zinc 68.

From Basu S, Kwee TC, Surti S, et al. Fundamentals of PET and PET/CT imaging. Ann N Y Acad Sci 2011;1228:1–18; with permission.

electrically neutral, subatomic particle with zero or negligible mass and half-integer spin, which escapes without interacting in the surrounding material. The positron, on the other hand, is highly interactive and travels a short distance (termed *positron range*), which is a function of its energy and is defined by the following equation:

Positron energy + neutrino energy = transition energy − 1.022 MeV.

While traveling, the electron clouds of the surrounding materials retards it until at last it completely loses its energy and combines with an electron to form an unstable system known as positronium, consisting of an electron and a positron, which annihilate each other in a fraction of a second (average lifetime of 125 picoseconds) to produce 2 gamma ray photons (termed *annihilation photons*) each of 511 keV (an energy equivalent to the combined rest mass of an electron and a positron); they are emitted in opposite directions at approximately 180° from each other (**Fig. 1**).

The annihilation photons emitted at nearly 180° are detected by opposing PET detectors with a principle of electronic collimation: They register the arrival of the annihilation photons as an event only when they arrive within a narrow timing window (of typically 3–15 nanoseconds). The requirement of detecting both photons within a time window forms the basis of *coincidence detection in PET* (see **Fig. 1**). In the PET detection principle, it is assumed that the interaction has taken place somewhere on the straight line drawn between the 2 detectors, the line being referred to as the *line of response* (LOR) or *coincidence line*.

With the availability in recent years of detectors with fast timing decay, high light output, and high stopping power, PET scanners have been investigated for the *time-of-flight* (TOF) capability, the principle of which relies on measuring the arrival time difference of the 2 annihilation photons, whereby it is possible to pinpoint the emission point along the LOR. TOF leads to better contrast PET images with resulting better sensitivity.[22] The TOF position uncertainty (denoted as Δx) along the LOR is defined and estimated by the coincidence time resolution by the following formula:

$$\Delta x = c^* \Delta t/2,$$

where c is the speed of light and Δt is the full-width-at-half-maximum time resolution of 2 coincidence detectors.

PET-SCANNER DESIGN

PET scanners are built from many small detectors that are placed in adjacent rings around the patient port. A clinical state-of-the-art PET system typically has a ring diameter of 60 to 90 cm and an axial extent of 10 to 25 cm and consists of up to 25,000 detectors. A single PET detector is a high-density scintillator crystal (eg, BGO, lutetium yttrium orthosilicate [LSO], or lutetium yttrium orthosilicate [LYSO]) that converts the energy of photons striking the detector into light. The scintillator is optically coupled to a device, most often a

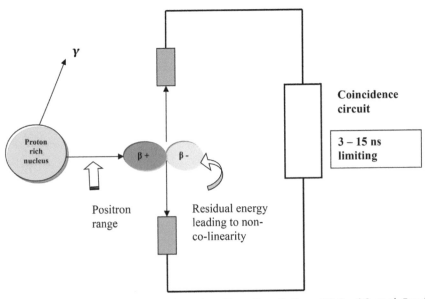

Fig. 1. Annihilation radiation and coincidence detection. (*From* Basu S, Kwee TC, Surti S, et al. Fundamentals of PET and PET/CT imaging. Ann N Y Acad Sci 2011;1228:2; with permission.)

photo multiplier tube (PMT), where the light is converted into an amplified electric signal. The signals from each detector are coupled to a coincidence circuit that tags each PET event by the detection time. Photons that are detected within the coincidence window of the system are accepted as coincidence events and assigned to the LOR connecting the 2 detectors, whereas other events are rejected.

Most PET systems acquire and save data over a given time frame in a list-mode file where each event is tagged with an LOR position and the time point of detection. Once the time frame has ended, tomographic images are reconstructed either directly from the list-mode file or from projections that are generated by sorting parallel LOR into sinograms. Classically, tomographic image reconstruction has been accomplished by analytical filtered back projection. However, better image quality can typically be obtained by statistical iterative reconstruction methods.[23] To simplify the reconstruction, each tomographic slice can be reconstructed independently by only accepting LOR within the given slice. This independent reconstruction can be obtained by inserting septa (thin lead or tungsten collimating rings) between crystal rings such that inter-ring coincidences are prevented. This method of imaging is called *2D PET*. A much higher sensitivity can be obtained if inter-ring coincidences are accepted, in which case the mode of imaging is termed *3D PET*. Historically, 2D PET has been preferred over 3D PET because of simpler data handling and image reconstruction. However, with the evolvement of faster computers and the development of better iterative reconstruction methods, the gains in sensitivity from 3D PET versus 2D PET have resulted in 3D PET becoming the preferred imaging mode in all modern clinical PET systems.

Ideally, PET images are quantitative in the sense that the reconstructed value in each image voxel can be calibrated to the in vivo absolute radioactivity concentration. In reality, this signature feature of PET can only be realized if images are corrected for inhomogeneity in detector output (normalization), dead-time effects, attenuation of coincidences, and if scattered and random coincidence events are subtracted. Normalization correction accounts for variations in the sensitivity of LOR across the PET detectors toward a homogenous source of annihilation photons. In practice, the sensitivity of an LOR that is angled on the detector surface is smaller than that of an LOR that hits the detector perpendicularly and, likewise, different PET crystals and PMTs may vary in sensitivity. Normalization correction factors are usually derived from a calibration scan of a known coincidence source. The 511-keV photons that arise from different annihilation events, but are detected by the PET system inside the coincidence window, are called *random coincidences*. The rate of random coincidences on a particular LOR is a function of the width of the coincidence window and the event rates in the detectors that define the LOR. As a consequence, the random coincidences may be modeled by the measured singles' rates in the PET detectors. Likewise, dead-time losses are related to the count rates in the PET system and can, therefore, also be modeled from these. The intensity of a beam of photons passing through the material is attenuated by interactions between the photons in the beam and electrons and atoms in the material. The impact of attenuation on PET quantification is huge. Along an LOR through a 30-cm object, the fraction of events that survive nonattenuated to detection can be as low as 5%. Correction for attenuation in PET is, therefore, very important. In a hybrid PET/CT system, CT measures the attenuation along projections through the scanned object. Attenuation correction is typically implemented directly inside the reconstruction algorithm and can be accomplished to a high degree of accuracy.[24]

More than 99% of all 511-keV photon interactions in PET are by Compton scattering (ie, inelastic scattering of photons on effectively free electrons). This process results in the production of new photons with lower energy than the original beam that are emitted at an oblique angle relative to the direction of the unscattered photons. Scattered coincidences are assigned an LOR that does not pass through the point of annihilation and, thus, uncorrected compromise quantitation and image contrast. Scatter is more difficult to correct than attenuation. PET scanners can, to a certain degree, correct scattered photons by only accepting photons that are detected with energy inside an energy discriminator window. The energy resolution in PET detectors is quite poor; the lower-level energy discriminator is, therefore, set quite low, typically at 425 keV on a 3D LYSO/LSO-based PET system. Approximately 50% of all single scattered photons are emitted with energies more than 425 keV, and the scatter fraction in clinical studies is more than 50%. Most modern PET/CT systems model scatter by the scaled single scatter simulation model proposed by Watson and colleagues.[25] In this model, the CT image is segmented into scatter points; scatter at these points is calculated inside the loop of an iterative reconstruction by a direct analytical implementation of the Klein-Nishina model to Compton single scatter. When necessary, corrections for multiple scattered events and scatter from outside the scanner field of view (FOV) can be implemented in the model (**Box 1**).

Novel Developments

Developments in PET instrumentation seek to improve the quantitative accuracy of the quantitation of small lesions by increasing the image contrast and reducing partial volume effects. Limitations on the PET reconstructed spatial resolution (approximately 5 mm) result in partial volume effects where the PET signal inside small lesions is reduced because of activity spill-out. The spatial resolution is related to the size of the detector crystals; some vendors, therefore, seek to improve spatial resolution be equipping their scanners with smaller crystals. In conventional PET designs, the light output from a particular crystal is shared among several PMTs. Improvements in spatial resolution can be realized in PET designs whereby there is a direct electronic readout of the light emitted by a given crystal. Such features are implemented in PET photon-counting detector designs[26] and in PET detectors using silicon photomultiplier detectors developed for PET/MR imaging.[27]

Partial volume effects are also affected by variations of the spatial resolution as a function of the radial distance from the center of the PET FOV. This effect arises because off-center LORs hit the crystals at an oblique angle, increasing the probability, therefore, of 511-keV photons penetrating a crystal in such a way that scintillation light is emitted in several crystals. One solution to this problem is to equip the PET system with more than one layer of crystals so the path of the 511-keV photons through the detector can be determined.[28] Another more common procedure is to measure the position dependent system response of a point source in water in the PET system. The impact on spatial resolution from the measured response, often called the *point-spread function*, can then be corrected inside an iterative reconstruction algorithm.

Modern PET systems are usually equipped with TOF capabilities. The big advantage of TOF-PET is that image contrast is improved and noise reduced by the better localization of the annihilation position. The better the TOF resolution is, the higher the gain is on the signal-to-noise ratio. New detector designs are expected to improve the TOF resolution further in the future. Improvements on signal-to-noise ratios may be used to reduce the patient dose by administering less activity or by reducing the scan time in each patient. Other designs accomplish a potential reduction in patient dose or PET scan time by improving the PET scanner sensitivity. This improvement can be obtained by increasing the axial extent of the PET detector.

The implementation of hybrid PET/CT has improved the value of PET imaging tremendously, not only because of the complementary diagnostic features of PET and CT but also because of the improvements on PET image quality that can be obtained from corrections derived from the CT images. Recently, clinical PET/MR imaging scanners have been introduced.[29] Such systems may have value, particularly in pediatric patients whereby patient dose reductions are desired and in areas where CT performance is inferior to MR imaging. The coupling of PET and MR imaging has turned out to be very challenging, and issues related to attenuation correction are still unsolved. Furthermore, the economic cost of PET/MR imaging is currently very high; the clinical application that justifies this cost is yet to be discovered.

PET RADIONUCLIDES AND PRODUCTION OF FDG

For several good reasons, ^{18}F is still the backbone of PET radiochemistry (**Box 2**). The ^{18}F is produced in a cyclotron by the nuclear reaction between oxygen 18 (^{18}O)–enriched water bombarded with protons releasing a neutron according to the aforementioned production equation ^{18}O(p,n)^{18}F. With regard to ^{68}Ga, the decay product of germanium 68 bound to column material in the generator can be eluded to yield the daughter isotope.

Automated synthesis modules have been designed and helped lead the synthesis of FDG into a standardized and fairly easy task. Hamacher and colleagues[30] developed the widely used method of today in 1986. Initially, FDG was

---

Box 1
Limits of the spatial resolution of PET can be attributed to a combination of the following factors

Detector size and intrinsic detector spatial resolution

Noncolinearity of the annihilation photons (related to residual momentum of the positron before it combines with the electron)

Positron range (related to positron energy and is characteristic of a particular positron-emitting radionuclide)

Penetration into the detector ring

Decoding errors in the detector modules

Data from Moses WW. Fundamental limits of spatial resolution in PET. Nucl Instrum Methods Phys Res A 2011;648(Suppl 1):S236–40.

Box 2
Characteristics of ¹⁸F making it the workhorse of PET imaging

The relatively long half-life of 110 minutes that allows synthesis and studies that can be extended over hours and transfer to distant centers

The low positron energy (640 keV) results in short tissue range (2.3 mm) resulting in relatively higher resolution and low radiation dose

¹⁸F synthesis can be accomplished in relatively high radioactive quantities (ie, curies)

¹⁸F has the advantages over the short-lived radioisotopes in rendering metabolite and plasma analysis (needed for quantification and dynamic studies) possible

---

synthesized by electrophilic fluorination with a low yield (8%) and long synthesis time (>2 hours). Subsequent developments led to improved routes of synthesis, but the use of electrophilic reactions remained the method of choice for the next decade despite continuous low yield and lengthy synthesis.[31] Thus, considerable efforts were used to develop a nucleophile substitution (S_N2); Hamacher and colleagues[30] succeeded in using Kryptofix 2.2.2, an amino polyether, together with potassium carbonate (K_2CO_3) to form the counter ion for the ¹⁸F ion, making ¹⁸F able to act as a nucleophile. This process increased the reactivity of ¹⁸F, and the reaction route devised by Hamacher and colleagues[30] had a consistent yield of greater than 50% and a synthesis time of less than 1 hour.

As mentioned earlier, ¹⁸F is produced in the target system in the cyclotron by proton bombardment of ¹⁸O-enriched water. The formed hydrogen fluoride (HF) in water is pushed to the synthesis module

and absorbed on the QMA column. The fluoride ions are eluded from the column into the reaction vial by kryptofix 2.2.2/K_2CO_3; after coevaporation with acetonitrile, the residual water is removed from the fluoride. A solution of mannose-triflate in acetonitrile is added to the reactive fluoride ions. The mixture is heated and the S_N2 reaction at the triflate-substituted carbon leads to an acetyl-protected FDG (FTAG). The reaction mixture is then passed through a silica cartridge column, which binds the FTAG; the unreacted fluoride is removed. Sodium hydroxide hydrolyses the protecting groups and the resulting ¹⁸F-FDG is purified through purification cartridges before sterile filtration and formulation into sodium chloride and ethanol (**Fig. 2**). The ¹⁸F-FDG is tested against the requirements set in the pharmacopeia before released for patient use.

THE FDG CONCEPT

Tumors consume more glucose than most other tissues because of the increased glycolysis (known as the Warburg effect), and this feature is exploited in PET using FDG as a tracer. FDG is a radiolabeled glucose analogue whereby the 2′ hydroxyl group has been substituted with ¹⁸F.

Cellular Uptake of FDG

Despite the chemical differences, cellular uptake of FDG is similar as for glucose. FDG passes the cellular membrane through facilitated transport mediated by the glucose transporters (GLUTs), of which more than 14 different isoforms have been identified in humans differing in their tissue distribution and affinity for glucose.[32] GLUT1 is the most common glucose transporter in humans and is, together with GLUT3, overexpressed in many tumors.[33] However, GLUT4 has also been

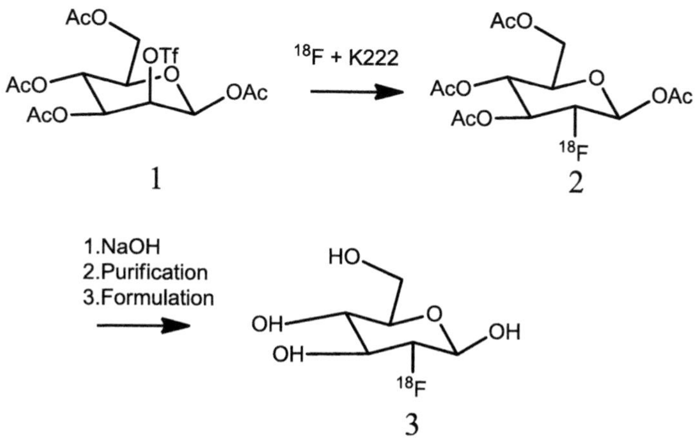

Fig. 2. Final steps in FDG synthesis: 1. Acetylated mannose triflate. 2. Acetylated FDG. 3. FDG. NaOH, sodium hydroxide. AcO, acetyl protecting group; OTF, triflate group.

suggested to be important in certain types of cancer (eg, breast cancer).[34] Furthermore, levels of GLUT1 expression correlate with tumor development and unfavorable prognosis.[35] Once inside the cell, FDG is phosphorylated by hexokinase yielding FDG-6-phosphate, which, unlike glucose, cannot be further metabolized because it lacks the necessary 2′ hydroxyl group and, when phosphorylated, cannot exit the cell. In mammals, there are 4 different hexokinase isoforms (HK1–4), again differing in their expression pattern and affinity for glucose; but mostly HK2 is expressed at high levels in many tumors.[36]

The only way FDG-phosphate can leave cells is by being dephosphorylated, in a reciprocal reaction of that catalyzed by hexokinases. The dephosphorylation is catalyzed by glucose-6-phosphatase and yields FDG that can leave the cell through facilitated diffusion via the GLUTs. Reduced levels of glucose-6-phosphatase in cancer cells (compared with normal cells) lead to the accumulation of FDG-phosphate in cancer cells (metabolic trapping) (Fig. 3).[37,38] It is also important to note that FDG is not specific for cancer and can accumulate at sites of infection and inflammation and also in normal tissues with a high glucose turnover.

Factors Influencing FDG Uptake

Several factors play a role in FDG uptake in cancer cells besides the abovementioned proteins. These factors include the number of viable tumor cells; histologic type; tumor grade; proliferative activity; and, importantly, a well-developed tumor vasculature, which is required for sufficient delivery of glucose and oxygen.[39] Inadequate vascularization of the tumor will lead to hypoxia, which, in terms of cancer, is defined as tumors having a lower partial pressure of oxygen compared with their respective normal tissue. The degree of tumor hypoxia varies in a solid tumor; the presence of hypoxic regions is associated with increased malignancy, poor prognosis, and therapy resistance.[40]

The hypoxic response is primarily mediated by hypoxia-inducible factor (HIF) because hypoxia leads to a nuclear accumulation of this DNA-binding transcription factor because of the lack of rapid degradation. HIF induces several target genes, including genes involved in increased glucose consumption (eg, GLUT1 and HK2).[41,42] Hence, the increased glucose metabolism in tumors is driven in part by tumor hypoxia through the activity of HIF; but increased proliferation will also increase glucose utilization.[43]

Correlation Between ^{18}F-FDG Accumulation and the Levels of GLUT, HK, HIF, and Glucose-6-Phosphatase

Because increased glucose metabolism in cancer depends on increased glycolysis, the expression levels of GLUT1, HK2, glucose-6-phosphatase,

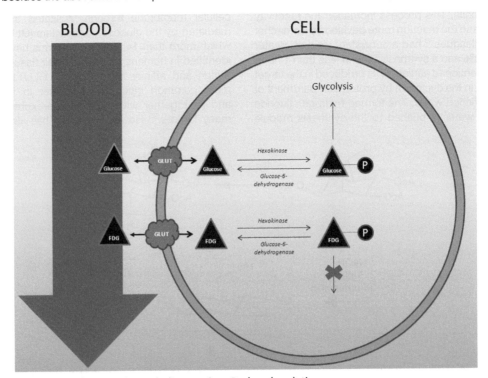

Fig. 3. The concept of FDG and metabolic trapping. P, phosphorylation.

and HIF have been correlated with the accumulation of FDG in vitro, in murine xenograft models, and also in several malignant human tumors. It is beyond the scope of this article to discuss all tumor types; hence, the emphasis is on non–small cell lung cancer (NSCLC), esophageal squamous cell carcinoma (ESCC), and oral squamous cell carcinoma (OSCC) because these tumor types have been investigated the most (**Table 2**).

The uptake of FDG (standardized uptake value [SUV]) correlated with the expression of GLUTs; hexokinases; glucose-6-phosphatase; and, in some cases, Ki67, a proliferation marker.[44] Expression analysis was performed by immunohistochemical staining. Note that most studies only examined the expression of one or a few of the proteins involved in FDG uptake. In each case, the proteins were either found to correlate significantly or no significant correlation was noted.

Most of the studies have focused on a correlation between FDG uptake (given by an SUV) and the expression of GLUT1 analyzed by immunohistochemical staining. However, no clear conclusion can be drawn from these studies, even though most of them show a significantly positive correlation between GLUT1 expression and FDG uptake (see **Table 2**). But in each tumor type, there are also studies showing that there is no significant correlation between levels of GLUT1 and FDG uptake.

Fewer studies have looked at a correlation between the expression of GLUT3, HIF, or HK2 and FDG; again, there are discrepancies within each tumor type because none of the proteins are solely found to either significantly correlate or not significantly correlate with the SUV (see **Table 2**). Only one group has looked for a correlation between SUV and the expression of glucose-6-phosphatase; however, no positive correlation was found in OSCC, even if this study found a positive correlation with GLUT1, HK2, and HIF.[38]

One explanation for the large degree of discrepancy between the investigated levels of proteins and FDG accumulation, not only in NSCLC, ESCC, and OSCC but also in other tumor types tested, could be the large intratumor heterogeneity.[65,66] Furthermore, the uptake of FDG probably does not depend solely on only one protein but rather the concerted action of several.

PATIENT PREPARATION, PHYSIOLOGIC UPTAKE, AND PITFALLS

As mentioned earlier, FDG is a glucose analogue; as such, distribution largely follows the body's physiologic glucose metabolism (**Fig. 4**). The

Table 2
Correlation between FDG uptake and protein expression

Tumor Type	N	Significant Correlation with SUV	No Significant Correlation with SUV	References
NSCLC	34	GLUT1	—	45
	32	—	GLUT1 and 3	46
	36	GLUT1, Ki67	—	47
	102	GLUT1, HIF	GLUT3, Ki67	48
	19	GLUT1 and 3	HK1, 2, and 3	49
	149	GLUT1	—	50
	25	GLUT1	—	51
	32	GLUT1	—	52
	73	—	GLUT1 and 3	53
ESCC	60	GLUT1	—	54
	43	GLUT1	Ki67	47
	57	GLUT1	—	55
	72	HK2	GLUT1	56
	80	GLUT	—	57
	67	GLUT1	—	58
OSCC	44	GLUT1	—	59
	47	—	GLUT1, HK2, HIF, Ki67	60
	36	GLUT1, HK2, HIF	Glucose-6-phosphatase	38
	37	HIF	GLUT1	61
	45	HIF, Ki67	—	62
	19	—	HK2	63
	19	—	GLUT1 and 3	64

Abbreviation: SUV, standardized uptake value.
Data from Refs.[38,45–62]

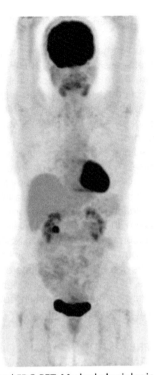

Fig. 4. Normal FDG-PET. Marked physiologic uptake in the brain and the heart and lesser physiologic uptake in the salivary glands. Tracer excretion is seen in the urinary tract with accumulation in the bladder.

spectrum of potential pitfalls in FDG-PET/CT is relatively broad and variable, but interpretive mistakes may be avoided with a thorough knowledge of both technical and patient-related factors. Thus, knowledge of the normal distribution, physiologic

uptake, and common normal variants is pivotal. This section briefly reviews some of the considerations necessary to facilitate the correct interpretation of PET findings including some basic but important issues of patient preparation.[67,68]

In general, hyperglycemia and hyperinsulinism impairs FDG uptake in tumors because of the competitive uptake of FDG and glucose. Therefore, patients are asked to fast for at least 4 to 6 hours before FDG injection to reduce insulin levels and facilitate the highest possible target-to-background ratio. Blood glucose levels should be within normal range, preferably less than 8 to 11 mmol/L (~150–200 mg/dL); with higher levels, scans should be rescheduled rather than performed after administering insulin to reduce blood glucose. Insulin-induced hypoglycemia reduces tumor uptake and facilitates physiologic uptake in muscles and fat, thereby overall decreasing the tumor-to-background ratio (**Figs. 5** and **6**). This decrease only seems to be an issue in malignant tissue and not inflammatory processes as described by Zhuang and colleagues[69] who found no effect on the SUV in benign lesions, even with blood glucose levels up to 14 mmol/L (~250 mg/dL). Higher levels may also be accepted in patients with type 2 diabetes because there is some evidence that chronic hyperglycemia (>11 mmol/L, ~200 mg/dL) only minimally influences FDG uptake.[70]

Despite fasting, high physiologic uptake is still seen in predominantly glycolytic organs, such as the brain and the heart. In the former, the uptake is usually especially marked and uniform in the cortex and basal ganglia, with lesser uptake in white

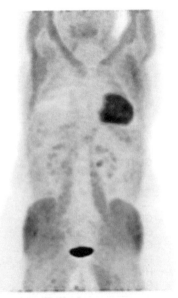
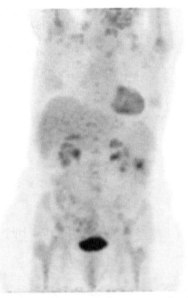

Fig. 5. Physiologic muscle uptake. The same patient scanned with 2 days apart, without proper fasting (*left*) and after proper 6 hours of fasting (*right*). Note the marked, diffuse uptake in skeletal muscles in the former.

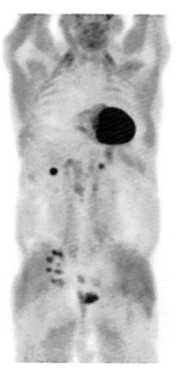
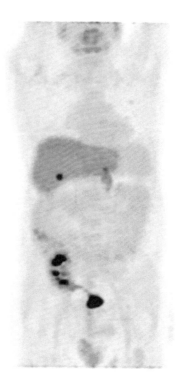

Fig. 6. Effect of insulin. The same patient scanned with 2 days apart. In the scan to the left, the patient had just self-administered fast-acting insulin because of a high plasma glucose level. The scan to the right was done a few days later under normal blood-glucose conditions. Note again the marked, diffuse FDG uptake in skeletal muscles in the first scan. Liver lesions were present in both scans as well as tracer excretion to a kidney graft.

matter and cerebrospinal fluid. Uptake in the myocardium is highly variable, from uniform and intense to virtually absent. This uptake pattern applies to the left ventricle, whereas the right ventricle and atria are usually devoid of FDG. Although a regimen of prolonged fasting (>18 hours) and a low-carbohydrate-high-fat diet may be considered to facilitate a substrate shift from glucose to free fatty acids, irregular uptake may remain because of a temporal and geographic nonuniformity of the decreased glycolytic activity. Uptake in the liver, spleen, and bone marrow is usually homogenous and low; but especially the bone marrow may be subject to diffusely increased uptake in systemic inflammation, prolonged bleeding, or following therapeutic interventions with chemotherapy or bone marrow stimulants (**Fig. 7**). This uptake pattern may mask osseous metastases or malignant bone marrow infiltration; but these conditions are usually readily distinguishable, with the latter being more intensely focal in appearance.

Skeletal muscles can be considered collectively as the largest glucose-consuming organ; physiologic uptake is, therefore, an important source of error throughout the body and should be minimized as much as possible. Under normal circumstances, skeletal muscle uptake is uniformly low but subject to considerable variability in voluntary muscle contractions; even subtle muscle activity may demonstrate high FDG uptake (eg, eye movements and talking during the injection phase). Patients are usually injected after a resting period in the supine position and remain lying for at least half an hour. Involuntary muscle activity may also sometimes be a problem, usually in anxious patients and most prominently in the paravertebral muscles of the neck and thorax. In severe cases, anxiolytic drugs may be considered. In the early days of stand-alone FDG-PET, a characteristic, symmetric uptake pattern in the supraclavicular region was also considered to be caused by skeletal muscles. However, with FDG-PET/CT, no corresponding structural explanations were present; this finding is now considered to be caused by metabolically active brown fat, a rudimentary thermogenetic tissue most abundant in children and young adults and most prominent in the cold months. Uptake may especially obscure pathologic uptake in lymphoma or head-and-neck cancers; as brown fat is sympathetically innervated, pretreatment with beta-blockers may be considered besides temperature controlled injection rooms and blankets for young patients (**Fig. 8**).

Physiologic FDG activity in the genitourinary system poses yet another challenge. Unlike glucose, FDG is not reabsorbed by the renal tubules; intense

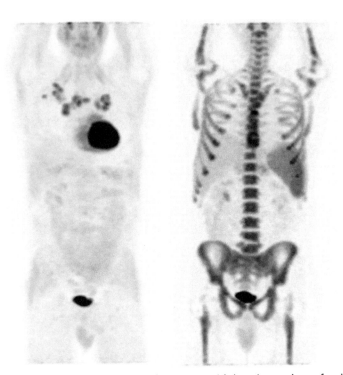

Fig. 7. Activated bone marrow. Baseline scan (*left*) of a patient with lymphoma shows focal FDG uptake in peri-clavicular and mediastinal lymph nodes. Treatment response-assessment after 3 cycles of chemotherapy (*right*) in the same patient; there is no longer FDG uptake in lymph nodes (complete metabolic remission) but marked, diffuse uptake in the bone marrow caused by effects of chemotherapy.

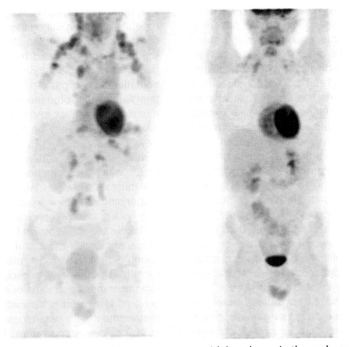

Fig. 8. Brown fat. Two scans in the same patient, a young man with lymphoma in the neck scanned during winter. At baseline (*left*) there is marked, focal FDG uptake in brown fat in the periclavicular region. A subsequent scan a few days later after pretreatment with beta-blocker and hot blankets during injection shows normalized distribution with faint uptake in lymph nodes in the neck.

activity is, therefore, often present throughout the urinary tract or in urine reservoirs. Hydration, the administration of diuretics, and bladder catheterization have been advocated but have not gained widespread acceptance and are not part of standard protocols at any of the authors' institutions. Moderate uptake in testicles is relatively commonly encountered and seemingly inversely related to age. Similarly, uptake in ovaries and uterine cavity may be present in premenopausal women during ovulation and menstruation, respectively, as well as in the glandular tissue of the breasts.

Finally, 2 areas in which physiologic uptake commonly give rise to suspicious incidental findings deserve special mention, namely, the thyroid gland and the gastrointestinal tract. Regarding the former, diffuse or focal uptake may be present in normal tissue as well as in goitrous glands or thyroiditis. However, such findings have been reported to represent malignancies or premalignant findings in as many as 33% of patients and should be further examined.[71] Similarly, uptake in the gastrointestinal tract is a common finding. It is highly variable and may be present in all parts of the gastrointestinal tract, albeit with some common regional characteristics: Esophageal uptake is rare unless inflammation or malignancy is present, whereas diffuse uptake in the gastric mucosa or smooth muscles is relatively common. Focal uptake may also be present at the gastroesophageal

junction (physiologic) or associated with ulcers, whereas uptake in the small intestine is usually limited. Physiologic colonic uptake is highly variable, from faint and diffuse to highly intense and focal; it may be present in all segments, although most commonly in the caecum and rectosigmoid and especially in patients undergoing treatment with metformin (**Fig. 9**). The exact underlying mechanism of intestinal uptake is not fully understood but is probably multifarious (ie, smooth muscle activity, metabolically active mucosa, luminal contents, or glycolytic bacteria). However, incidental findings of focal colonic uptake may be malignant or premalignant in as many as 65% of all cases.[72]

CONCLUDING REMARKS

As shown in this introductory article, PET/CT imaging with FDG (and other tracers) is based on a complex set of basic physiologic and pathophysiologic, chemical and radiochemical, physical and radiophysical, and technical concepts and processes, which, in the eyes of many, probably make these imaging methods less attractive and more difficult to understand and handle than the more common and more widespread structural imaging modalities as conventional radiography and CT. On the other hand, these conditions are the realities one has to deal with and understand to be able to exploit fully the treasure chest of

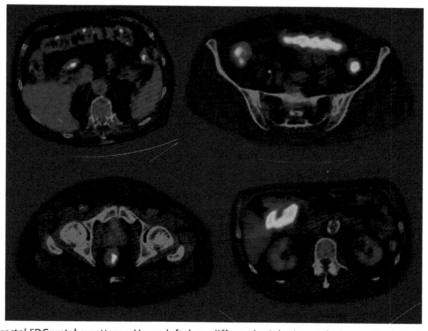

Fig. 9. Colorectal FDG uptake patterns. Upper left: low, diffuse physiologic uptake in a patient treated with metformin. Upper right: More marked uptake in a colon segment with wall thickening; biopsy confirmed colitis. Lower left: marked, focal uptake in the rectum; colonoscopy identified a small, benign polyp. Lower right: marked, focal uptake in the ascending colon; biopsy confirmed adenocarcinoma of the colon.

possibilities that can be achieved with these methods only and that one needs to master to use and be part of twenty-first-century imaging, which is molecular and not structural and will bring medical science and health care in general a very significant leap forward in decades to come.

REFERENCES

1. Mankoff DA. A definition of molecular imaging. J Nucl Med 2007;48:18N, 21N.
2. Hess S, Blomberg BA, Zhu H, et al. The pivotal role of FDG-PET/CT in modern medicine. Acad Radiol 2014;21:232–49.
3. Joliot-Curie F, Curie I. Artificial production of a new kind of radio-element. Nature 1934;133:201.
4. Ter-Pogossian M. The origins of positron emission tomography. Semin Nucl Med 1992;22(3):140–9.
5. Rich DA. A brief history of positron emission tomography. J Nucl Med Technol 1997;25(1):4–11.
6. Wagner HW Jr. A brief history of positron emission tomography (PET). Semin Nucl Med 1998;28(3):213–20.
7. Ter-Pogossian M, Powers WE. The use of radioactive oxygen-15 in the determination of oxygen content in malignant neoplasms. Radioisotopes in scientific research, vol. 3. Proceedings of the 1st UNESCO International Conference, Paris 1957. New York: Pergamon; 1958.
8. Wrenn FR, Good ML, Handler P. The use of positron-emitting radioisotopes for the localization of brain tumours. Science 1951;113:525–7.
9. Brownell GL, Sweet WH. Localization of brain tumours with positron emitters. Nucleonics 1953;11:40–5.
10. Rankowitz S, Robertson JS, Higgenbotham WA, et al. Positron scanner for locating brain tumours. IRE Int Conv Rec 1962;9:49–56.
11. Kuhl DE, Edwards RQ. Image separation radioisotope scanning. Radiology 1963;80:653–61.
12. Phelps ME, Hoffmann EJ, Mullani NA, et al. Application of annihilation coincidence detection to transaxial reconstruction tomography. J Nucl Med 1975;16:210–24.
13. Ter-Pogossian MM, Phelps ME, Hoffmann EJ, et al. Positron-emission transaxial tomography for nuclear imaging (PETT). Radiology 1975;114:89–98.
14. Cho ZH, Chan JK, Eriksson L. Circular ring transverse axial positron camera for three-dimensional reconstruction of radionuclides distribution. IEEE Trans Nucl Sci 1976;NS-23:613–22.
15. Cho ZH, Farukhi MR. Bismuth germinate as a potential scintillation detector in positron cameras. J Nucl Med 1977;18:840–4.
16. Ter-Pogossian MM, Mullani NA, Ficke DC, et al. Photon time-of-flight-assisted positron emission tomography. J Comput Assist Tomogr 1981;5:227–39.
17. Ter-Pogossian MM, Raichle ME, Sobel BE. Positron-emission tomography. Sci Am 1980;243:170–81.
18. Hess S, Høilund-Carlsen PF, Alavi A. Historic images in nuclear medicine 1976: the first issue of clinical nuclear medicine and the first human FDG study. Clin Nucl Med 2014;39:701–3.
19. Alavi A, Reivich M. The conception of FDG-PET imaging. Semin Nucl Med 2002;XXXII(1):2–5.
20. Ido T, Wan CN, Casella V, et al. Labeled 2-deoxy-D-glucose analogs. Fluorine-18-labeled 2-deoxy-2-fluoro-D-glucose, 2-deoxy-2-fluoro-D-mannose, and C-14-2-deoxy-2-fluoro-D-glucose. J Labelled Comp Radiopharm 1978;14:175–82.
21. Reivich M, Kuhl D, Wolf A, et al. The [18F]fluorodeoxyglucose method for the measurement of local cerebral glucose utilization in man. Circ Res 1979;44:127–37.
22. Karp JS, Surti S, Daube-Witherspoon ME, et al. Benefit of time-of-flight in PET: experimental and clinical results. J Nucl Med 2008;49(3):462–70.
23. Hudson HM, Larkin RS. Accelerated image reconstruction using ordered subsets of projection data. IEEE Trans Med Imaging 1994;13(4):601–9.
24. Kinahan PE, Hasegawa BH, Beyer T. X-ray-based attenuation correction for positron emission tomography/computed tomography scanners. Semin Nucl Med 2003;33(3):166–79.
25. Watson CC, Newport D, Casey ME, et al. Evaluation of simulation-based scatter correction for 3-D PET cardiac imaging. IEEE Trans Nucl Sci 1997;44(1):90–7.
26. Miller M, Griesmer J, Jordan D, et al. Initial characterization of a prototype digital photon counting PET system. J Nucl Med 2014;55:658.
27. Wong WH, Li H, Zhang Y, et al. A high-resolution time-of-flight clinical PET detection system using the PMT-quadrant-sharing technology. J Nucl Med 2014;55:657.
28. Sossi V, de Jong HW, Barker WC, et al. The second generation HRRT: a multi-centre scanner performance investigation. IEEE Nucl Sci Symp Conf Rec 2005;4:2195–9.
29. Delso G, Fürst S, Jakoby B, et al. Performance measurements of the Siemens mMR integrated whole-body PET/MR scanner [Erratum appears in J Nucl Med 2012;53(3):507]. J Nucl Med 2011;52(12):1914–22. http://dx.doi.org/10.2967/jnumed.111.092726.
30. Hamacher K, Coenen HH, Stocklin G. Efficient stereospecific synthesis of no-carrier-added 2-[18F]-fluoro-2-deoxy-D-glucose using aminopolyether supported nucleophilic substitution. J Nucl Med 1986;27(2):235–8.
31. Fowler JS, Ido T. Initial and subsequent approach for the synthesis of 18FDG. Semin Nucl Med 2002;XXXII(1):6–12.

32. Macheda ML, Rogers S, Best JD. Molecular and cellular regulation of glucose transporter (GLUT) proteins in cancer. J Cell Physiol 2005;202:654–62.

33. Ganapathy V, Thangaraju M, Prasad PD. Nutrient transporters in cancer: relevance to Warburg hypothesis and beyond. Pharmacol Ther 2009;121:29–40.

34. Moadel RM, Weldon RH, Katz EB, et al. Positherapy: targeted nuclear therapy of breast cancer with 18F-2-deoxy-2-fluoro-D-glucose. Cancer Res 2005;65:698–702.

35. Szablewski L. Expression of glucose transporters in cancers. Biochim Biophys Acta 2013;1835:164–9.

36. Mathupala SP, Ko YH, Pedersen PL. Hexokinase-2 bound to mitochondria: cancer's stygian link to the "Warburg Effect" and a pivotal target for effective therapy. Semin Cancer Biol 2009;19:17–24.

37. Nelson CA, Wang JQ, Leav I, et al. The interaction among glucose transport, hexokinase, and glucose-6-phosphatase with respect to 3H-2-deoxyglucose retention in murine tumor models. Nucl Med Biol 1996;23:533–41.

38. Yamada T, Uchida M, Kwang-Lee K, et al. Correlation of metabolism/hypoxia markers and fluorodeoxyglucose uptake in oral squamous cell carcinomas. Oral Surg Oral Med Oral Pathol Oral Radiol 2012;113:464–71.

39. Bos R, van Der Hoeven JJ, van Der Wall E, et al. Biologic correlates of (18)fluorodeoxyglucose uptake in human breast cancer measured by positron emission tomography. J Clin Oncol 2002;20:379–87.

40. Bertout JA, Patel SA, Simon MC. The impact of O2 availability on human cancer. Nat Rev Cancer 2008;8:967–75.

41. Iyer NV, Kotch LE, Agani F, et al. Cellular and developmental control of O2 homeostasis by hypoxia-inducible factor 1 alpha. Genes Dev 1998;12:149–62.

42. Ryan HE, Lo J, Johnson RS. HIF-1 alpha is required for solid tumor formation and embryonic vascularization. EMBO J 1998;17:3005–15.

43. Avril N, Menzel M, Dose J, et al. Glucose metabolism of breast cancer assessed by 18F-FDG PET: histologic and immunohistochemical tissue analysis. J Nucl Med 2001;42:9–16.

44. Scholzen T, Gerdes J. The Ki-67 protein: from the known and the unknown. J Cell Physiol 2000;182:311–22.

45. Usuda K, Sagawa M, Aikawa H, et al. Correlation between glucose transporter-1 expression and 18F-fluoro-2-deoxyglucose uptake on positron emission tomography in lung cancer. Gen Thorac Cardiovasc Surg 2010;58:405–10.

46. Suzawa N, Ito M, Qiao S, et al. Assessment of factors influencing FDG uptake in non-small cell lung cancer on PET/CT by investigating histological differences in expression of glucose transporters 1 and 3 and tumour size. Lung Cancer 2011;72:191–8.

47. Kaida H, Kawahara A, Hayakawa M, et al. The difference in relationship between 18F-FDG uptake and clinicopathological factors on thyroid, esophageal, and lung cancers. Nucl Med Commun 2014;35:36–43.

48. van Baardwijk A, Dooms C, van Suylen RJ, et al. The maximum uptake of (18)F-deoxyglucose on positron emission tomography scan correlates with survival, hypoxia inducible factor-1alpha and GLUT-1 in non-small cell lung cancer. Eur J Cancer 2007;43:1392–8.

49. de Geus-Oei LF, van Krieken JH, Aliredjo RP, et al. Biological correlates of FDG uptake in non-small cell lung cancer. Lung Cancer 2007;55:79–87.

50. Taylor MD, Smith PW, Brix WK, et al. Fluorodeoxyglucose positron emission tomography and tumor marker expression in non-small cell lung cancer. J Thorac Cardiovasc Surg 2009;137:43–8.

51. Chung JK, Lee YJ, Kim SK, et al. Comparison of [18F]fluorodeoxyglucose uptake with glucose transporter-1 expression and proliferation rate in human glioma and non-small-cell lung cancer. Nucl Med Commun 2004;25:11–7.

52. Higashi K, Ueda Y, Sakurai A, et al. Correlation of Glut-1 glucose transporter expression with [18F]FDG uptake in non-small cell lung cancer. Eur J Nucl Med 2000;27:1778–85.

53. Marom EM, Aloia TA, Moore MB, et al. Correlation of FDG-PET imaging with Glut-1 and Glut-3 expression in early-stage non-small cell lung cancer. Lung Cancer 2001;33:99–107.

54. Hiyoshi Y, Watanabe M, Imamura Y, et al. The relationship between the glucose transporter type 1 expression and F-fluorodeoxyglucose uptake in esophageal squamous cell carcinoma. Oncology 2009;76:286–92.

55. Kobayashi M, Kaida H, Kawahara A, et al. The relationship between GLUT-1 and vascular endothelial growth factor expression and 18F-FDG uptake in esophageal squamous cell cancer patients. Clin Nucl Med 2012;37:447–52.

56. Tohma T, Okazumi S, Makino H, et al. Relationship between glucose transporter, hexokinase and FDG-PET in esophageal cancer. Hepatogastroenterology 2005;52:486–90.

57. Kita Y, Okumura H, Uchikado Y, et al. Clinical significance of ^{18}F-fluorodeoxyglucose positron emission tomography in superficial esophageal squamous cell carcinoma. Ann Surg Oncol 2013;20:1646–52.

58. Taylor MD, Smith PW, Brix WK, et al. Correlations between selected tumor markers and fluorodeoxyglucose maximal standardized uptake values in

esophageal cancer. Eur J Cardiothorac Surg 2009; 35:699–705.

59. Kato H, Takita J, Miyazaki T, et al. Correlation of 18-F-fluorodeoxyglucose (FDG) accumulation with glucose transporter (Glut-1) expression in esophageal squamous cell carcinoma. Anticancer Res 2003;23:3263–72.

60. Schreurs LM, Smit JK, Pavlov K, et al. Prognostic impact of clinicopathological features and expression of biomarkers related to 18F-FDG uptake in esophageal cancer. Ann Surg Oncol 2014. [Epub ahead of print].

61. Miyawaki A, Ikeda R, Hijioka H, et al. SUVmax of FDG-PET correlates with the effects of neoadjuvant chemoradiotherapy for oral squamous cell carcinoma. Oncol Rep 2010;23:1205–12.

62. Shimomura H, Sasahira T, Yamanaka Y, et al. [18F] fluoro-2-deoxyglucose-positron emission tomography for the assessment of histopathological response after preoperative chemoradiotherapy in advanced oral squamous cell carcinoma. Int J Clin Oncol 2014. [Epub ahead of print].

63. Tian M, Zhang H, Higuchi T, et al. Hexokinase-II expression in untreated oral squamous cell carcinoma: comparison with FDG PET imaging. Ann Nucl Med 2005;19:335–8.

64. Tian M, Zhang H, Nakasone Y, et al. Expression of Glut-1 and Glut-3 in untreated oral squamous cell carcinoma compared with FDG accumulation in a PET study. Eur J Nucl Med Mol Imaging 2004;31:5–12.

65. Tixier F, Le Rest CC, Hatt M, et al. Intratumor heterogeneity characterized by textural features on baseline 18F-FDG PET images predicts response to concomitant radiochemotherapy in esophageal cancer. J Nucl Med 2011;52:369–78.

66. Tixier F, Hatt M, Valla C, et al. Visual versus quantitative assessment of intratumor 18F-FDG PET uptake heterogeneity: prognostic value in non-small cell lung cancer. J Nucl Med 2014. pii:jnumed.113.133389.

67. Gorospe L, Raman S, Echeveste J, et al. Whole-body PET/CT: spectrum of physiological variants, artifacts and interpretative pitfalls in cancer patients. Nucl Med Commun 2005;26(8):671–87.

68. Cook GJ, Wegner EA, Fogelman I. Pitfalls and artifacts in 18FDG PET and PET/CT oncologic imaging. Semin Nucl Med 2004;34(2):122–33.

69. Zhuang HM, Cortes-Blanco A, Pourdehnad M, et al. Do high glucose levels have different effect on FDG uptake in inflammatory and malignant disorders? Nucl Med Commun 2001;22:1123–8.

70. Hara T, Higashi T, Nakamoto Y, et al. Significance of chronic marked hyperglycemia on FDG-PET: is it really problematic for clinical oncologic imaging? Ann Nucl Med 2009;23:657–69.

71. Shie P, Cardarelli R, Sprawls K, et al. Systematic review: prevalence of malignant incidental thyroid nodules identified on fluorine-18 fluorodeoxyglucose positron emission tomography. Nucl Med Commun 2009;30(9):742–8.

72. Treglia G, Calcagni ML, Rufini V, et al. Clinical significance of incidental focal colorectal 18F-fluorodeoxyglucose uptake: our experience and a review of the literature. Colorectal Dis 2011;14: 174–80.

Fluorodeoxyglucose PET in Neurology and Psychiatry

Michael Schöll, PhD[a,b,*], Andrés Damián, MD[c],
Henry Engler, MD, PhD[c,d]

KEYWORDS

- Fluorodeoxyglucose positron emission tomography • [18F]-Fluorodeoxyglucose • Neurology
- Psychiatry • Dementia

KEY POINTS

- Molecular imaging with [18F]fluoro-D-deoxyglucose (FDG) PET can assist in the differential diagnosis of neurologic and psychiatric disorders, particularly in their early stages.
- FDG PET has the potential to describe the course of neurologic and psychiatric disease.
- Pitfalls should be known by nuclear medicine physicians to obtain a correct diagnosis.
- Combining FDG PET with a recent magnetic resonance image and performing integrated multimodality interpretation can add important complementary information.
- The combination of FDG with other PET tracers can enhance accuracy in differential diagnoses.

INTRODUCTION

The synthesis of 2-deoxy-2-[18F]fluoro-D-glucose (FDG) at the Brookhaven National Laboratory in 1976 was a groundbreaking development in nuclear medicine imaging.[1]

FDG has developed since then into the most widely available tracer for PET and is used extensively in clinical and research settings.

The first application of FDG PET in humans was to measure glucose metabolism in the brain,[2] and although most clinical FDG PET examinations are performed in oncology, its application in the assessment of disorders of the central nervous system (CNS) is of cardinal importance.

In neurology and psychiatry, focal lesions in the highly plastic CNS can lead to complex symptoms, and neuroimaging by means of computed tomography (CT) and magnetic resonance (MR) imaging plays an important role in the in vivo detection of structural lesions. However, it was with the advent of PET that the ability was provided to understand the underlying molecular mechanisms that often precede structural changes, allowing an early diagnosis as well as targeted treatment management based on functional rather than structural measures.

The great diversity of existing PET tracers allows the study of numerous brain functions in normal and pathologic conditions, such as the measurement of regional blood flow, glucose metabolism, enzyme activity, protein accumulation, or receptor density in the CNS. However, in this article, the focus is on selected established and eligible applications of FDG PET in neurology and psychiatry (**Box 1**).

Disclosures: The authors have no relations to disclose.
[a] MedTech West and the Department of Clinical Neuroscience and Rehabilitation, University of Gothenburg, Blå stråket 5, 6th Floor, Gothenburg 413 45, Sweden; [b] Department NVS, Center for Alzheimer Research, Translational Alzheimer Neurobiology, Karolinska Institute, Novum 5th Floor, Stockholm 14186, Sweden; [c] Uruguayan Centre of Molecular Imaging (CUDIM), Av. Dr. Américo Ricaldoni 2010, Montevideo 11600, Uruguay; [d] Department of Medical Sciences, Uppsala University, Box 256, Uppsala 75105, Sweden
* Corresponding author. MedTech West, Sahlgrenska University Hospital, Blå stråket 5, 6th Floor, Gothenburg 413 45, Sweden
E-mail address: michael.scholl@neuro.gu.se

PET Clin 9 (2014) 371–390
http://dx.doi.org/10.1016/j.cpet.2014.07.005

- Dementia: assessment of patients with symptoms of dementia. Early diagnosis of dementia. FDG PET can be useful in the differential diagnosis between different dementing disorders including Alzheimer disease, dementia with Lewy bodies, frontotemporal lobe dementia, and vascular dementia.
- Epilepsy: FDG PET is useful in the presurgical evaluation of refractory epilepsy to lateralize and localize the functionally impaired region, especially in patients with normal MR imaging findings.
- Parkinsonian disorders: differential diagnosis of parkinsonisms. FDG PET is useful in the evaluation of Parkinson disease, and in the diagnosis of atypical parkinsonisms, including corticobasal degeneration, multiple system atrophy, and progressive supranuclear palsy.
- Psychiatry: FDG PET has been proved useful in the study of patients with psychiatric disorders such as depression, bipolar disorder, and schizophrenia.
- Stroke and assessment of neuronal plasticity.

IMAGING TECHNIQUE

The technical aspects of FDG PET and its application are covered in the article "The basic principles of FDG-PET/CT imaging" in this issue and are thus only sketchily described here.

FDG PET in the study of the CNS is safe for the patient and a straightforward procedure, which generally is as follows (for European Association for Nuclear Medicine [EANM] guidelines, see Ref.[3]): the patient does not need any preparation except for at least 4 hours of fasting and abstention from coffee, tea, alcohol, and nicotine, and in case of diabetes, normalization of glycemia. A dose of approximately 3.0 MBq/kg (**Box 2** for detailed information) of FDG is administered intravenously once the patient is in a condition of neurosensory relaxation, lying on a bed in a dimmed room with eyes closed and no external auditory stimuli. If a patient is unable to cooperate, mild sedation may be used shortly before image acquisition. After 30 to 60 minutes under these conditions, images are acquired with the patient supine and the head stabilized in the center of the field of detection. In three-dimensional acquisition mode of modern PET scanners, offering a spatial resolution of 3 to 6 mm, a static emission scan commonly lasts about 30 minutes, including transmission scans for tissue attenuation correction, whereas dynamic

Recommended FDG PET patient preparation and image acquisition:

- Patient preparation: fasting for 4 to 6 hours. Measure of blood glucose level before FDG injection (low-quality images can be expected with blood glucose levels higher than 160 mg/dL). Patient positioning in a quiet area 15 minutes before FDG injection and during the established uptake period, especially in the first minutes. Intravenous cannulation 15 minutes before tracer injection. Bladder voiding before FDG administration and acquisition.
- Injection: 185 to 740 MBq in adults (typically 300–600 MBq in 2D mode, 125–250 MBq in 3D mode).[3,161] In children refer to the European Association of Nuclear Medicine dosage card v.1.5.2008, (class B radiotracer). Effective dose: 19 µSv/MBq in adults. Highest absorbed dose in bladder: 0.13–0.16 mGy/MBq in adults.
- Positioning: patients should be instructed to avoid or minimize head movements. Head fixation may be useful. The orbitomeatal line in parallel to the detector rings can be used for standardization of the positioning.
- Acquisition: attenuation correction can be performed with CT. Inspect images to detect patient motion between CT and PET acquisition. Standardized acquisition times after injection (eg, 30, 40, or 60 minutes after FDG administration). List mode acquisition and dynamic acquisition with short frames can be useful for movement corrections. Reconstruction with ordered-subsets expectation maximization or filtered back projection.
- Quantification: semiquantitative analysis comparing patients with age-matched normal control individuals can be used to assist visual analysis. Standardized uptake values (SUVs) help in the assessment of uptake patterns. Ideally, SUV ratios are created using an unaffected reference region. Quantification of CMRglc can be performed using arterial or arterialized blood input. Regional analysis should use manual or atlas-based regions of interest or voxel-based analysis, ideally created on coregistered MR images.
- Report: include the acquisition protocol. Characteristic disease patterns should be explicitly stated. Include differential diagnoses. If possible inform in conjunction with neuroradiology specialist.

imaging, meaning the collection of a temporal series of frames, can last up to 90 minutes. In addition to studies of resting state, acquisition can also be performed in the course of a pharmacologic or cognitive stimulation.

Attenuation correction is obligatory and can be performed using either measured data from transmission scans, acquired with an external radiation source or the embedded CT camera, mathematical estimations, or hybrid correction using short transmission measurements followed by theoretically derived corrections based on image segmentation algorithms. The images are finally reconstructed from the acquired sinograms through an iterative algorithm or filtered back projection.

Image Analysis and Data Acquisition

For visual image assessment, coregistered and fused structural images by means of CT or MR imaging scans can improve anatomic accuracy and assist in making a diagnosis. In addition to a mere visual assessment of the images, semiquantitative measures such as the calculation of standardized uptake values (SUV, computed from dividing the ratio of region of interest [ROI]/volume of interest [VOI]–derived radioactivity and injected activity by body weight) help in estimating and comparing levels of cerebral glucose metabolism. However, other factors, such as blood glucose levels, body composition, and pharmaceuticals, influence this parameter and are not taken in account. Longitudinal studies and intersubject comparisons benefit from normalizing VOI or voxel SUVs to the activity in either a reference region where activity is relatively stable and suggested to be independent of disease stage or pharmaceutical effects or to global activity, thus creating SUV ratios (SUVR).

Furthermore, FDG PET offers the possibility not only to visualize but also to quantify the cerebral metabolic rate of glucose (CMRglc, expressed as μmol/100 g/min) by compartmental or graphical kinetic modeling[4–6] and the application of a lumped constant to correct for differences between FDG and glucose.[7] This method requires invasive sampling of arterial or arterialized venous blood to measure the concentration of glucose in plasma, and although the approximated information about CMRglc is valuable for instance in the evaluation of treatment effects, this renders the procedure less feasible for clinical routine examinations.

Computer-aided and automated methods for regional FDG PET image analysis are so far mainly used in research settings but have gained importance also for clinical use. Voxel by voxel–based comparisons as implemented in free software packages such as Statistical Parametric Mapping (SPM, Wellcome Trust Center for Neuroimaging, University College London, UK),[8–10] Neurostat/3D-SSP (Department of Radiology, University of Washington, Seattle, WA, USA),[11,12] or commercially available programs such as PMOD (PMOD Technologies Ltd., Zurich, Switzerland),[13] deliver useful information when differences between 2 patients or a patient and control group are sought after. Segmentation of brain MR imaging using atlas-based methods such as MAPER (Multi-Atlas Propagation with Enhanced Registration),[14] FreeSurfer,[15] FSL (Functional MRI of the Brain Software Library),[16] or other tools result in maps of anatomically highly accurate regions that can be applied to coregistered FDG PET images for the extraction of regional metabolic data and thus make use of the detailed anatomic information in MR images (**Fig. 1**).

NORMAL ANATOMY

In the healthy brain, the cortical gray matter and at a subcortical level, the caudate nuclei, the putamina, and the thalami show highest FDG uptake. Cerebellar cortical and brainstem uptake is usually lower than that of the cerebral neocortex, the basal ganglia, and the thalami. White matter generally shows low uptake and can hardly be visually distinguished from the adjacent ventricular system (**Fig. 2**).[17] Cortical and subcortical uptake patterns

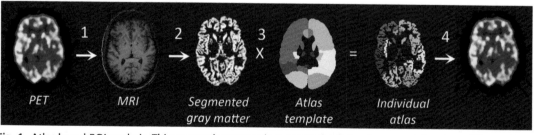

Fig. 1. Atlas-based ROI analysis. This approach commonly requires the following processing steps: (1) coregistration of PET and MR images. (2) Segmentation of MR image. (3) Multiplication of a binary map created from the segmented gray matter MR imaging with a predefined brain atlas. (4) Application of the resulting individual atlas on to the coregistered PET image and extraction of regional values.

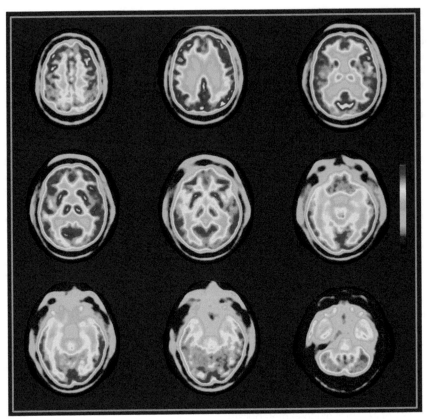

Fig. 2. Normal distribution of FDG uptake in the brain. Axial images of a healthy volunteer.

are mostly symmetric. Auditory or visual stimuli, as well as motor activity, 10 to 20 minutes after administration of FDG can increase uptake in the respective brain areas.

Because of the high variability of SUVs of FDG, the use of relative values (ratios, SUVR) is recommended. Overall FDG uptake may be altered by medications such as benzodiazepines, corticosteroids, and barbiturates, as well as by caffeine and nicotine.[18]

IMAGING FINDINGS/PATHOLOGY
Dementia

Dementia is a group of disorders causing progressive cognitive impairment. Affecting an estimated 29 million patients worldwide, it ranks among the major causes of death and constitutes a considerable burden for health care systems.[19] The prevalence of dementia is strongly related to age, with a rate of 33% in individuals aged 85 years or older.[20] The 4 major types of dementia are Alzheimer disease (AD), frontotemporal dementia (FTD), vascular dementia (VaD), and dementia with Lewy bodies (DLB) (**Box 3**, **Table 1**). A recent article compared the sensitivity and specificity of mere visual evaluation of FDG PET images for

these 4 disorders, which ranged from 93.4% for AD, 92.3% for other dementias, including VaD, and 88.8% for FTD, to 66.6% for DLB.[21] When compared with single-photon CT (SPECT), a recent review reported an overall higher sensitivity of FDG PET for the differential diagnosis of AD (84%–96% vs 63%–86%), FTD (97%–99% vs 71%–80%), and DLB (83%–99% vs 65%–85%), whereas specificity was comparable (**Boxes 4 and 5**).[22]

Alzheimer's disease (AD)

The most common form of dementia is AD, accounting for 50% to 70% of all cases.[23] Along with the global increase in life expectancy, the prevalence of AD has been predicted to increase globally to 80 million patients within the next 40 years.[24] AD is a lethal, progressive neurodegenerative disorder, with a clinical picture of gradually deteriorating memory with subsequent onset of other cognitive, behavioral, and neuropsychiatric changes that impair social interactions and activities of daily living, until the afflicted person is completely dependent on caregivers.[25] No cure has been discovered, and only symptomatic treatment is available for the treatment of AD.

Box 3
Diagnostic criteria for FDG PET in neurology and psychiatry

Typical FDG PET patterns in selected neurodegenerative diseases:

- AD: hypometabolism in parietal, medial, and posterolateral temporal cortex and posterior cyngulum. Frontal hypometabolism may also be present with the progression of the disease. These changes are often bilateral but can be unilateral. Preserved metabolism in occipital, sensory-motor cortex, basal ganglia, and cerebellum.

- FTD: hypometabolism in frontal cortex, anterior cyngulum, and anterolateral temporal cortex. The hypometabolism can affect the caudate nuclei. The cortical hypometabolism may vary in different forms of FTD.

- DLB: parietal and temporolateral hypometabolism similar to the pattern observed in AD. The occipital and primary visual cortex involvement is important for the differential diagnosis. Hypometabolism may also be present in the basal ganglia.

- Creutzfeldt-Jakob disease (CJD): distinct hypometabolism in large areas of the brain involving the right or the left hemisphere, the whole frontal lobe or both parietal lobes and occipital cortex, as in the Heidenheim variant of the disease. Temporal lobes are less frequently affected.

- Parkinson dementia: hypometabolism in the parietal and temporolateral cortices similar to the pattern described in AD. Preserved glucose uptake in the basal ganglia.

- Atypical parkinsonism: in multiple system atrophy, the hypometabolism affects the caudate nuclei and the putamina. Cerebellar and pons hypometabolism may be present. In the corticobasal degeneration, the hypometabolism is observed unilaterally in the frontal or the parietal cortex, the basal ganglia, and the thalami. In PSP, the frontal bilateral hypometabolism predominates.

FDG PET has been used to evaluate deterioration in the AD brain for almost 30 years[26–28] and is certainly the best-evaluated PET tracer in AD research. Since the US Food and Drug Administration (FDA) approved FDG PET in 2004 for the diagnostic evaluation of dementia, it has increasingly been implemented in the clinical examination of patients with suspected AD. The application of FDG PET in combination with other biomarkers has recently also been recommended by the National Institute on Aging–Alzheimer's Association workgroup on diagnostic guidelines for the

Table 1
FDG PET patterns in dementia

Dementia Type	Typical Hypometabolic Brain Regions
AD	Parietotemporal association cortices Medial temporal cortex Posterior cingulate Frontal cortex (at later stages)
FTD	Anterior cingulate Frontal cortex Anterior temporal cortex
DLB	Parietal and posterior temporal cortices Posterior cingulate Occipital cortex (primary visual cortex)
VaD	Multifocal (related to infarct foci in multi-infarct VaD) (Basal ganglia Cerebellum)
Creutzfeldt-Jakob	Parietal, frontal, temporal, and occipital cortical regions

investigation of the preclinical, the symptomatic predementia, and the dementia phase of AD.[29–31] Against a background of global hypometabolism, numerous studies have reported a specific decrease in glucose metabolism in the parietotemporal association cortex, the angular gyrus, and

Box 4
Pitfalls and variants

- Patient's condition at the time of the study: pharmacologic treatment altering brain metabolism (psychotropic treatment, antipsychotic or corticosteroid medication, drug abuse). Activation (sensorial or motor activation during uptake period may significantly change FDG uptake). Anesthesia or sedation may significantly change radiotracer uptake and distribution. Recent therapy (postsurgical inflammation, previous chemotherapy or radiotherapy) Hyperglycemia.

- Acquisition artifacts (metal artifacts in attenuation correction images, patient movement during image acquisition, attenuation correction in misregistered PET and CT scans); inappropriate processing (attenuation correction, reduced frontal activity in hyperostosis frontalis).

- Lack of absolute metabolic quantification may result in imprecise interpretation of the acquired data.

the posterior cingulate cortex, as well as in the medial temporal lobe, including structures such as the hippocampus and entorhinal cortex, whereas regions like the cerebellum, pons, striatum, sensorimotor, and primary visual cortices remain spared in patients with AD (**Figs. 3** and **4**).[12,32,33] This pattern can vary with age of disease onset and disease severity. One study[9] showed more severe hypometabolism in parietal, frontal,

and several subcortical areas, whereas in another study,[34] greater impairment in parietal and posterior cingulate cortices and precuneus was reported in early onset AD when compared with late onset AD. The diagnostic accuracy of FDG PET as regards a definite AD diagnosis has been shown to be more than 90% in terms of sensitivity in pathologically confirmed AD, exceeding previous clinical diagnostic accuracy significantly.[35,36]

The decrease in CMRglc in AD is closely related to cognitive decline[37–39] and hence has consistently been shown to be a reliable predictor for the progression from healthy aging to mild cognitive impairment (MCI) and from MCI to AD. Hypometabolism mainly in the posterior cingulate cortex and medial temporal lobe, more precisely the hippocampus but also in the parietotemporal cortex, has figured as a robust measure of disease progression.[40–45] Furthermore, CMRglc reductions in the angular, left midtemporal, and left middle frontal gyri have been shown to be associated with faster cognitive decline among cognitively healthy individuals.[46] (see Refs.[47–49] for detailed reviews).

Likewise, hypometabolism, albeit mild, has been observed in the same regions as in clinically affected patients with AD in nondemented individuals carrying at least 1 *ApoE* ε4 allele compared with noncarriers and has been shown to be progressive and to correlate with cognitive performance in these individuals.[50–53]

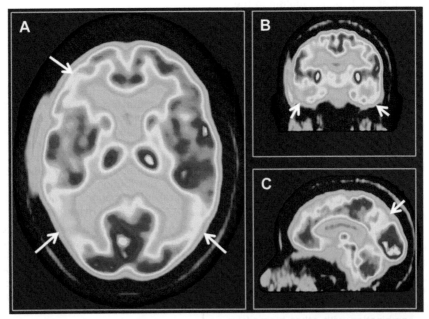

Fig. 3. FDG PET of a 56-year-old woman presenting with early onset dementia without family history of AD. FDG PET images showing bilateral posterior parietal, posterior cingulum, and temporal hypometabolism (*white arrows*) in axial (*A*), coronal (*B*), and sagittal (*C*) orientation. This uptake pattern is suggestive of AD with frontal involvement.

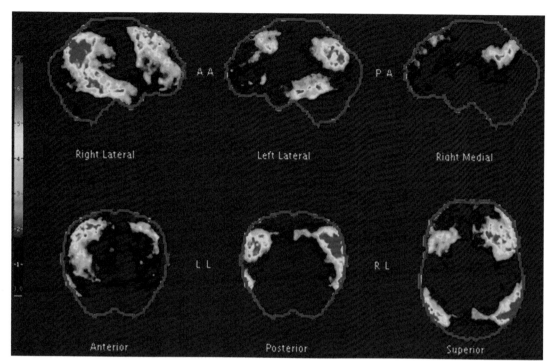

Fig. 4. Typical FDG uptake pattern in a patient with advanced AD. The image shows a z-score map representing hypometabolic regions in a patient with AD compared with healthy control individuals. The z-score defines the deviation of a sample (patient with AD) with respect to the mean of a distribution (healthy controls (z = (x − m)/s)). Images show bilateral posterior parietotemporal hypometabolism and hypometabolism in the posterior cingulum, the precuneus, and in the bilateral frontal cortex. LL, left lateral; RL, right lateral.

Several studies have assessed hypometabolism in presymptomatic carriers of autosomal dominant early onset familial AD mutations, all of which showed regional abnormalities many years before the development of cognitive impairment. A decrease was often accompanied by global CMRglc impairment later on in the disease course, observed in parietal, parietotemporal, temporal, posterior cingulate, and entorhinal cortical regions but also in subcortical structures, such as the hippocampus and the thalamus.[54–62] These findings are of particular interest because they suggest that FDG PET can detect pathologic changes leading to AD at early presymptomatic stages.

An interesting connection to mitochondrial dysfunction was established by the finding of declining glucose metabolism in brain regions typically affected in AD in individuals with a maternal, rather than paternal, family history of AD.[63,64] This concept has further been validated by the observed correlation between postmortem mitochondrial dysfunction and in vivo hypometabolism in the posterior cingulate cortex.[65,66]

FDG PET has furthermore been shown to be a valuable outcome measure in treatment studies,[67,68] permitting a substantial decrease in the required sample size in treatment trials.[39,69]

The deposition of β-amyloid into amyloid plaques is one of the major pathologic hallmarks of AD, and hence, the advent of PET ligands visualizing cerebral fibrillar amyloid burden has been a key event in AD research.[70,71] A substantial body of literature has been created during the past 10 years (see Refs.[72–74] for reviews), reporting excellent ability of these ligands to distinguish AD from controls, also at early disease stages, and to identify patients who are likely to progress to AD (see Ref.[75] for review).

Although amyloid PET ligands show good diagnostic and prognostic accuracy, they do not share the ability of FDG PET to depict longitudinal disease progression, which is also shown by the poor correlation between the 2 modalities.[76–79]

Frontotemporal dementia (FTD)
Although AD is the most common form of dementia among the elderly, FTD is the leading cause of dementia in middle age. A group of clinical syndromes have been termed FTD: the behavioral variant of FTD (bvFTD), previously also called Pick disease, and the language variants progressive nonfluent aphasia and semantic dementia, which can be grouped together as primary progressive aphasia.

Diseases leading to FTD syndromes are summarized under the term frontotemporal lobar degeneration, which includes not only the disorders mentioned earlier but also other neurodegenerative disorders such as progressive supranuclear palsy (PSP) and corticobasal degeneration (CBD, see later discussion) that are Parkinson-plus syndromes, meaning that they share some of the symptoms of Parkinson disease but may also cause changes in memory and cognitive function, as in FTD.

Clinically, FTD is characterized by changes in personality and behavior, for instance disinhibition and apathy, and, depending on the subtype, language abilities, whereas memory impairment may be less prominent or even absent.[80,81] Also, enhanced artistic creativity has been reported.[82,83]

The characteristic pattern of FDG uptake in FTD involves frontal and anterior temporal, as well as anterior cingulate cortical hypometabolism, clearly different from the more posterior impairment seen in typical AD (**Fig. 5**).[11,80,84–86] Analogously, these areas appear atrophied on structural MR images.[87] However, the different clinical subtypes of FTD can present with different patterns of hypometabolism (see Ref.[88] for review).[85,89]

The recently revised diagnostic criteria for bvFTD (Frontotemporal Dementia Consensus Criteria) now involve the use MR imaging and FDG PET for the diagnosis of probable bvFTD, which has been shown to improve sensitivity and specificity significantly when compared with the antecedent criteria.[90] However, not all individuals with bvFTD present with structural abnormalities as visualized by MR imaging. Kerklaan and colleagues[91] reported that FDG PET could identify almost half of the cases that had remained undetected by MR imaging. FDG PET has further been shown to detect anterior hypometabolic changes in presymptomatic carriers of progranulin (*GRN*) mutations causing the rare familial variants of FTD.[92]

Dementia with lewy bodies (DLB)

In patients older than 65 years, DLB constitutes the second most common type of dementia after AD, accounting for up to 30% of all cases.[93] Typical clinical symptoms include visual hallucinations, pronounced fluctuation of attention levels and cognitive alertness, memory loss, and spontaneous parkinsonism.[94]

The diagnosis of DLB is aggravated by the substantial overlap of clinical symptoms and pathologic hallmarks with AD[95] and to some extent also with Parkinson disease dementia.[96] FDG PET imaging shows a pattern of bilateral parietal and posterior temporal as well as posterior cingulate cortical hypometabolism, similar to what is seen in AD.[97–99] However, in DLB there can appear involvement of the occipital lobe, often the primary visual cortex,

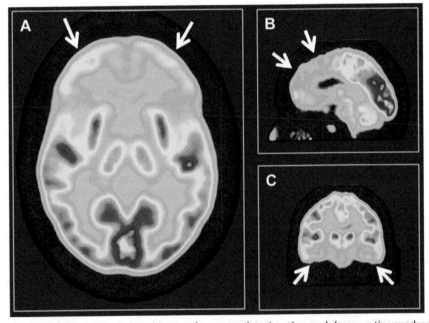

Fig. 5. A 54-year-old woman with a 2-year history of memory deterioration and dysexecutive syndrome. Brain CT was normal. Images show a bilateral frontal and temporal hypometabolism (*white arrows*) in axial (*A*), sagittal (*B*), and coronal (*C*) images, a characteristic pattern for FTD.

which is typically preserved in AD.[100–102] This preferential occipital hypometabolism is compatible with a clinical diagnosis of DLB; if the occipital involvement is not present, the diagnosis is more likely to be AD (**Fig. 6**).

Fujishiro and colleagues,[103] furthermore, reported in a longitudinal study that hypometabolism in the primary visual cortex is present in patients with prodromal DLB and, together with parietal involvement, can be predictive of a progression to DLB.

Vascular dementia (VaD)

VaD is part of a group of vascular cognitive disorders including vascular cognitive impairment, cerebrovascular disease, and mixed AD,[104] accounting for approximately 5% of dementia in individuals aged 65 years or older.[105] Clinical symptoms can overlap with AD, naturally the case in mixed AD, but may be more characterized by deficits in executive functions such as reasoning, judgment, or planning than by prominent memory defects.

Multi-infarct dementia is the most common form of VaD. The pattern of reductions in CMRglc is characterized by multifocal cortical hypometabolism, coinciding with the location of infarcts, without limitation to specific brain structures

(**Fig. 7**).[106] In other cases, instead of multiple cortical lesions, VaD may be associated with small lacunar infarcts in the basal ganglia and periventricular white matter. Then, a marked decrease of FDG uptake in the basal ganglia and the cerebellum, as well as a diffuse decrease in cortical glucose metabolism, can be observed.[107,108]

In VaD hypometabolism, the subcortical areas and primary sensorimotor cortex are more pronounced, whereas the associated areas are typically less affected when compared with AD.[105,109]

Creutzfeldt-Jakob disease (CJD)

The human forms of the transmissible spongiform encephalopathies (TSE), sporadic Creutzfeldt-Jakob disease (sCJD), familial CJD, fatal familial insomnia, Gerstmann-Sträussler-Scheinker syndrome, variant CJD (vCJD), related to bovine spongiform encephalopathy and kuru, are all neuropathologically characterized by neuronal loss, astrocytosis, spongiform changes, and deposits in the brain of a protease-resistant prion protein (called PrPres or PrPSc). Clinical diagnosis may be difficult, because the symptoms are not always specific. Suspicion of the disease may emerge in patients with rapidly progressive dementia and multifocal signs. It is of utmost importance to

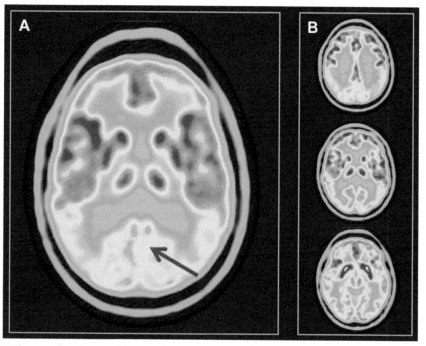

Fig. 6. FDG PET image of a 69-year-old man with cognitive impairment, parkinsonism, and visual hallucinations. The patient was referred to distinguish AD from DLB. Images show occipital (*A, red arrow*), parietotemporal, and posterior cingulate cortical hypometabolism (*B*). The extension of hypometabolism to the primary visual cortex is suggestive of DLB.

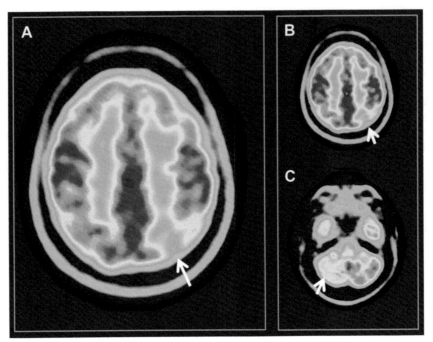

Fig. 7. FDG PET image of a 64-year-old patient with a 2-year history of memory impairment. FDG PET was indicated to rule out AD. Images show a focal area of hypometabolism in the left parietal cortex (*A* and *B*), and mild hypometabolism (*C*) in the contralateral hemicerebellar cortex (*white arrows*). The pattern is suggestive of a VaD with cerebellar diaschisis. Follow-up of the patient confirmed the vascular cause of the lesion.

obtain a diagnosis as early as possible, because some types of rapidly progressive dementia may be associated with treatable diseases (autoimmune, paraneoplastic, or viral encephalitis).[110–113]

The diagnosis of definite CJD is at present possible only through neuropathologic examination of brain tissue according to international (World Health Organization and European Union) consensus and evidence of the presence of the PrPres. A noninvasive diagnostic test with high sensitivity and specificity could improve the accuracy in diagnosing CJD. In recent years, MR imaging, CT, PET, and SPECT have been used in the evaluation of CJD. CT findings have been shown to be vague and often normal even in the advanced stages of the disease.[114]

In a recent study, Caobelli and colleagues[115] reviewed 34 studies comprising 945 patients with CJD. Thirty-nine patients were evaluated with PET imaging, 15 with SPECT, 24 both with PET and MR imaging, and 867 with MR imaging only.

Concerning the studies with PET, Caobelli and colleagues[115] evaluated 3 studies. The first study by Henkel and colleagues[116] included 8 patients. In this study, the investigators show the presence of glucose hypometabolism in parietal, temporal, frontal, and occipital lobes, the thalamus, and basal ganglia. In 1 patient, also the cerebellum was involved. In most patients, alterations

occurred in more than 1 site and were asymmetric. PET alterations were shown to appear earlier than corresponding MR hyperintensities, thus suggesting a higher sensitivity for PET in the early stages of the disease.

The second study was performed by Engler and colleagues[117] as a multitracer PET study using FDG and N-[11C-methyl]-L deuterodeprenyl (DED), a monoamine oxidase B inhibitor labeled with 11C able to assess astrocytosis in the brain, and 15O-labeled water, a tracer for brain perfusion. In this study, FDG PET findings were identified different from what is usually observed in AD or FTD. Moreover, a strong correlation between the reduction in glucose metabolism and astrocytosis, as shown by DED PET, was reported. In particular, patients with definite or probable CJD showed a simultaneously high DED binding and low FDG uptake, affecting various regions of the brain and the cerebellum but not the temporal lobes (**Fig. 8**). Cerebral perfusion reduction also showed a direct relation with DED uptake in all brain regions.

The third study was performed recently by Kim and colleagues[118] as a semiquantitative study of FDG uptake in patients with sporadic and variant CJD using SPM analysis. Patients with sCJD showed glucose hypometabolism in bilateral parietal, frontal, and occipital cortices and middle, as well as in superior, temporal gyri with a right-sided

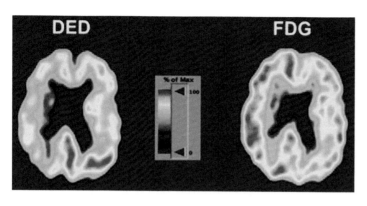

Fig. 8. DED and FDG PET images showing a typical pattern of CJD with increased DED binding (astrocytosis) and decreased glucose metabolism predominant in the left hemisphere. (*Data from* Masullo C, Macchi G. Resistance of the hippocampus in Creutzfeldt-Jakob disease. Clin Neuropathol 1997;16(1):37–44; and Engler H, Nennesmo I, Kumlien E, et al. Imaging astrocytosis with PET in Creutzfeldt-Jakob disease: case report with histopathological findings. Int J Clin Exp Med 2012;5(2):201–7.)

predominance. Conversely, patients with vCJD showed glucose hypometabolism in bilateral occipital and parietal areas with a right-sided predominance and in right middle frontal and superior temporal gyri. The results of this study seem to indicate that many cortical areas present glucose hypometabolism in an asymmetrical pattern, whereas basal ganglia and thalamus, which are often affected on diffusion-weighted imaging, appear to be preserved.

Concerning the PET studies in CJD, Caobelli and colleagues[115] conclude that the study by Engler and colleagues,[117] combining complementing information provided by multiple tracers, elucidates some metabolic changes occurring in patients with CJD. Patients with definite or probable CJD showed strong correlations between the clinical symptoms and PET/CT pattern of hypometabolism, which were also strictly correlated with astrocytosis/gliosis, as shown by DED binding (**Fig. 9**).

Corticobasal Degeneration (CBD)

CBD is a rare, progressive neurodegenerative disorder affecting cortical and deep brain structures. Patients suffering from this Parkinson-plus syndrome present with atypical parkinsonism and, in some cases, alien limb syndrome. A clinical diagnosis can be difficult, because of the symptomatic similarity of CBD and other parkinsonian disorders, PSP, and DLB. Zhang and colleagues[119] even reported a case of CJD mimicking CBD. Typical regions showing glucose hypometabolism in a distinct asymmetric manner are the parietotemporal, frontal, and motor cortex, as well as the basal ganglia and the thalamus (**Fig. 10**).[120,121]

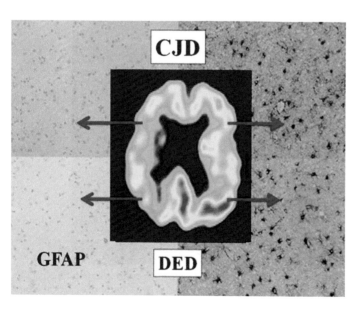

Fig. 9. The pattern of high DED/FDG ratio found in patients with CJD could be investigated in an autopsy in relation to the results of the DED PET examination, showing a clear correlation between the astrocytosis detected with the glial fibrillary acidic protein (GFAP) and increased DED binding (*image center*). PET indicates increased DED binding in the left hemisphere. Histopathology of the frontal and parietal cortices shows GFAP-positive astrocytes in the sites with high DED binding. (*Data from* Engler H, Nennesmo I, Kumlien E, et al. Imaging astrocytosis with PET in Creutzfeldt-Jakob disease: case report with histopathological findings. Int J Clin Exp Med 2012;5(2):201–7; and Engler H, Lundberg PO, Ekbom K, et al. Multitracer study with positron emission tomography in Creutzfeldt-Jakob disease. Eur J Nucl Med Mol Imaging 2003;30(1):85–95.)

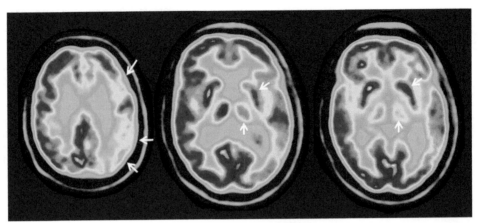

Fig. 10. FDG PET of a 65-year-old man with a history of cognitive impairment with memory loss, and an extrapyramidal syndrome. Axial images show a left parietal and frontal hypometabolism, with a left caudate, putamen, and thalamic hypometabolism (*white arrows*). This pattern is suggestive of a corticobasal degeneration.

Epilepsy

Epilepsy is a common neurologic condition affecting approximately 70 million people worldwide, with an estimated incidence of 50.4/100,000/y.[122,123] Poor response to pharmacologic treatment is seen in almost one-third of the patients with epilepsy. Surgery has proved to be effective in many of these patients, with seizure control in almost 60% of the patients after 1 year.[124] FDG PET has proved to be effective in the lateralization and regional localization of the epileptogenic foci, providing functional information to the diagnostic assessment of the patients with refractory epilepsy.

The protracted time course of FDG uptake in the brain differs from the brief nature of epileptic seizures, which can last just a few minutes. This factor determines some constraints in the evaluation of a purely ictal period, which has led to a more generalized use of FDG PET for the interictal assessment of brain metabolism (**Fig. 11**).[125]

Temporal lobe epilepsy

Temporal lobe epilepsy (TLE) is one of the most common causes of refractory epilepsy. Interictal studies of patients with nonlesional TLE have shown a consistent cortical hypometabolism in

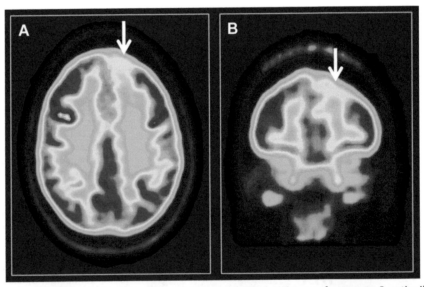

Fig. 11. FDG PET of a 16-year-old woman with a history of frontal epilepsy refractory to 3 antiepileptic drugs. Recent MR imaging was unremarkable. Video EEG showed frontal lobe seizures. A hypometabolic cortical region is visible in the left frontal cortex (*white arrow*) in axial (*A*) and coronal (*B*) images. This area was found to be related to the epileptogenic region.

relation to the epileptogenic region.[126] In most patients, the extension of hypometabolism is larger than the epileptogenic focus itself, reflecting cortical functional deficits and possibly primary spread.[127,128]

The main usefulness of FDG PET in patients with TLE is the lateralization and overall localization of the epileptogenic foci.[129] This information can be used to plan invasive electroencephalographic (EEG) recordings.[130] Several studies have proved that in patients with TLE and discordant findings on MR imaging and video EEG, FDG PET provides substantial clinical information and is cost-benefit effective.[131] FDG PET can be especially useful in patients with TLE and normal MR imaging.[129,132–134] The reported sensitivity of FDG PET in TLE is as high as 92% to 96%.[135] However, FDG PET has also been reported to detect hypometabolism in 67.8% of the patients with nonlesional refractory childhood epilepsy.[136]

Gaillard and colleagues[137] postulated that the magnitude of cortical hypometabolism may be correlated with the evolution of the disease and the severity of the seizures in terms of frequency and duration. Children with new-onset partial epilepsy may have less severe abnormalities.

Epileptic patients with TLE can present other hypometabolic areas besides the focal hypometabolism in the cortical epileptogenic region,[138] even contralateral to seizure focus, reflecting the functional bilateral connections between both hemispheres.[129] In this regard, Tepmongkol and colleagues[139] showed that patients with less than 48 hours since the last seizure had a higher proportion of bilateral temporal hypometabolism. These investigators propose that this information can be used to plan acquisitions to avoid bilateral metabolic abnormalities.

Some of the findings of FDG PET may correlate with seizure-free outcome after surgery. Recently, Takahashi and colleagues[140] compared brain metabolism in postsurgical seizure-free patients with TLE against non–seizure-free patients with TLE after surgery. These investigators found that the extent of metabolic impairment in the hippocampal, thalamic, and frontal areas was significantly higher in the seizure-free patients compared with the non–seizure-free. Struck and colleagues[141] showed that in TLE, the use of MR imaging, FDG PET, and EEG could predict surgical candidacy, but that only FDG PET was able to predict favorable seizure control after surgery.

The coregistration of MR images and PET images may provide additional information to that obtained by each modality separately.[142] This information may be useful to review an MR image that was previously reported as unremarkable, to find small areas of cortical dysplasia, which may have previously gone unnoticed.

Extratemporal epilepsy

In extratemporal epilepsy, FDG PET may not perform as well in the localization of the hypometabolic epileptogenic region as in TLE. The reported sensitivity for FDG PET in extratemporal epilepsy can be less than 60%.[143,144] Kim and colleagues[8] reported a sensitivity of 36% in patients with frontal lobe epilepsy with normal MR imaging, and 73% in patients with known abnormalities on MR imaging.

In a similar fashion to TLE, patients with extratemporal epilepsy can show hypometabolic areas not restricted to the epileptogenic region. Knopman and colleagues[145] described that patients with occipital lobe epilepsy presented temporal lobe hypometabolism in addition to the metabolic impairment of the occipital cortex.

Cortical hypometabolism can also predict outcome after surgery in extratemporal epilepsy. Wong and colleagues[146] showed that in neocortical epilepsy, the amount of cortical hypometabolism remote to the primary epileptogenic zone may be associated with a non–seizure-free outcome.

Schizophrenia and Bipolar Disorder

Schizophrenia and bipolar disease are essentially different disorders, yet they are frequently confused because of a relative overlap in (negative) signs and symptoms and certain common causes and pathophysiologic pathways.[147]

Schizophrenia is a chronic and often debilitating psychotic disease, which often starts in adolescence. The wide-ranging positive and negative symptoms, disorganization, and cognitive deficits have been suggested to derive from neuropathologic processes during early brain development.[148,149]

FDG PET has been widely used in the study of schizophrenia. In 1982, Buchsbaum and colleagues[150] showed for the first time global CMRglc decrease in patients with schizophrenia compared with controls. Negative schizophrenic symptoms, including changes in abstraction, verbal fluency, mental flexibility, processing speed, and anhedonia, have been associated with frontal, prefrontal, and anterior cingulate cortical hypoactivity and hypometabolism.[151–155] Productive positive symptoms such as hallucinations and delusions have been linked to hypermetabolism in the temporolimbic system, including amygdala, the basal ganglia, and temporal cortical regions.[153,156,157]

Bipolar disorder, also known as manic-depressive illness, is more common in the population than schizophrenia. It is characterized by alternating mood episodes lasting weeks or even months and may feature psychotic episodes during manic episodes. Studies with FDG PET have shown a pattern of corticolimbic metabolic dysregulation at rest, involving hypermetabolic rates in limbic structures including the anterior temporal cortex, the parahippocampal gyrus, and amygdala accompanied by hypometabolism in frontal cortical regions such as the dorsolateral prefrontal and the anterior cingulate cortex.[158] A recent meta-analysis of functional neuroimaging in bipolar disorder confirmed this pattern of dysregulation.[159]

The patterns of gray matter CMRglc thus seem to be relatively comparable between schizophrenia and bipolar disorder. Both share, based on FDG PET studies, a common dissociative frontotemporolimbic metabolic pattern. Therefore, a recent FDG PET study examined if differences in white matter CMRglc could distinguish the 2 disorders. The investigators found decreased metabolism in large cerebral and cerebellar white matter tracts in the schizophrenic patients compared with those with bipolar disorder.[160]

SUMMARY

Examinations with FDG PET have become a standard technique during the past 20 years and are now available at many sites. The long-standing tradition of using FDG PET in the research of neurologic and psychiatric disorders has resulted in a massive body of evidence, which has cleared the way for many clinical applications, although FDG PET is not yet part of the clinical routine for many of these diseases.

In this review, relevant examples from the plethora of application areas for FDG PET within neurology and psychiatry are presented. A particularly important feature of FDG PET is its ability to detect pathophysiologic changes at early disease stages, as in neurodegenerative disorders. This finding and the possibility to visualize the course of many diseases render FDG PET a favorable tool for treatment planning and management.

As with all biomarkers, FDG PET benefits from the combination with other diagnostic modalities, including imaging with other PET ligands and structural imaging.

This modality provides an exciting opportunity but is also associated with serious challenges. In particular, the interpretation and analysis of FDG PET images is a dynamic field. Software improving diagnostic accuracy has yet to reach clinical practice.

FDG PET has made a lasting impact on nuclear medicine but also on neurology/psychiatry, and it is likely to play an increasing role in patient management.

ACKNOWLEDGMENTS

The authors are grateful to Adriana Quagliata, MD, who helped with acquiring the images in this article. All images were provided by and belong to the Uruguayan Center of Molecular Imaging (CUDIM) and may not be reproduced without permission.

REFERENCES

1. Ido T, Wan C, Casella V, et al. Labeled 2-deoxy-D-glucose analogs: 18F-labeled 2-deoxy-2-fluoro-D-glucose, 2-deoxy-2-fluoro-D-mannose and 14C-2-deoxy-2-fluoro-D-glucose. J Labelled Comp Radiopharm 1978;24:174–83.
2. Reivich M, Kuhl D, Wolf A, et al. The [18F]fluorodeoxyglucose method for the measurement of local cerebral glucose utilization in man. Circ Res 1979;44(1):127–37.
3. Varrone A, Asenbaum S, Vander Borght T, et al. EANM procedure guidelines for PET brain imaging using [18F]FDG, version 2. Eur J Nucl Med Mol Imaging 2009;36(12):2103–10.
4. Phelps ME, Huang SC, Hoffman EJ, et al. Tomographic measurement of local cerebral glucose metabolic rate in humans with (F-18)2-fluoro-2-deoxy-D-glucose: validation of method. Ann Neurol 1979;6(5):371–88.
5. Sokoloff L, Reivich M, Kennedy C, et al. The [14C] deoxyglucose method for the measurement of local cerebral glucose utilization: theory, procedure, and normal values in the conscious and anesthetized albino rat. J Neurochem 1977;28(5):897–916.
6. Patlak CS, Blasberg RG, Fenstermacher JD. Graphical evaluation of blood-to-brain transfer constants from multiple-time uptake data. J Cereb Blood Flow Metab 1983;3(1):1–7.
7. Gjedde A, Wienhard K, Heiss WD, et al. Comparative regional analysis of 2-fluorodeoxyglucose and methylglucose uptake in brain of four stroke patients. With special reference to the regional estimation of the lumped constant. J Cereb Blood Flow Metab 1985;5(2):163–78.
8. Kim YK, Lee DS, Lee SK, et al. (18)F-FDG PET in localization of frontal lobe epilepsy: comparison of visual and SPM analysis. J Nucl Med 2002;43(9):1167–74.
9. Kim EJ, Cho SS, Jeong Y, et al. Glucose metabolism in early onset versus late onset Alzheimer's disease: an SPM analysis of 120 patients. Brain 2005;128(Pt 8):1790–801.
10. Signorini M, Paulesu E, Friston K, et al. Rapid assessment of regional cerebral metabolic

abnormalities in single subjects with quantitative and nonquantitative [18F]FDG PET: a clinical validation of statistical parametric mapping. NeuroImage 1999;9(1):63–80.

11. Foster NL, Heidebrink JL, Clark CM, et al. FDG-PET improves accuracy in distinguishing frontotemporal dementia and Alzheimer's disease. Brain 2007; 130(Pt 10):2616–35.

12. Minoshima S, Giordani B, Berent S, et al. Metabolic reduction in the posterior cingulate cortex in very early Alzheimer's disease. Ann Neurol 1997;42(1):85–94.

13. Herholz K, Salmon E, Perani D, et al. Discrimination between Alzheimer dementia and controls by automated analysis of multicenter FDG PET. NeuroImage 2002;17(1):302–16.

14. Heckemann RA, Hajnal JV, Aljabar P, et al. Automatic anatomical brain MRI segmentation combining label propagation and decision fusion. NeuroImage 2006;33(1):115–26.

15. Fischl B, Salat DH, Busa E, et al. Whole brain segmentation: automated labeling of neuroanatomical structures in the human brain. Neuron 2002;33(3): 341–55.

16. Smith SM, Jenkinson M, Woolrich MW, et al. Advances in functional and structural MR image analysis and implementation as FSL. NeuroImage 2004;23(Suppl 1):S208–19.

17. Loessner A, Alavi A, Lewandrowski KU, et al. Regional cerebral function determined by FDG-PET in healthy volunteers: normal patterns and changes with age. J Nucl Med 1995;36(7):1141–9.

18. Dager SR, Friedman SD. Brain imaging and the effects of caffeine and nicotine. Ann Med 2000;32(9): 592–9.

19. Wimo A, Winblad B, Jonsson L. An estimate of the total worldwide societal costs of dementia in 2005. Alzheimers Dement 2007;3(2):81–91.

20. Ferri CP, Prince M, Brayne C, et al. Global prevalence of dementia: a Delphi consensus study. Lancet 2005;366(9503):2112–7.

21. Tripathi M, Tripathi M, Damle N, et al. Differential diagnosis of neurodegenerative dementias using metabolic phenotypes on F-18 FDG PET/CT. Neuroradiol J 2014;27(1):13–21.

22. Davison CM, O'Brien JT. A comparison of FDG-PET and blood flow SPECT in the diagnosis of neurodegenerative dementias: a systematic review. Int J Geriatr Psychiatry 2014;29(6):551–61.

23. Querfurth HW, LaFerla FM. Alzheimer's disease. N Engl J Med 2010;362(4):329–44.

24. Brookmeyer R, Johnson E, Ziegler-Graham K, et al. Forecasting the global burden of Alzheimer's disease. Alzheimers Dement 2007;3(3):186–91.

25. Cummings JL. Alzheimer's disease. N Engl J Med 2004;351(1):56–67.

26. de Leon MJ, Ferris SH, George AE, et al. Positron emission tomographic studies of aging and

Alzheimer disease. AJNR Am J Neuroradiol 1983; 4(3):568–71.

27. Foster NL, Chase TN, Fedio P, et al. Alzheimer's disease: focal cortical changes shown by positron emission tomography. Neurology 1983; 33(8):961–5.

28. Friedland RP, Budinger TF, Ganz E, et al. Regional cerebral metabolic alterations in dementia of the Alzheimer type: positron emission tomography with [18F]fluorodeoxyglucose. J Comput Assist Tomogr 1983;7(4):590–8.

29. Albert MS, DeKosky ST, Dickson D, et al. The diagnosis of mild cognitive impairment due to Alzheimer's disease: recommendations from the National Institute on Aging-Alzheimer's Association workgroups on diagnostic guidelines for Alzheimer's disease. Alzheimers Dement 2011;7(3): 270–9.

30. McKhann GM, Knopman DS, Chertkow H, et al. The diagnosis of dementia due to Alzheimer's disease: recommendations from the National Institute on Aging-Alzheimer's Association workgroups on diagnostic guidelines for Alzheimer's disease. Alzheimers Dement 2011;7(3):263–9.

31. Sperling RA, Aisen PS, Beckett LA, et al. Toward defining the preclinical stages of Alzheimer's disease: recommendations from the National Institute on Aging-Alzheimer's Association workgroups on diagnostic guidelines for Alzheimer's disease. Alzheimers Dement 2011;7(3):280–92.

32. Herholz K. PET studies in dementia. Ann Nucl Med 2003;17(2):79–89.

33. Mosconi L. Brain glucose metabolism in the early and specific diagnosis of Alzheimer's disease. FDG-PET studies in MCI and AD. Eur J Nucl Med Mol Imaging 2005;32(4):486–510.

34. Sakamoto S, Ishii K, Sasaki M, et al. Differences in cerebral metabolic impairment between early and late onset types of Alzheimer's disease. J Neurol Sci 2002;200(1-2):27–32.

35. Jagust W, Reed B, Mungas D, et al. What does fluorodeoxyglucose PET imaging add to a clinical diagnosis of dementia? Neurology 2007;69(9): 871–7.

36. Silverman DH, Small GW, Chang CY, et al. Positron emission tomography in evaluation of dementia: regional brain metabolism and long-term outcome. JAMA 2001;286(17):2120–7.

37. Herholz K, Nordberg A, Salmon E, et al. Impairment of neocortical metabolism predicts progression in Alzheimer's disease. Dement Geriatr Cogn Disord 1999;10(6):494–504.

38. Desgranges B, Baron JC, Lalevee C, et al. The neural substrates of episodic memory impairment in Alzheimer's disease as revealed by FDG-PET: relationship to degree of deterioration. Brain 2002;125(Pt 5):1116–24.

39. Landau SM, Harvey D, Madison CM, et al. Associations between cognitive, functional, and FDG-PET measures of decline in AD and MCI. Neurobiol Aging 2011;32(7):1207–18.

40. Arnaiz E, Jelic V, Almkvist O, et al. Impaired cerebral glucose metabolism and cognitive functioning predict deterioration in mild cognitive impairment. Neuroreport 2001;12(4):851–5.

41. Chetelat G, Desgranges B, de la Sayette V, et al. Mild cognitive impairment: can FDG-PET predict who is to rapidly convert to Alzheimer's disease? Neurology 2003;60(8):1374–7.

42. de Leon MJ, Convit A, Wolf OT, et al. Prediction of cognitive decline in normal elderly subjects with 2-[(18)F]fluoro-2-deoxy-D-glucose/poitron-emission tomography (FDG/PET). Proc Natl Acad Sci U S A 2001;98(19):10966–71.

43. Drzezga A, Lautenschlager N, Siebner H, et al. Cerebral metabolic changes accompanying conversion of mild cognitive impairment into Alzheimer's disease: a PET follow-up study. Eur J Nucl Med Mol Imaging 2003;30(8):1104–13.

44. Nestor PJ, Fryer TD, Smielewski P, Hodges JR. Limbic hypometabolism in Alzheimer's disease and mild cognitive impairment. Ann Neurol 2003; 54(3):343–51.

45. Mosconi L, Mistur R, Switalski R, et al. FDG-PET changes in brain glucose metabolism from normal cognition to pathologically verified Alzheimer's disease. Eur J Nucl Med Mol Imaging 2009;36(5): 811–22.

46. Jagust W, Gitcho A, Sun F, et al. Brain imaging evidence of preclinical Alzheimer's disease in normal aging. Ann Neurol 2006;59(4):673–81.

47. Herholz K. FDG PET and differential diagnosis of dementia. Alzheimer Dis Assoc Disord 1995;9(1):6–16.

48. Herholz K, Heiss WD. Positron emission tomography in clinical neurology. Mol Imaging Biol 2004; 6(4):239–69.

49. Mosconi L. Glucose metabolism in normal aging and Alzheimer's disease: methodological and physiological considerations for PET studies. Clin Transl Imaging 2013;1(4):217–33.

50. Small GW, Mazziotta JC, Collins MT, et al. Apolipoprotein E type 4 allele and cerebral glucose metabolism in relatives at risk for familial Alzheimer disease. JAMA 1995;273(12):942–7.

51. Reiman EM, Caselli RJ, Yun LS, et al. Preclinical evidence of Alzheimer's disease in persons homozygous for the epsilon 4 allele for apolipoprotein E. N Engl J Med 1996;334(12):752–8.

52. Small GW, Ercoli LM, Silverman DH, et al. Cerebral metabolic and cognitive decline in persons at genetic risk for Alzheimer's disease. Proc Natl Acad Sci U S A 2000;97(11):6037–42.

53. Mosconi L, De Santi S, Brys M, et al. Hypometabolism and altered cerebrospinal fluid markers in normal apolipoprotein E E4 carriers with subjective memory complaints. Biol Psychiatry 2008;63(6): 609–18.

54. Kennedy AM, Newman SK, Frackowiak RS, et al. Chromosome 14 linked familial Alzheimer's disease. A clinico-pathological study of a single pedigree. Brain 1995;118(Pt 1):185–205.

55. Kennedy AM, Frackowiak RS, Newman SK, et al. Deficits in cerebral glucose metabolism demonstrated by positron emission tomography in individuals at risk of familial Alzheimer's disease. Neurosci Lett 1995;186(1):17–20.

56. Mosconi L, Sorbi S, de Leon MJ, et al. Hypometabolism exceeds atrophy in presymptomatic early-onset familial Alzheimer's disease. J Nucl Med 2006;47(11):1778–86.

57. Wahlund LO, Basun H, Almkvist O, et al. A follow-up study of the family with the Swedish APP 670/671 Alzheimer's disease mutation. Dement Geriatr Cogn Disord 1999;10(6):526–33.

58. Ringman JM, Gylys KH, Medina LD, et al. Biochemical, neuropathological, and neuroimaging characteristics of early-onset Alzheimer's disease due to a novel PSEN1 mutation. Neurosci Lett 2011;487(3):287–92.

59. Perani D, Graasi F, Sorbi S, et al. PET study in subjects from two Italian FAD families with APP717 Val to Ileu mutation. Eur J Neurosci 1997;4:214–20.

60. Schöll M, Almkvist O, Axelman K, et al. Glucose metabolism and PIB binding in carriers of a His163Tyr presenilin 1 mutation. Neurobiol Aging 2011;32(8):1388–99.

61. Schöll M, Almkvist O, Bogdanovic N, et al. Time course of glucose metabolism in relation to cognitive performance and postmortem neuropathology in Met146Val PSEN1 mutation carriers. J Alzheimers Dis 2011;24(3):495–506.

62. Benzinger TL, Blazey T, Jack CR Jr, et al. Regional variability of imaging biomarkers in autosomal dominant Alzheimer's disease. Proc Natl Acad Sci U S A 2013;110(47):E4502–9.

63. Mosconi L, Brys M, Switalski R, et al. Maternal family history of Alzheimer's disease predisposes to reduced brain glucose metabolism. Proc Natl Acad Sci U S A 2007;104(48):19067–72.

64. Mosconi L, Mistur R, Switalski R, et al. Declining brain glucose metabolism in normal individuals with a maternal history of Alzheimer disease. Neurology 2009;72(6):513–20.

65. Valla J, Berndt JD, Gonzalez-Lima F. Energy hypometabolism in posterior cingulate cortex of Alzheimer's patients: superficial laminar cytochrome oxidase associated with disease duration. J Neurosci 2001;21(13):4923–30.

66. Valla J, Yaari R, Wolf AB, et al. Reduced posterior cingulate mitochondrial activity in expired young adult carriers of the APOE epsilon4 allele, the major

late-onset Alzheimer's susceptibility gene. J Alzheimers Dis 2010;22(1):307–13.

67. Keller C, Kadir A, Forsberg A, et al. Long-term effects of galantamine treatment on brain functional activities as measured by PET in Alzheimer's disease patients. J Alzheimers Dis 2011;24(1):109–23.

68. Kadir A, Andreasen N, Almkvist O, et al. Effect of phenserine treatment on brain functional activity and amyloid in Alzheimer's disease. Ann Neurol 2008;63(5):621–31.

69. Alexander GE, Chen K, Pietrini P, et al. Longitudinal PET evaluation of cerebral metabolic decline in dementia: a potential outcome measure in Alzheimer's disease treatment studies. Am J Psychiatry 2002; 159(5):738–45.

70. Klunk WE, Engler H, Nordberg A, et al. Imaging brain amyloid in Alzheimer's disease with Pittsburgh Compound-B. Ann Neurol 2004;55(3):306–19.

71. Klunk WE, Wang Y, Huang GF, et al. The binding of 2-(4'-methylaminophenyl)benzothiazole to postmortem brain homogenates is dominated by the amyloid component. J Neurosci 2003;23(6):2086–92.

72. Cohen AD, Klunk WE. Early detection of Alzheimer's disease using PiB and FDG PET. Neurobiol Dis 2014. pii:S0969-9961(14)00110-7.

73. Jack CR Jr, Barrio JR, Kepe V. Cerebral amyloid PET imaging in Alzheimer's disease. Acta Neuropathol 2013;126(5):643–57.

74. Rowe CC, Villemagne VL. Amyloid imaging with PET in early Alzheimer disease diagnosis. Med Clin North Am 2013;97(3):377–98.

75. Frisoni GB, Bocchetta M, Chetelat G, et al. Imaging markers for Alzheimer disease: which vs how. Neurology 2013;81(5):487–500.

76. Forsberg A, Almkvist O, Engler H, et al. High PIB retention in Alzheimer's disease is an early event with complex relationship with CSF biomarkers and functional parameters. Curr Alzheimer Res 2010;7(1):56–66.

77. Furst AJ, Rabinovici GD, Rostomian AH, et al. Cognition, glucose metabolism and amyloid burden in Alzheimer's disease. Neurobiol Aging 2012;33(2):215–25.

78. Kadir A, Almkvist O, Forsberg A, et al. Dynamic changes in PET amyloid and FDG imaging at different stages of Alzheimer's disease. Neurobiol Aging 2012;33(1):198.e1–14.

79. Rabinovici GD, Furst AJ, Alkalay A, et al. Increased metabolic vulnerability in early-onset Alzheimer's disease is not related to amyloid burden. Brain 2010;133(Pt 2):512–28.

80. Neary D, Snowden JS, Gustafson L, et al. Frontotemporal lobar degeneration: a consensus on clinical diagnostic criteria. Neurology 1998;51(6):1546–54.

81. Kertesz A, Munoz D. Pick's disease, frontotemporal dementia, and Pick complex: emerging concepts. Arch Neurol 1998;55(3):302–4.

82. Drago V, Foster PS, Trifiletti D, et al. What's inside the art? The influence of frontotemporal dementia in art production. Neurology 2006;67(7):1285–7.

83. Miller BL, Boone K, Cummings JL, et al. Functional correlates of musical and visual ability in frontotemporal dementia. Br J Psychiatry 2000;176:458–63.

84. Diehl-Schmid J, Grimmer T, Drzezga A, et al. Decline of cerebral glucose metabolism in frontotemporal dementia: a longitudinal 18F-FDG-PET-study. Neurobiol Aging 2007;28(1):42–50.

85. Drzezga A, Grimmer T, Henriksen G, et al. Imaging of amyloid plaques and cerebral glucose metabolism in semantic dementia and Alzheimer's disease. Neurolmage 2008;39(2):619–33.

86. Jeong Y, Cho SS, Park JM, et al. 18F-FDG PET findings in frontotemporal dementia: an SPM analysis of 29 patients. J Nucl Med 2005;46(2):233–9.

87. Kanda T, Ishii K, Uemura T, et al. Comparison of grey matter and metabolic reductions in frontotemporal dementia using FDG-PET and voxel-based morphometric MR studies. Eur J Nucl Med Mol Imaging 2008;35(12):2227–34.

88. Brown RK, Bohnen NI, Wong KK, et al. Brain PET in suspected dementia: patterns of altered FDG metabolism. Radiographics 2014;34(3):684–701.

89. Diehl J, Grimmer T, Drzezga A, et al. Cerebral metabolic patterns at early stages of frontotemporal dementia and semantic dementia. A PET study. Neurobiol Aging 2004;25(8):1051–6.

90. Rascovsky K, Hodges JR, Knopman D, et al. Sensitivity of revised diagnostic criteria for the behavioural variant of frontotemporal dementia. Brain 2011; 134(Pt 9):2456–77.

91. Kerklaan BJ, Berckel BN, Herholz K, et al. The added value of 18-fluorodeoxyglucose-positron emission tomography in the diagnosis of the behavioral variant of frontotemporal dementia. Am J Alzheimers Dis Other Demen 2014. [Epub ahead of print].

92. Jacova C, Hsiung GY, Tawankanjanachot I, et al. Anterior brain glucose hypometabolism predates dementia in progranulin mutation carriers. Neurology 2013;81(15):1322–31.

93. Warr L, Walker Z. Identification of biomarkers in Lewy-body disorders. Q J Nucl Med Mol Imaging 2012;56(1):39–54.

94. Mosimann UP, McKeith IG. Dementia with Lewy bodies–diagnosis and treatment. Swiss Med Wkly 2003;133(9-10):131–42.

95. Nervi A, Reitz C, Tang MX, et al. Comparison of clinical manifestations in Alzheimer disease and dementia with Lewy bodies. Arch Neurol 2008; 65(12):1634–9.

96. Yong SW, Yoon JK, An YS, et al. A comparison of cerebral glucose metabolism in Parkinson's disease, Parkinson's disease dementia and dementia with Lewy bodies. Eur J Neurol 2007;14(12):1357–62.

97. Higuchi M, Tashiro M, Arai H, et al. Glucose hypo-metabolism and neuropathological correlates in brains of dementia with Lewy bodies. Exp Neurol 2000;162(2):247–56.

98. Kono AK, Ishii K, Sofue K, et al. Fully automatic differential diagnosis system for dementia with Lewy bodies and Alzheimer's disease using FDG-PET and 3D-SSP. Eur J Nucl Med Mol Imaging 2007; 34(9):1490–7.

99. Okamura N, Arai H, Higuchi M, et al. [18F] FDG-PET study in dementia with Lewy bodies and Alzheimer's disease. Prog Neuropsychopharmacol Biol Psychiatry 2001;25(2):447–56.

100. Cordery RJ, Tyrrell PJ, Lantos PL, et al. Dementia with Lewy bodies studied with positron emission tomography. Arch Neurol 2001;58(3):505–8.

101. Imamura T, Ishii K, Hirono N, et al. Occipital glucose metabolism in dementia with Lewy bodies with and without Parkinsonism: a study using positron emission tomography. Dement Geriatr Cogn Disord 2001;12(3):194–7.

102. Perneczky R, Drzezga A, Boecker H, et al. Cerebral metabolic dysfunction in patients with dementia with Lewy bodies and visual hallucinations. Dement Geriatr Cogn Disord 2008;25(6):531–8.

103. Fujishiro H, Iseki E, Kasanuki K, et al. A follow up study of non-demented patients with primary visual cortical hypometabolism: prodromal dementia with Lewy bodies. J Neurol Sci 2013;334(1-2):48–54.

104. Roman GC, Sachdev P, Royall DR, et al. Vascular cognitive disorder: a new diagnostic category updating vascular cognitive impairment and vascular dementia. J Neurol Sci 2004;226(1-2):81–7.

105. Heiss WD, Zimmermann-Meinzingen S. PET imaging in the differential diagnosis of vascular dementia. J Neurol Sci 2012;322(1-2):268–73.

106. Meguro K, Yamaguchi S, Yamazaki H, et al. Cortical glucose metabolism in psychiatric wandering patients with vascular dementia. Psychiatry Res 1996;67(1):71–80.

107. Sabri O, Hellwig D, Schreckenberger M, et al. Correlation of neuropsychological, morphological and functional (regional cerebral blood flow and glucose utilization) findings in cerebral microangiopathy. J Nucl Med 1998;39(1):147–54.

108. De Reuck J, Decoo D, Marchau M, et al. Positron emission tomography in vascular dementia. J Neurol Sci 1998;154(1):55–61.

109. Kerrouche N, Herholz K, Mielke R, et al. 18FDG PET in vascular dementia: differentiation from Alzheimer's disease using voxel-based multivariate analysis. J Cereb Blood Flow Metab 2006;26(9): 1213–21.

110. Gultekin SH, Rosenfeld MR, Voltz R, et al. Paraneoplastic limbic encephalitis: neurological symptoms, immunological findings and tumour association in 50 patients. Brain 2000;123(Pt 7):1481–94.

111. Meyer MA, Hubner KF, Raja S, et al. Sequential positron emission tomographic evaluations of brain metabolism in acute herpes encephalitis. J Neuroimaging 1994;4(2):104–5.

112. Provenzale JM, Barboriak DP, Coleman RE. Limbic encephalitis: comparison of FDG PET and MR imaging findings. AJR Am J Roentgenol 1998; 170(6):1659–60.

113. Weiner SM, Otte A, Schumacher M, et al. Alterations of cerebral glucose metabolism indicate progress to severe morphological brain lesions in neuropsychiatric systemic lupus erythematosus. Lupus 2000;9(5):386–9.

114. Kovanen J, Erkinjuntti T, Iivanainen M, et al. Cerebral MR and CT imaging in Creutzfeldt-Jakob disease. J Comput Assist Tomogr 1985;9(1):125–8.

115. Caobelli F, Cobelli M, Pizzocaro C, et al. The role of neuroimaging in evaluating patients affected by Creutzfeldt-Jakob disease: a systematic review of the literature. J Neuroimaging 2014. [Epub ahead of print].

116. Henkel K, Zerr I, Hertel A, et al. Positron emission tomography with [(18)F]FDG in the diagnosis of Creutzfeldt-Jakob disease (CJD). J Neurol 2002; 249(6):699–705.

117. Engler H, Lundberg PO, Ekbom K, et al. Multitracer study with positron emission tomography in Creutzfeldt-Jakob disease. Eur J Nucl Med Mol Imaging 2003;30(1):85–95.

118. Kim EJ, Cho SS, Jeong BH, et al. Glucose metabolism in sporadic Creutzfeldt-Jakob disease: a statistical parametric mapping analysis of (18)F-FDG PET. Eur J Neurol 2012;19(3):488–93.

119. Zhang Y, Minoshima S, Vesselle H, et al. A case of Creutzfeldt-Jakob disease mimicking corticobasal degeneration: FDG PET, SPECT, and MRI findings. Clin Nucl Med 2012;37(7):e173–5.

120. Hosaka K, Ishii K, Sakamoto S, et al. Voxel-based comparison of regional cerebral glucose metabolism between PSP and corticobasal degeneration. J Neurol Sci 2002;199(1-2):67–71.

121. Teune LK, Bartels AL, de Jong BM, et al. Typical cerebral metabolic patterns in neurodegenerative brain diseases. Mov Disord 2010;25(14):2395–404.

122. Ngugi AK, Bottomley C, Kleinschmidt I, et al. Estimation of the burden of active and life-time epilepsy: a meta-analytic approach. Epilepsia 2010; 51(5):883–90.

123. Ngugi AK, Kariuki SM, Bottomley C, et al. Incidence of epilepsy: a systematic review and meta-analysis. Neurology 2011;77(10):1005–12.

124. Wiebe S, Blume WT, Girvin JP, et al. A randomized, controlled trial of surgery for temporal-lobe epilepsy. N Engl J Med 2001;345(5):311–8.

125. Kim S, Mountz JM. SPECT imaging of epilepsy: an overview and comparison with F-18 FDG PET. Int J Mol Imaging 2011;2011:813028.

126. Lamusuo S, Jutila L, Ylinen A, et al. [18F]FDG-PET reveals temporal hypometabolism in patients with temporal lobe epilepsy even when quantitative MRI and histopathological analysis show only mild hippocampal damage. Arch Neurol 2001; 58(6):933–9.

127. Garibotto V, Picard F. Nuclear medicine imaging in epilepsy. Epileptologie 2013;30:109–31.

128. Nelissen N, Van Paesschen W, Baete K, et al. Correlations of interictal FDG-PET metabolism and ictal SPECT perfusion changes in human temporal lobe epilepsy with hippocampal sclerosis. NeuroImage 2006;32(2):684–95.

129. Kumar A, Chugani HT. The role of radionuclide imaging in epilepsy, Part 1: sporadic temporal and extratemporal lobe epilepsy. J Nucl Med 2013; 54(10):1775–81.

130. Chiron C, Hertz-Pannier L. Structural and functional imaging: particularities in children. Neurochirurgie 2008;54(3):212–8 [in French].

131. Hinde S, Soares M, Burch J, et al. The added clinical and economic value of diagnostic testing for epilepsy surgery. Epilepsy Res 2014;108(4):775–81.

132. Heinz R, Ferris N, Lee EK, et al. MR and positron emission tomography in the diagnosis of surgically correctable temporal lobe epilepsy. AJNR Am J Neuroradiol 1994;15(7):1341–8.

133. O'Brien TJ, Hicks RJ, Ware R, et al. The utility of a 3-dimensional, large-field-of-view, sodium iodide crystal–based PET scanner in the presurgical evaluation of partial epilepsy. J Nucl Med 2001;42(8):1158–65.

134. Willmann O, Wennberg R, May T, et al. The contribution of 18F-FDG PET in preoperative epilepsy surgery evaluation for patients with temporal lobe epilepsy. A meta-analysis. Seizure 2007;16(6): 509–20.

135. Knowlton RC, Laxer KD, Ende G, et al. Presurgical multimodality neuroimaging in electroencephalographic lateralized temporal lobe epilepsy. Ann Neurol 1997;42(6):829–37.

136. Rubi S, Setoain X, Donaire A, et al. Validation of FDG-PET/MRI coregistration in nonlesional refractory childhood epilepsy. Epilepsia 2011;52(12):2216–24.

137. Gaillard WD, Kopylev L, Weinstein S, et al. Low incidence of abnormal (18)FDG-PET in children with new-onset partial epilepsy: a prospective study. Neurology 2002;58(5):717–22.

138. Henry TR, Mazziotta JC, Engel J Jr. Interictal metabolic anatomy of mesial temporal lobe epilepsy. Arch Neurol 1993;50(6):582–9.

139. Tepmongkol S, Srikijvilaikul T, Vasavid P. Factors affecting bilateral temporal lobe hypometabolism on 18F-FDG PET brain scan in unilateral medial temporal lobe epilepsy. Epilepsy Behav 2013; 29(2):386–9.

140. Takahashi M, Soma T, Kawai K, et al. Voxel-based comparison of preoperative FDG-PET between mesial temporal lobe epilepsy patients with and without postoperative seizure-free outcomes. Ann Nucl Med 2012;26(9):698–706.

141. Struck AF, Hall LT, Floberg JM, et al. Surgical decision making in temporal lobe epilepsy: a comparison of [(18)F]FDG-PET, MRI, and EEG. Epilepsy Behav 2011;22(2):293–7.

142. Salamon N, Kung J, Shaw SJ, et al. FDG-PET/MRI coregistration improves detection of cortical dysplasia in patients with epilepsy. Neurology 2008;71(20):1594–601.

143. da Silva EA, Chugani DC, Muzik O, et al. Identification of frontal lobe epileptic foci in children using positron emission tomography. Epilepsia 1997; 38(11):1198–208.

144. Swartz BW, Khonsari A, Vrown C, et al. Improved sensitivity of 18FDG-positron emission tomography scans in frontal and "frontal plus" epilepsy. Epilepsia 1995;36(4):388–95.

145. Knopman AA, Wong CH, Stevenson RJ, et al. The cognitive profile of occipital lobe epilepsy and the selective association of left temporal lobe hypometabolism with verbal memory impairment. Epilepsia 2014. http://dx.doi.org/10.1111/epi.12623. [Epub ahead of print].

146. Wong CH, Bleasel A, Wen L, et al. Relationship between preoperative hypometabolism and surgical outcome in neocortical epilepsy surgery. Epilepsia 2012;53(8):1333–40.

147. Maier W, Zobel A, Wagner M. Schizophrenia and bipolar disorder: differences and overlaps. Curr Opin Psychiatry 2006;19(2):165–70.

148. Heckmatt J. Schizophrenia. Lancet 2004; 364(9442):1313.

149. Mueser KT, McGurk SR. Schizophrenia. Lancet 2004;363(9426):2063–72.

150. Buchsbaum MS, Ingvar DH, Kessler R, et al. Cerebral glucography with positron tomography. Use in normal subjects and in patients with schizophrenia. Arch Gen Psychiatry 1982;39(3):251–9.

151. Soares JC, Innis RB. Neurochemical brain imaging investigations of schizophrenia. Biol Psychiatry 1999;46(5):600–15.

152. Epstein J, Stern E, Silbersweig D. Mesolimbic activity associated with psychosis in schizophrenia. Symptom-specific PET studies. Ann N Y Acad Sci 1999;877:562–74.

153. Fujimoto T, Takeuch K, Matsumoto T, et al. Abnormal glucose metabolism in the anterior cingulate cortex in patients with schizophrenia. Psychiatry Res 2007;154(1):49–58.

154. Haznedar MM, Buchsbaum MS, Hazlett EA, et al. Cingulate gyrus volume and metabolism in the schizophrenia spectrum. Schizophr Res 2004; 71(2-3):249–62.

155. Park HJ, Lee JD, Chun JW, et al. Cortical surface-based analysis of 18F-FDG PET: measured

metabolic abnormalities in schizophrenia are affected by cortical structural abnormalities. NeuroImage 2006;31(4):1434–44.

156. Seethalakshmi R, Parkar SR, Nair N, et al. Regional brain metabolism in schizophrenia: an FDG-PET study. Indian J psychiatry 2006;48(3):149–53.

157. Fernandez-Egea E, Parellada E, Lomena F, et al. 18FDG PET study of amygdalar activity during facial emotion recognition in schizophrenia. Eur Arch Psychiatry Clin Neurosci 2010;260(1):69–76.

158. Brooks JO 3rd, Hoblyn JC, Woodard SA, et al. Corticolimbic metabolic dysregulation in euthymic older adults with bipolar disorder. J Psychiatr Res 2009;43(5):497–502.

159. Kupferschmidt DA, Zakzanis KK. Toward a functional neuroanatomical signature of bipolar disorder: quantitative evidence from the neuroimaging literature. Psychiatry Res 2011;193(2):71–9.

160. Altamura AC, Bertoldo A, Marotta G, et al. White matter metabolism differentiates schizophrenia and bipolar disorder: a preliminary PET study. Psychiatry Res 2013;214(3):410–4.

161. Waxman AD, Herholz K, Lewis DH, et al. Society of Nuclear Medicine procedure guideline for FDG PET brain imaging. Version 1.0. Society of Nuclear Medicine; February 8, 2009. Available at: https://www.snmmi.org/ClinicalPractice/content.aspx?ItemNumber=6414. Accessed July, 2014.

[18F]Fluorodeoxyglucose PET in Thoracic Malignancies

Mie Holm Vilstrup, MD[a], Drew A. Torigian, MD, MA, FSAR[b],*

KEYWORDS

- Fluorodeoxyglucose (FDG) • Thoracic malignancy • Lung cancer • Malignant pleural mesothelioma
- Esophageal cancer • Thymic tumors

KEY POINTS

- [18F]Fluorodeoxyglucose (FDG) PET/computed tomography (CT) is useful for the characterization of lung nodules, and is currently recommended when a solid indeterminate lung nodule greater than 8 to 10 mm in diameter is present in the setting of a low to moderate pretest probability of malignancy or when a persistent part-solid indeterminate nodule greater than 8 to 10 mm in diameter is present.
- FDG-PET/CT is recommended for the staging of patients with lung cancer, and is also useful for prognostication of clinical outcome, pretreatment planning, response assessment, and restaging.
- FDG-PET/magnetic resonance imaging and FDG-PET/CT virtual bronchoscopy are emerging techniques that may one day play a greater role in the staging of patients with lung cancer.
- Dual time-point FDG-PET/CT may be useful in selected patients to improve lesion characterization and disease staging, although further prospective investigation is warranted before routine clinical implementation.
- FDG-PET/CT plays a major role in the diagnostic workup and management of patients with malignant pleural mesothelioma, esophageal cancer, and thymic epithelial tumors.

INTRODUCTION

[18F]Fluorodeoxyglucose (FDG) PET is a robust quantitative molecular imaging technique that is currently most often performed in hybrid fashion with computed tomography (CT) or magnetic resonance (MR) imaging. This article reviews the utility of FDG-PET in the evaluation of patients with thoracic malignancy, with an emphasis on non–small cell lung cancer (NSCLC), although applications of FDG-PET in small cell lung cancer (SCLC), malignant pleural mesothelioma (MPM), esophageal cancer, and thymic epithelial tumors are also discussed. In particular, the use of FDG-PET for lung nodule characterization, cancer staging, prognosis assessment, pretreatment planning, response prediction, response monitoring, and restaging is discussed. Also reviewed is the role of dual time-point (DTP) FDG-PET in the thoracic oncologic setting.

LUNG NODULE CHARACTERIZATION

A lung nodule is defined as a rounded opacity measuring 3 cm or less in diameter surrounded by lung parenchyma.[1] Although chest CT is currently the mainstay for detecting lung nodules given its high sensitivity, these nodules are often unable to be accurately characterized on CT alone as benign or malignant, as structural imaging

---

The authors have no disclosures to make for this article.
[a] Department of Nuclear Medicine, Odense University Hospital, Sdr. Boulevard 29, Odense 5000, Denmark;
[b] Department of Radiology, Hospital of the University of Pennsylvania, 3400 Spruce Street, Philadelphia, PA 19104, USA
* Corresponding author.
E-mail address: Drew.Torigian@uphs.upenn.edu

PET Clin 9 (2014) 391–420
http://dx.doi.org/10.1016/j.cpet.2014.06.002
1556-8598/14/$ – see front matter © 2014 Elsevier Inc. All rights reserved.

pet.theclinics.com

features are often nonspecific.[2] FDG-PET may be useful to improve the characterization of lung nodules, given the assumption that malignant nodules exhibit increased FDG uptake owing to the presence of increased glucose uptake and metabolism (**Figs. 1** and **2**).

In a meta-analysis of 40 studies including 1474 focal pulmonary lesions, Gould and colleagues[3] reported sensitivity and specificity of 97% and 78%, respectively, and a maximum joint sensitivity and specificity of 91% (95% confidence interval [CI] 89%–93%) of FDG-PET for detection of pulmonary malignancy. In another meta-analysis of 44 studies (22 of which included FDG-PET), Cronin and colleagues[4] reported a pooled sensitivity, specificity, positive predictive value (PPV), negative predictive value (NPV), accuracy, and diagnostic odds ratio (DOR) of 95% (95% CI 93%–98%), 82% (95% CI 77%–88%), 91% (95% CI 88%–93%), 90% (95% CI 85%–94%), 94% (83%–98%), and 97.31

(95% CI 6.26–188.37) for FDG-PET in the evaluation of the solitary pulmonary nodule (SPN). No significant difference in diagnostic performance was noted between FDG-PET and dynamic contrast-enhanced CT, dynamic contrast-enhanced MR imaging, and [^{99m}Tc]depreotide single-photon emission CT (SPECT). Fletcher and colleagues[5] prospectively studied 532 patients with 344 SPN with FDG-PET and CT. The sensitivity, specificity, and accuracy for FDG-PET were 92%, 82%, and 93%, respectively, compared with 96%, 41%, and 82% for CT. Moreover, FDG-PET had superior intraobserver and interobserver reliability compared with CT, and resulted in far fewer indeterminate test results.

In a multicenter prospective study of 81 patients with 10- to 30-mm peripheral lung nodules who underwent thin-section CT along with FDG-PET, Kubota and colleagues[6] reported that the specificity of FDG-PET plus CT for distinguishing

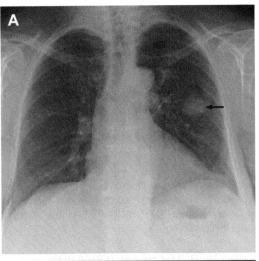
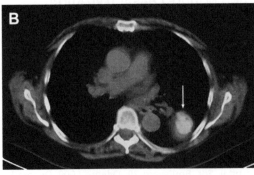
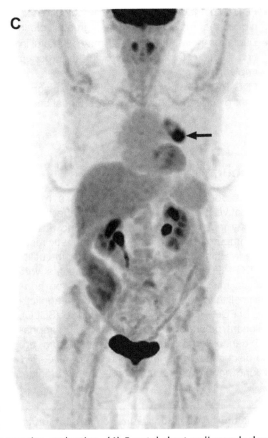

Fig. 1. A 74-year-old woman undergoing routine preoperative evaluation. (*A*) Frontal chest radiograph shows incidentally detected 2.5-cm nodule (*arrow*) in left mid-lung. (*B*) Axial fused FDG-PET/CT image shows avid FDG uptake (SUV$_{max}$ 9.9) in left lower lobe nodule (*arrow*). (*C*) Coronal PET maximum-intensity projection (MIP) image from same study again reveals FDG-avid lung nodule (*arrow*) and no other FDG-avid sites. Subsequent surgical resection revealed poorly differentiated lung adenocarcinoma along with 5 of 15 metastatic left peribronchial and hilar nodes.

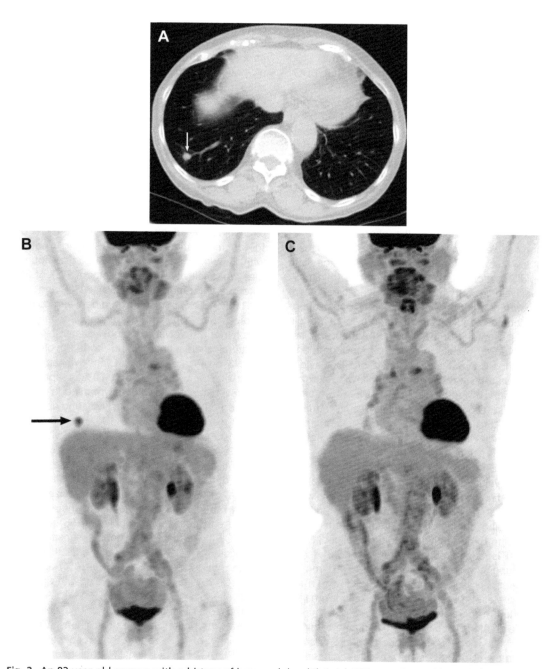

Fig. 2. An 83-year-old woman with a history of lung nodules. (*A*) Axial CT image shows 11-mm right lower lobe solid nodule (*arrow*), previously 5 mm on prior CT 5 months prior (not shown). (*B*) Coronal PET MIP image from baseline FDG-PET/CT shows FDG uptake (SUV_{max} 4.4) in nodule (*arrow*) and no other FDG-avid sites, most consistent with stage IA lung adenocarcinoma. (*C*) Coronal PET MIP image from FDG-PET/CT after stereotactic body radiation therapy reveals complete metabolic response of nodule.

malignant from benign causes was 91% (95% CI 76%–98%), which was significantly improved in comparison with 68% (95% CI 50%–83%) for CT alone and 79% (95% CI 62%–91%) for PET alone. The accuracy of FDG-PET plus CT was 92% (95% CI 83%–97%), which was significantly higher than that of CT or PET alone (both 81%; 95% CI 70%–88%), whereas the sensitivities (92% vs 90% vs 81%, respectively) were not significantly different. Jeong and colleagues[7] retrospectively studied 100 patients with an SPN, and reported sensitivity, specificity, and accuracy of 88%, 77%, and

81%, respectively, for FDG-PET/CT, significantly more specific than either CT or PET alone. Yi and colleagues[8] prospectively evaluated 100 patients with an SPN, and reported that FDG-PET/CT had sensitivity, specificity, PPV, NPV, and accuracy of 96%, 88%, 94%, 92%, and 93%, respectively, compared with 81%, 93%, 96%, 71%, and 85% for dynamic contrast-enhanced CT. Several other studies have reported a similarly high diagnostic performance of FDG-PET/CT for lung nodule evaluation, and interestingly that qualitative visual assessment is sufficient for lung nodule characterization.[9–11]

However, FDG-PET may sometimes provide false-negative results in the characterization of lung nodules as malignant, particularly when there is low tumor metabolic activity, such as with lepidic-predominant adenocarcinomas (minimally invasive or in situ, which often appear as persistent subsolid nodules on CT images), mucinous adenocarcinomas, and carcinoid tumors, or a nodule size less than 8 to 10 mm.[12–20] Although false-negative PET results may occur more commonly with subsolid nodules, absence of FDG avidity portends a favorable prognosis following surgical resection.[21–25] Furthermore, FDG-PET may sometimes also provide false-positive results attributable to the presence of active infection or noninfectious inflammation, such as in the setting of tobacco use or sarcoidosis.[13,26,27]

FDG-PET may be most cost-effective for lung nodule evaluation when clinical pretest probability and CT findings are discordant, especially when the pretest probability is relatively low and the CT imaging characteristics are indeterminate.[28] According to currently available guidelines, FDG-PET/CT is recommended when a solid indeterminate lung nodule greater than 8 to 10 mm in diameter is present in the setting of a low to moderate pretest probability (5%–65%) of malignancy or when a persistent part-solid indeterminate nodule greater than 8 to 10 mm in diameter is present.[2,29–31] The DTP technique (see later discussion) may also further improve the diagnostic performance of FDG-PET in characterizing pulmonary nodules.

STAGING OF NON–SMALL CELL LUNG CANCER

Accurate staging of lung cancer is critical for optimization of the treatment approach to be used, whether for curative or palliative intent, and in particular to select those patients who may benefit from surgical resection. FDG-PET, and in particular FDG-PET/CT, has improved the diagnostic performance of regional nodal (N) staging and

distant metastatic (M) staging in patients with NSCLC (**Figs. 3** and **4**), and is now considered as a standard component of the staging workup of patients with NSCLC.[32–36] Several studies have recently reported that FDG-PET is cost-effective for the staging of patients with NSCLC.[36,37]

N Staging

FDG-PET is very useful in improving the accuracy of N staging in NSCLC, as demonstrated by several representative studies. In a meta-analysis by Gould and colleagues[38] including 39 studies examining the diagnostic performance of FDG-PET for mediastinal lymph node staging in patients with known or suspected NSCLC, they found a median sensitivity and specificity of PET of 85% (interquartile range [IQR] 66%–89%) and 90% (IQR 82%–96%) to discriminate between no nodal involvement (N0) and hilar/intrapulmonary (N1) lymph node involvement and ipsilateral or contralateral mediastinal lymph node involvement (N2/N3) disease. The median sensitivity and specificity of CT were 61% and 79%, respectively. Moreover, in patients without lymph node enlargement on CT, the median sensitivity and specificity of PET were 82% (IQR 65%–100%) and 93% (IQR 92%–100%), respectively, compared with 100% (IQR 90%–100%) and 78% (IQR 68%–100%), respectively in patients with lymph node enlargement, demonstrating that the diagnostic performance of PET depended on the size of the lymph nodes.[38] In a more recent meta-analysis by Wu and colleagues[39] including 56 studies of NSCLC, the patient-level pooled sensitivity and specificity of FDG-PET/CT for mediastinal nodal staging was 72% (95% CI 65%–78%) and 91% (95% CI 86%–94%), respectively, with an accuracy of 88% (95% CI 85%–91%). A meta-analysis of 14 studies by Lv and colleagues[40] reported a patient-level pooled sensitivity and specificity of 76% and 88%, respectively, for FDG-PET/CT in mediastinal N staging for NSCLC. Another meta-analysis of 18 studies by Toloza and colleagues[41] reported a pooled sensitivity and specificity of 84% and 89%, respectively, for FDG-PET/CT in mediastinal N staging for NSCLC, compared with 57% and 82% for contrast-enhanced CT. In a multicenter prospective study of 81 patients with NSCLC and enlarged mediastinal lymph nodes on contrast-enhanced CT who underwent pretreatment FDG-PET, Kubota and colleagues[42] reported that the specificity for diagnosis of mediastinal lymph node metastases significantly improved from 56% (95% CI 43%–68%) for CT alone to 81% (95% CI 70%–89%)

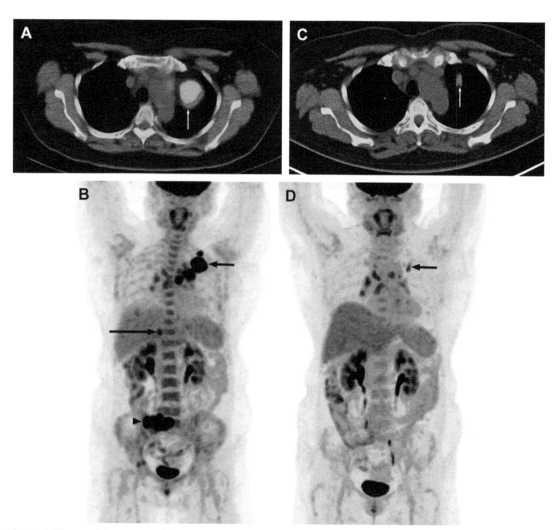

Fig. 3. A 65-year-old woman with lung adenocarcinoma undergoing staging assessment. (*A*) Axial fused baseline FDG-PET/CT image shows 3.8-cm left upper lobe mass (*arrow*) with avid FDG uptake (SUV$_{max}$ 30.7) caused by lung cancer. (*B*) Coronal PET MIP image from same study again shows FDG-avid uptake in mass (*short arrow*) along with FDG-avid subjacent left supraclavicular, bilateral hilar and mediastinal lymphadenopathy, right adrenal metastasis (*long arrow*), and right sacral bone marrow metastasis (*arrowhead*), consistent with stage IV disease. (*C*) Axial fused FDG-PET/CT image after chemotherapy reveals interval decrease in size and FDG uptake (SUV$_{max}$ 4.8) of left upper lobe mass (*arrow*). (*D*) Coronal PET MIP image from same study again shows interval improvement in mass (*arrow*) and in regional nodal metastases along with interval resolution of distant metastases, consistent with partial metabolic response.

for CT plus PET, and that the accuracy significantly improved from 62% (95% CI 52%–72%) to 79% (95% CI 70%–87%), respectively.

The main limitations of FDG-PET for N staging of lung cancer are false-negative results attributable to microscopic lymph node involvement or low tumor metabolic activity, and false-positive results owing to the presence of infection or noninfectious inflammation.[43] Occult lymph node metastases have been reported to more likely to occur with increasing T stage, centrally located tumors, adenocarcinoma histology, and a higher primary tumor standardized uptake value (SUV).[44–46] Also, the specificity of FDG-PET/CT for thoracic mediastinal lymph node involvement in NSCLC is diminished in areas endemic for granulomatous disease.[39,47] As such, histopathologic confirmation with invasive mediastinal lymph node sampling is still generally performed before treatment with curative intent, with the possible exception of patients who have small peripheral tumors and no imaging findings of regional lymphadenopathy. In a meta-analysis of 14 studies of patients with NSCLC, de Langen and colleagues[48] reported that the likelihood for malignancy in an FDG-nonavid lymph node was 5% when 10 to 15 mm in diameter versus 21% when greater than 15 mm, whereas the likelihood for in an FDG-avid node was 62% when 10 to 15 mm versus 90% when greater than 15 mm in diameter.

M Staging

Overall, FDG-PET decreases the number of futile thoracotomies in a significant proportion of patients with lung cancer, and leads to changes in therapeutic management in up to 40%.[49,50] For example, in a recent retrospective study of 976

veterans with newly diagnosed NSCLC who underwent surgical resection, Zeliadt and colleagues[51] reported that preoperative staging FDG-PET prevented unnecessary surgery in 38% of patients. In a study of 592 patients with NSCLC, Takeuchi and colleagues[52] reported that FDG-PET/CT changed disease stage in 29% of patients, by upstaging in 16% and downstaging in 12%, significantly affecting management in 37% of patients overall, because FDG-PET improves the accuracy of detection and characterization of sites of distant metastatic disease. In a meta-analysis by Wu and colleagues,[39] the pooled sensitivity and specificity of FDG-PET/CT was

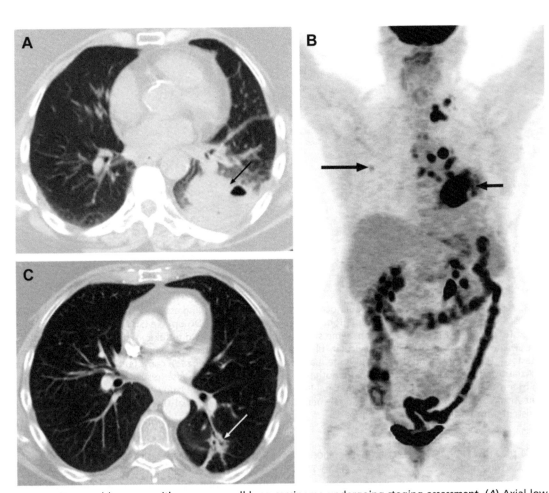

Fig. 4. A 67-year-old woman with squamous cell lung carcinoma undergoing staging assessment. (*A*) Axial low-dose CT image from baseline FDG-PET/CT shows 4.1-cm mass (*arrow*) in left lower lobe of lung. (*B*) Coronal PET MIP image from same study shows avid FDG uptake (SUV$_{max}$ 26.2) in mass (*short arrow*) along with FDG-avid left supraclavicular, mediastinal, and left hilar regional lymphadenopathy and mildly FDG-avid nodule in contralateral lung (*long arrow*), consistent with stage IV disease. (*C*) Axial CT image after chemotherapy reveals marked interval decrease in size of mass with residual scar remaining (*arrow*). Regional lymphadenopathy and right lung nodule also resolved (not shown). (*D*) Axial CT imaging performed 5 months later for restaging shows new 1.8-cm nodule (*arrow*) in site of prior left lower lobe scar, suspicious for recurrent tumor. (*E*) Coronal PET MIP image from same study shows avid FDG uptake (SUV$_{max}$ 17.3) in nodule (*arrow*), confirming recurrent lung cancer. No other FDG-avid sites were seen.

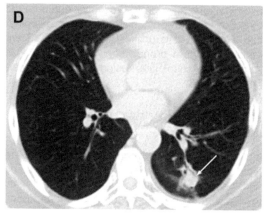

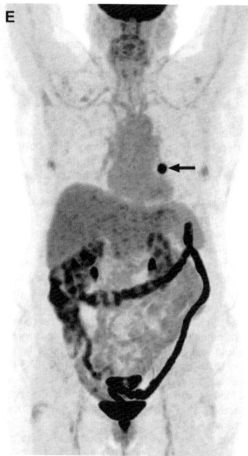

Fig. 4. (continued)

77% (95% CI 47%–93%) and 95% (95% CI 92%–97%), respectively, for extrathoracic metastatic disease, and 91% (95% CI 80%–97%) and 98% (95% CI 94%–99%), respectively, for osseous metastatic disease in NSCLC. In another meta-analysis of 9 studies by Li and colleagues,[53] the sensitivity, specificity, positive likelihood ratio (PLR), and negative likelihood ratio (NLR) of FDG-PET/CT for M staging in lung cancer were

93% (95% CI 88%–96%), 96% (95% CI 95%–96%), 28.4 (95% CI 14.0–57.5), and 0.08 (95% CI 0.02–0.37), respectively, indicating excellent diagnostic performance. FDG-PET may not be necessary to perform for M staging in patients who have obvious widespread metastatic disease based on CT or other diagnostic imaging tests.

With regard to adrenal gland assessment, a retrospective study by Lu and colleagues[54] of 87 patients with lung cancer with 110 adrenal masses showed that FDG-PET/CT had sensitivity, specificity, PPV, NPV, and accuracy of 97%, 94%, 95%, 94%, and 95%, respectively, for the detection of adrenal metastatic disease based on qualitative image assessment. In a retrospective study of 94 patients with lung cancer and 113 adrenal masses, Kumar and colleagues[55] reported that FDG-PET had sensitivity, specificity, PPV, NPV, and accuracy of 93%, 90%, 94%, 88%, and 92%, respectively, for the detection of adrenal metastatic disease based on qualitative image assessment.

For bone marrow assessment, in a meta-analysis of 14 studies of patients with lung cancer, Liu and colleagues[56] reported that FDG-PET was found to be the best modality to detect bone marrow metastases, on both a per-patient and per-lesion basis, whereas MR imaging had the highest specificity on a per-lesion basis. In a meta-analysis of 17 studies including 2940 patients with lung cancer, Qu and colleagues[57] reported pooled sensitivities for detection of bone marrow metastases using FDG-PET/CT, FDG-PET, MR imaging, and bone scintigraphy of 92% (95% CI 88%–95%), 87% (95% CI 81%–92%), 77% (95% CI 65%–87%), and 86% (95% CI 82%–89%), respectively, and pooled specificities of 98% (95% CI 97%–98%), 94% (95% CI 92%–96%), 92% (95% CI 88%–95%), and 88% (95% CI 86%–89%), respectively.

However, FDG-PET/CT has a low sensitivity of detection of brain metastases resulting from lung cancer. In particular, Kruger and colleagues[58] reported that FDG-PET/CT had sensitivity, specificity, PPV, and NPV of 27%, 98%, 75%, and 83%, respectively, for a diagnosis of brain metastasis in lung cancer, with significantly fewer brain metastases detected in comparison with brain MR imaging. Similarly, Lee and colleagues[59] reported sensitivity, specificity, and accuracy of 24%, 100%, and 91%, respectively, for FDG-PET/CT diagnosis of brain metastases in NSCLC compared with 88%, 98%, and 97%, respectively, for brain MR imaging. In a prospective study of 442 patients with lung adenocarcinoma who underwent pretreatment FDG-PET/CT and brain MR imaging, Lee and colleagues[59] reported that MR imaging had significantly higher sensitivity for the detection of brain metastases than PET/CT (88% vs 24%). In a prospective study of 104 neurologic asymptomatic patients with lung cancer who underwent pretreatment cerebral FDG-PET/CT and MR imaging, Kruger and colleagues[58] reported that MR imaging is more accurate than PET/CT for the detection of multiple and smaller brain metastases.

New FDG-PET Techniques for Lung Cancer Staging

PET/MR imaging is a new hybrid imaging technique that may prove to be useful for the staging of lung cancer.[60] For example, in a study of 22 patients with NSCLC, Heusch and colleagues[61] reported that FDG-PET/CT and FDG-PET/MR imaging both correctly staged patients in 100% when compared with histopathology, and were not significantly different in terms of staging for NSCLC. In a study of 160 patients with lung cancer (mostly adenocarcinoma) by Usuda and colleagues,[62] significantly higher sensitivity (64% vs 39%) and accuracy (96% vs 94%) for N staging were observed through use of diffusion-weighted (DW) imaging compared with FDG-PET/CT alone, which may indicate a potential role for FDG-PET/MR imaging for staging patients with NSCLC. This finding is similarly demonstrated in a study of 48 NSCLC patients by Kim and colleagues,[63] who reported sensitivity, specificity, PPV, NPV, and accuracy of 69%, 93%, 71%, 93%, and 89%, respectively for FDG-PET/CT in combination with separately acquired DW and T2-weighted MR images, compared with 46%, 96%, 75%, 88%, and 87%, respectively for FDG-PET/CT alone. Kohan and colleagues[64] reported that FDG-PET/CT and FDG-PET/MR imaging had comparable diagnostic performance for N staging in 11 patients with lung cancer, and that FDG-PET/MR imaging had substantial interobserver agreement for N staging.

PET/CT virtual bronchoscopy (VB) is another technique that may someday play a greater role in the staging of lung cancer. In a multicenter prospective study of 261 patients with lung cancer who underwent FDG-PET/CT VB, CT VB, and reference standard fiberoptic bronchoscopy (FOB), Yildirim and colleagues[65] reported sensitivity, specificity, PPV, NPV, and accuracy of PET/CT VB to determine segmental involvement by malignancy of 95%, 97%, 99%, 87%, and 96%, respectively, compared with 91%, 83%, 94%, 77%, and 89%, respectively for CT VB. The investigators therefore recommend the use of FDG-PET/CT VB in routine lung cancer examinations, as it provides similar outcomes to those of FOB and cytohistopathologic examination. However, it is unlikely that PET/CT VB will replace standard bronchoscopy, because tissue sampling of suspicious lesions cannot be performed via VB.

PROGNOSTICATION OF CLINICAL OUTCOME IN NSCLC

In patients with lung cancer, 2 major factors are typically associated with prognosis: disease stage and performance status. With the current shift toward a more individualized treatment approach to such patients, there is a need for additional biomarkers of risk stratification in this patient population.

The degree of FDG uptake measured on PET imaging, reflecting the rate and amount of cellular glucose uptake and phosphorylation, is one such biomarker. A recent systematic review and meta-analysis of 21 studies by Paesmans and colleagues[66] summarized the prognostic value of pretherapeutic FDG-PET for survival, and reported that a high primary tumor SUV portends a poor overall survival (OS) with an overall combined hazard ratio of 2.08. In a prospective study of 610 patients with stage IA lung adenocarcinoma who underwent pretreatment FDG-PET/CT and high-resolution CT, Uehara and colleagues[67] reported that high tumor maximum SUV (SUV_{max}) and a low ground-glass opacity ratio reflected tumor invasiveness, presence of nodal metastasis, and tumor recurrence, and were significant prognostic factors for recurrence-free survival (RFS) and cancer-specific survival on multivariate analyses. In a retrospective study of 222 patients with pathologic stage I lung adenocarcinoma, Kadota and colleagues[68] reported that a high tumor SUV_{max} (≥ 3.0) on pretreatment FDG-PET was associated with high-grade histology and an increased risk of recurrence. In another retrospective study of 103 patients with locally advanced NSCLC, Ulger and colleagues[69] reported that primary tumor FDG uptake has predictive value independent of tumor size, with a 3-year OS of 42% versus 23% in low (SUV_{max} <10.7) versus high (SUV_{max} $\geq$10.7) FDG-uptake groups. In a retrospective study of 354 NSCLC patients, Muto and colleagues[70] reported that primary tumor SUV_{max} on pretreatment FDG-PET/CT was significantly lower in those tumors without associated lymph node involvement compared with those with lymph node involvement, but does not allow for prediction of the extent of lymph node involvement. In a retrospective study of 440 patients with lung cancer (mostly NSCLC),

Ishibashi and colleagues[71] reported that primary tumor SUV_{max} on pretreatment FDG-PET was significantly lower in lesions without intratumoral vessel invasion compared with those with vascular invasion. In addition, presence of intratumoral vessel invasion was associated with a significantly higher probability of regional lymph node metastases.

Metabolic tumor volume (MTV) and total lesional glycolysis (TLG) (defined as the sum of the products of lesion volume and lesion SUV across all lesions in the body) measured from FDG-PET/CT are additional potentially useful biomarkers to prognosticate outcome in patients with lung cancer and to guide pretreatment planning. In a retrospective study of 106 patients with lung adenocarcinoma, Chung and colleagues[72] reported that high total MTV and high TLG on pretreatment FDG-PET/CT were independent prognostic factors for poor progression-free survival (PFS) and OS in patients with stage III or IV disease, although not in patients with stage I or II disease. In another retrospective study of 104 patients with NSCLC who underwent pretreatment FDG-PET/CT, Zhang and colleagues[73] reported that high total MTV and TLG were significantly associated with decreased OS, independent of clinical stage and other prognostic factors, although tumor SUV_{max} and SUV_{mean} were not significantly associated with clinical outcome. In a retrospective study of 61 patients with NSCLC, Lee and colleagues[74] reported that a high total MTV on pretreatment FDG-PET/CT was significantly associated with a worse OS on multivariate analysis. In a prospective study of 105 patients with NSCLC, Chen and colleagues[75] reported that a high TLG on pretreatment FDG-PET/CT was significantly associated with a worse PFS on multivariate analysis.

DUAL TIME-POINT FDG-PET FOR EVALUATION OF LUNG NODULES AND LUNG CANCER

There may be substantial overlap in the FDG avidity of both malignant and benign thoracic lesions on routine single time-point (STP) PET imaging, limiting the specificity and accuracy of diagnosis. However, DTP FDG-PET imaging, which entails the acquisition of 2 sets of PET images following FDG administration, has been suggested as a straightforward method to overcome this limitation. This approach is based on the observation that malignant and nonmalignant lesions typically have different patterns of FDG uptake over time. For example, Hamberg and colleagues[76] reported in 8 patients with stage III lung cancer that tumor FDG uptake did not reach

a plateau within 90 minutes of PET imaging. Through use of a 3-compartment model, they showed that the average time to reach 95% of the FDG plateau value was 298 ± 42 minutes (range 130–500 minutes). Other studies have similarly shown that FDG uptake in malignant cells tends to increase over time, whereas the FDG uptake within normal and chronic inflammatory cells tends to remain stable or decrease with time after approximately 60 minutes.[77,78] Retention index (RI) (defined as [the difference in lesion SUV_{max} measured on delayed and early time-point PET images]/[lesion SUV_{max} on the early time-point PET images] $\times$ 100%) is the typical parameter that is measured and calculated from DTP FDG-PET images to quantitatively evaluate lesions of interest.

Lung Nodule Characterization

Several studies have reported results regarding the use of DTP FDG-PET to improve the characterization of pulmonary nodules. In a recent prospective study of 43 patients who underwent pretreatment FDG-PET/CT (with 45 malignant lesions [mostly NSCLC] and 43 benign lesions), Cheng and colleagues[79] reported that malignant lesions had an average RI (from 1 to 2 hours) of 25% (vs −2% for benign lesions) and an average RI (from 1 to 3 hours) of 39% (vs 4% for benign lesions). The optimal cutoff values for SUV_{max} to differentiate malignant from benign lesions were 3.24, 3.67, and 4.21 at 1-, 2-, and 3-hour time-point images, respectively, with the 3-hour value providing the best accuracy of 89%. Lesion-to-background ratios also improved on delayed time-point PET images, improving image quality. Inflammatory granulomatous lesions were also noted to have increased FDG uptake on delayed time-point imaging, and could not be differentiated from malignant thoracic lesions by using either SUV_{max} or RI measures.

However, in a retrospective study of 77 patients with 34 benign (including both tuberculous and nontuberculous) pulmonary lesions and 47 lung cancers (mostly NSCLC), all with size greater than 1 cm and SUV_{max} greater than 2.5, Kaneko and colleagues[80] reported that benign and malignant pulmonary lesions showed similarly high RIs (from 1 to 2 hours) based on FDG-PET or PET/CT. A similar observation was also reported by Sathekge and colleagues[26] in another tuberculosis-endemic area. Moreover, Kadaria and colleagues[81] reported that DTP FDG-PET/CT was not useful in differentiating benign from malignant intrathoracic lesions in a study of 72 patients from an area endemic for histoplasmosis infection and with a high prevalence of sarcoidosis, although the presence of a negative RI reliably indicated nonmalignant disease.

Three recent meta-analyses comparing the diagnostic performance of STP with that of DTP FDG-PET found substantial heterogeneity in the results of the included studies attributable to varying study populations, PET scanning protocols (including interscan delay times), threshold values for a positive result, and lesion sizes.[82–84] Despite this, they found no significant difference in the diagnostic performance between STP and DTP FDG-PET for pulmonary nodule assessment, although one study reported that the specificity may improve with the DTP technique.

Lung Cancer Staging

Studies have also reported on the utility of DTP FDG-PET in improving lung cancer staging, with mixed results, some of which are summarized here.

In a prospective study of 104 patients with NSCLC (53 with pulmonary comorbidity and 49 without) who underwent pretreatment DTP FDG-PET/CT, Hu and colleagues[85] reported that in patients with pulmonary comorbidity, the sensitivity, specificity, PPV, NPV, and accuracy of DTP PET/CT at the patient level were 94%, 68%, 76%, 56, and 96%, respectively, compared with 88%, 60%, 68%, 48%, and 92%, respectively, for STP PET/CT. No significant difference in diagnostic performance was observed in patients without pulmonary comorbidity. In a retrospective study of 31 patients with NSCLC and pleural effusion, Alkhawaldeh and colleagues[86] reported that DTP FDG-PET/CT can improve the diagnostic accuracy of differentiating benign from malignant pleural disease, and has sensitivity, specificity, and accuracy of 100%, 94%, and 97%, respectively, when using the criterion of SUV_{max} 2.4 or higher and/or RI (from 1 to 2 hours) of 9% or higher. In a prospective study of 80 patients with suspected lung cancer, Demura and colleagues[87] reported that DTP FDG-PET significantly improved the ability to characterize thoracic lesions as malignant (sensitivity, specificity, and accuracy of 98%, 67%, and 86%, respectively), and improved the specificity (from 63% to 91%) and accuracy (from 70% to 92%) of mediastinal lymph node staging. In addition, tumor RI (from 1 to 3 hours) was significantly inversely correlated with the degree of tumor differentiation. Uesaka and colleagues[88] prospectively studied 150 patients with lung cancer (mostly NSCLC) with known or suspected regional lymph node involvement or distant metastatic disease, and reported that DTP FDG-PET (from 1 to 3 hours) significantly improved the diagnostic performance for N and M staging in comparison with STP FDG-PET.

In contradistinction, Kim and colleagues[89] found that DTP FDG-PET/CT was not useful in predicting the presence of N1-positive disease in a retrospective study of 70 patients with NSCLC. Furthermore, Yen and colleagues[90] reported that DTP FDG-PET was not useful in improving N staging in 96 NSCLC patients from a tuberculosis-endemic region. Similarly, Li and colleagues[91] reported in a prospective study of 80 NSCLC patients from a tuberculosis-endemic region that DTP FDG-PET/CT did not significantly differentiate benign from malignant lymph nodes. Kasai and colleagues[92] retrospectively studied 129 patients with NSCLC using DTP FDG-PET/CT (from 1 to 2 hours), and reported that STP FDG-PET/CT was sufficiently useful for N staging.

Lung Cancer Tumor Biology and Patient Outcome

The RI of lung cancer lesions determined from DTP FDG-PET may also serve as a biomarker of tumor biology and patient outcome. Tsuchida and colleagues[93] prospectively assessed 44 patients with lung cancer who underwent pretreatment multiple time-point PET/CT at 1, 2, and 3 hours after FDG administration. The RI (from 2 to 3 hours) differed significantly between squamous cell carcinoma, well-differentiated adenocarcinoma, and poorly/moderately differentiated adenocarcinoma subtypes, and the RIs (from 1 to 2 hours and from 1 to 3 hours) were significantly higher in squamous cell carcinoma than in well-differentiated adenocarcinoma. In another retrospective study of 187 patients with NSCLC who underwent DTP FDG-PET/CT, Chen and colleagues[94] reported that an absolute change in tumor SUV_{max} from 1 to 2 hours had the best discriminative yield for PFS, whereby 3-year PFS and OS were 62% and 88%, respectively, in patients with an SUV change of 1 or less, compared with 21% and 46%, respectively, in patients with an SUV change of greater than 1. Furthermore, in stage I NSCLC patients treated with surgery alone, the absolute change in tumor SUV_{max} on DTP FDG-PET/CT was the only significant prognostic factor. Similarly, in a retrospective study of 100 patients with lung adenocarcinoma who underwent DTP FDG-PET, Houseni and colleagues[95] reported that tumor RI (from 1 to 1.5 hours) of 25% or more had a median OS of 15 months, compared with 39 months when tumor RI was less than 25%. In a prospective study of 57 patients with stage I NSCLC who underwent pretreatment DTP FDG-PET/CT and subsequent stereotactic body RT (SBRT), Satoh and colleagues[96] reported that a high tumor RI (from 1 to 2 hours) is a significant predictor of recurrent distant metastatic disease on multivariate analysis. However, Kim and colleagues[97] reported no prognostic value of tumor RI (from 1 to 2 hours) on DTP FDG-PET/CT for OS and disease-free survival (DFS) in a retrospective study of 66 patients with surgically resected early-stage NSCLC.

Although DTP FDG-PET is not currently used routinely in clinical practice, it may be useful in selected cases with equivocal results when warranted to improve diagnostic accuracy. Further prospective investigation with regard to the optimal timing of the delayed time-point PET images, the cost-effectiveness of the technique (particularly in light of the added scanner time that is required), and the identification of those particular patients who will gain the most diagnostically from DTP FDG-PET imaging is warranted before implementation in routine clinical practice.

RADIATION THERAPY PRETREATMENT PLANNING AND RESPONSE ASSESSMENT IN NSCLC

Incorporation of FDG-PET into the radiation therapy (RT) planning process affects treatment delivery in a significant number of patients by altering treatment volumes, decreasing interobserver variability, and excluding patients with previously unsuspected advanced disease from receiving definitive RT. In a prospective study by Mac Manus and colleagues,[98] 30% of patients with unresectable NSCLC intended for definitive RT by conventional staging were converted to palliative therapies after FDG-PET (18% because of distant metastatic disease and 12% because of extensive locoregional disease). Similarly, in a prospective study of 100 patients with stage I to III NSCLC referred for curative RT, Kolodziejczyk and colleagues[99] reported that only 75% were suitable to undergo definitive RT based on pretreatment FDG-PET/CT, because of distant metastatic disease or extensive locoregional disease.

In recent years, the use of 3-dimensional conformal RT, intensity-modulated RT (IMRT), and SBRT for the curative treatment of NSCLC has emerged to enable delivery of high radiation doses to tumor sites while sparing normal tissues as much as possible to minimize toxicity. However, accurate delineation of tumor sites before RT is essential if local tumor control is to be achieved and patient outcome improved. Studies have shown that FDG-PET improves the delineation of lung cancer by improving N staging, M staging, and separation of tumor from atelectatic lung tissue, leading to dose sparing of uninvolved tissues.

In a prospective phase II multicenter trial of FDG-PET/CT in RT planning of 47 patients with NSCLC, Bradley and colleagues[100] reported that gross tumor volume (GTV) and median lung doses were significantly smaller for PET/CT-derived volumes than for CT-derived volumes, and nodal contours were altered by PET/CT in 51% of patients. In addition, only 1 patient developed an elective nodal failure, suggesting that PET/CT-assisted RT planning may negate the need for elective nodal irradiation. In a prospective study of 91 patients with NSCLC who underwent pretreatment FDG-PET or PET/CT, Nawara and colleagues[101] reported that PET provided additional diagnostic information over CT alone in 20%, leading to a change in planning target volume in 9%.

FDG-PET is also useful in patients with NSCLC to predict response before RT in addition to patient outcome. In a prospective study of 88 patients with stage I NSCLC who underwent FDG-PET/CT before SBRT, Satoh and colleagues[102] reported that primary tumor SUV_{max}, MTV, and TLG were significantly associated with DFS, whereas only MTV and TLG were predictive of DFS for tumors larger than 3 cm. However, in a retrospective study of 50 patients with stage I NSCLC who underwent FDG-PET/CT before SBRT, SUV_{max}, MTV, and TLG were not correlated with OS.[103] In a retrospective study of 95 patients with localized NSCLC, Takeda and colleagues[104] reported that primary tumor SUV_{max} on FDG-PET was a significant predictor of the local recurrence rate after SBRT on multivariate analysis. In a prospective study of 163 patients with medically inoperable early-stage NSCLC who underwent pretreatment FDG-PET/CT before RT, Nair and colleagues[105] reported that a primary tumor SUV_{max} of 7 or greater was associated with a worse regional RFS and distant metastasis–free survival.

FDG-PET is superior to CT for early response assessment and outcome assessment of patients with lung cancer following RT (see **Fig. 2**), and is useful in predicting the development of radiation-induced lung toxicity.[106–110] In prospective study of patients with medically inoperable early-stage NSCLC who underwent pre-SBRT (82 patients) and post-SBRT (62 patients) FDG-PET/CT, Clarke and colleagues[111] reported that a baseline primary tumor SUV_{max} greater than 5, a posttreatment tumor SUV_{max} of 2 or more, and a posttreatment reduction in tumor SUV_{max} of less than 2.55 were significantly associated with a higher risk of distant failure on multivariate analysis. In a prospective study of 51 patients with either stage I NSCLC, recurrent lung cancer, or a solitary lung metastasis who underwent pre-SBRT and post-SBRT FDG-PET/CT, Coon and colleagues[112] reported an average decrease in tumor SUV of 94%, 48%, 28%, and 0.4% in association with complete response, partial response, stable disease (SD), and progressive disease (PD), respectively. In a prospective study of 88 patients with NSCLC who underwent pre- and post-(chemo)radiation FDG-PET, Mac Manus and colleagues[113] reported a statistically significant median OS of 31 months for patients with complete metabolic response (CMR) compared with 11 months for those without a CMR. In addition, patients without CMR had higher rates of local failure and distant metastatic disease compared with those with a CMR. In another prospective study of 73 patients with NSCLC who underwent pre- and post-(chemo)radiation FDG-PET, Mac Manus and colleagues[106] reported that 2-year OS was significantly associated with PET response, and that PET and CT posttreatment findings were discordant in 40%.

In a recent multicenter prospective trial of 173 patients with stage III NSCLC who underwent FDG-PET before and approximately 14 weeks after concurrent platinum-based chemoradiation therapy, Machtay and colleagues[114] reported that pretreatment tumor SUV was not associated with OS, whereas high posttreatment tumor SUV was associated with a worse OS, although no clear cutoff value of SUV for routine clinical use was able to be specified. In a prospective study assessing the use of FDG-PET/CT versus CT 3 months after treatment with curative intent using (chemo)RT in 100 NSCLC patients, van Loon and colleagues[115] reported that 24 patients had PD. Of these patients, 16 were symptomatic and could not receive curative treatment, whereas 3 of the remaining 8 asymptomatic patients had PD potentially amenable to radical therapy only detected with PET. The investigators therefore concluded that selective use of FDG-PET/CT for response assessment may be effective in asymptomatic patients with NSCLC.

van Loon and colleagues[116] have recently reported in a prospective study of 100 NSCLC patients that FDG-PET/CT obtained 3 months after treatment with (chemo)RT for curative intent is potentially cost-effective, and more cost-effective than CT alone. However, more research is required to evaluate the cost-effectiveness of FDG-PET for follow-up evaluation of patients with NSCLC.

SYSTEMIC THERAPY RESPONSE ASSESSMENT IN NSCLC

Accurate early response assessment to systemic therapy is desirable to allow for timely adjustment of therapy when there is no response, such that unnecessary therapeutic side effects may be diminished and patient outcomes may be improved. FDG-PET can potentially be useful for this purpose in patients with NSCLC (see **Fig. 3**), as changes in tumor cellular metabolism occur more rapidly than changes in tumor volume, and a reduction in tumor FDG retention is more likely to be associated with both a pathologic response and improved survival.[107]

In a prospective study of 53 patients with stage IV NSCLC, Tiseo and colleagues[117] found that all patients with progressive metabolic disease (PMD) on FDG-PET/CT 2 days after epidermal growth factor receptor tyrosine kinase inhibition with erlotinib therapy had confirmed progression at 45 to 60 days as assessed by response evaluation criteria in solid tumors (RECIST), and that patients with early partial metabolic response (PMR) and stable metabolic disease had significantly longer PFS and OS than patients with PMD. Zander and colleagues,[118] in a phase II study of 34 patients with stage IV NSCLC treated with erlotinib, reported that changes in tumor FDG uptake after 1 week of therapy predicted nonprogression after 6 weeks of therapy with 75% accuracy. Patients with an early metabolic response had a significantly longer PFS and OS. Bengtsson and colleagues[119] similarly found that FDG-PET provided information about patient OS in NSCLC patients after 2 weeks of treatment with erlotinib. In a recent meta-analysis of 13 studies including 414 NSCLC patients by Zhang and colleagues,[120] the pooled sensitivity, specificity, PPV, and NPV for FDG-PET to predict response to neoadjuvant treatment were 83% (95% CI 76%–89%), 84% (95% CI 79%–88%), 74% (95% CI 67%–81%), and 91% (95% CI 87%–94%), respectively. The predictive value of FDG-PET to predict pathologic response to neoadjuvant therapy was reported to be superior to that of CT.

However, the lack of reproducibility and standardization of response measures, the variability of response criteria, and the uncertainty with regard to the optimal timing for therapeutic response assessment still need to be addressed before FDG-PET can be used effectively in clinical practice for early response assessment in NSCLC.[107]

RESTAGING OF NSCLC

Many patients with lung cancer who receive curative treatment will have tumor recurrence. Follow-up assessment with FDG-PET is useful for the detection of early disease recurrence (see **Fig. 4**), as it may be difficult to distinguish posttreatment changes from tumor recurrence on CT. In patients with NSCLC, early diagnosis of local recurrence may allow for a curative attempt by surgery or RT.

In a prospective study of 62 patients with suspected recurrent NSCLC after surgical therapy, Hellwig and colleagues[121] reported that FDG-PET has sensitivity, specificity, and accuracy of 93%, 89%, and 92%, respectively, for the detection of recurrent disease. In addition, recurrent tumor SUV_{max} was noted to have significant and independent prognostic value, whereby lower FDG uptake predicted a longer median OS (46 months for SUV_{max} <11 vs 3 months for SUV_{max} ≥11) in patients subsequently treated by surgery. Keidar and colleagues[122] prospectively studied 42 patients with suspected recurrent NSCLC, and found that FDG-PET/CT had sensitivity, specificity, PPV, and NPV of 96%, 82%, 89%, and 93%, respectively for detection of recurrent disease, compared with 96%, 53%, 75%, and 90% for FDG-PET. PET/CT changed the PET lesion classification in 52% of patients by determining the precise localization of sites of increased FDG uptake, and changed management in 29% of patients. In a study of 100 patients with stage I NSCLC undergoing surveillance with FDG-PET/CT and noncontrast chest CT 1 year after lobectomy, Dane and colleagues[123] reported that the sensitivity and specificity of PET/CT for the detection of recurrent disease were 100% and 93%, respectively, compared with 56% and 96%, respectively, for noncontrast CT. In another study of 101 patients with NSCLC who underwent surveillance FDG-PET/CT after potentially curative surgery, Toba and colleagues[124] reported that FDG-PET/CT had sensitivity, specificity, PPV, NPV, and accuracy of 94%, 98%, 90%, 99%, and 97%, respectively for the detection of asymptomatic recurrent disease. In a recent meta-analysis of 13 studies including 1035 patients with lung cancer by He and colleagues,[125] the pooled sensitivity, specificity, and accuracy for FDG-PET/CT to detect recurrent disease were 90% (95% CI 84%–95%), 90% (95% CI 87%–93%), and 95%, respectively. Moreover, FDG-PET/CT and FDG-PET were found to be superior modalities for the detection of recurrent lung cancer, and PET/CT was noted to be superior to PET.

Despite the potential of FDG-PET/CT for the detection of recurrent NSCLC, it is not currently recommended for routine surveillance after curative-intent therapy.[34,126] Further research will be required to determine its cost-effectiveness in this clinical setting.

OTHER SPECIFIC THORACIC MALIGNANCIES
Small Cell Lung Cancer

SCLC accounts for approximately 15% to 20% of lung cancers, and is characterized by neuroendocrine differentiation, early metastatic spread, and high initial sensitivity to chemotherapy and RT.

Although limited-stage SCLC (defined as disease confined to one hemithorax which can be safely covered by a radiation field, and which occurs in approximately one-third of patients) is potentially curable, most patients experience disease relapse and the OS remains poor. The TNM staging system used for NSCLC and the Veterans Administration system of limited-stage versus extensive-stage disease apply to SCLC, and FDG-PET/CT is currently recommended as a standard part of the staging workup of patients with SCLC, particularly in patients with clinically limited-stage disease, although further prospective studies are needed to fully define its role.[33,127–129]

Studies have reported a high diagnostic performance of FDG-PET for the staging of SCLC (Fig. 5), leading to a change in management in a significant proportion of patients that results from either upstaging or downstaging of disease.[129–143] For example, Sohn and colleagues[135] recently reported that FDG-PET/CT detected unexpected distant metastases in 25% of patients with SCLC who were thought to have limited-stage disease, leading to a treatment change in 77% of those patients who were upstaged by PET/CT. In particular, FDG-PET is superior to conventional imaging in both sensitivity and specificity for most metastatic disease sites, although it is inferior to MR imaging for the detection of brain metastases.[129–143]

FDG-PET/CT is also useful in prognosticating clinical outcome before treatment. Pandit and colleagues[144] retrospectively studied 46 SCLC patients, and reported that a high tumor SUV_{max} was significantly associated with a poor OS. In a prospective study of 119 patients with stage I to III SCLC who were treated with concurrent chemoradiation therapy, Reymen and colleagues[145] reported that a high GTV on FDG-PET/CT was associated with a worse OS on multivariate analysis. In another prospective study of 106 patients with SCLC, Oh and colleagues[146] reported that a high total MTV on baseline FDG-PET/CT was an independent predictor for worse PFS and OS on multivariate analysis, and that total MTV was more useful for providing improved prognostic information than that based on disease stage alone. In a retrospective study of 98 patients with SCLC, Zhu and colleagues[147] reported that a high total MTV on pretreatment FDG-PET/CT was significantly associated with a worse PFS and OS, whereas primary tumor SUV_{max} was not correlated with PFS or OS. In addition, patients with limited-stage disease and a larger MTV had a significantly shorter median OS and PFS in comparison with those with a smaller MTV. A similar observation was also noted for those with extensive-stage disease.

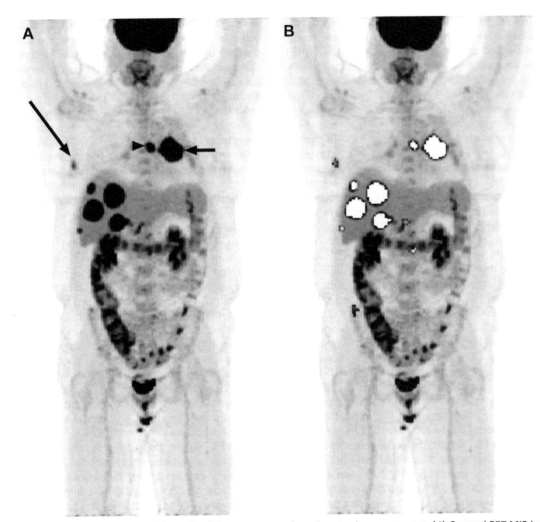

Fig. 5. A 55-year-old woman with small cell lung cancer undergoing staging assessment. (*A*) Coronal PET MIP image from baseline FDG-PET/CT shows FDG-avid (SUV$_{max}$ 21.8) 4.5-cm mass in left upper lobe (*short arrow*) along with FDG-avid subcarinal lymph node metastasis (*arrowhead*), liver metastases, and bone marrow metastases, including site in right scapula (*long arrow*), consistent with stage IV or extensive-stage disease. (*B*) Same coronal PET MIP image with color overlay highlighting segmented sites of malignancy. The total metabolic tumor volume is 133 cm^3, and the mean total lesional glycolysis is 1595 cm^3.

Lastly, FDG-PET may be useful for pretreatment planning for RT and early response assessment. van Loon and colleagues[148] retrospectively studied 21 patients with limited-stage SCLC, and found that FDG-PET changed the RT treatment plan in 24% of patients in comparison with CT. Subsequently, in another prospective study of 60 patients with limited-stage SCLC by van Loon and colleagues,[149] FDG-PET–based selective nodal irradiation resulted in a low rate of isolated nodal failures (3%), in contrast to an unexpectedly high rate of isolated nodal failures (11%) following CT-based selective nodal irradiation. Yamamoto and colleagues[150] prospectively studied 12 SCLC patients before and after 1 cycle

of chemotherapy with FDG-PET, and observed that an early metabolic response was associated with a subsequent response based on RECIST. Onitilo and colleagues[151] retrospectively assessed 22 patients with limited-stage SCLC who underwent FDG-PET within 4 months after chemotherapy. A significantly higher PFS of 10.5 months was reported for PET-negative patients compared with 4.3 months for PET-positive patients, and a higher OS of 29.2 months for PET-negative patients compared with 10.3 months for PET-positive patients.

Despite these promising results, the utility of FDG-PET for early response assessment of SCLC may be less impactful because of the rapidly visible response on CT.[152] Its role in pre-treatment RT planning and restaging also requires further study.

Malignant Pleural Mesothelioma

FDG-PET is useful to distinguish benign from malignant pleural disease, which at times is not possible on CT because of nonspecificity of structural imaging features. Orki and colleagues[153] retrospectively evaluated 83 patients with pleural lesions who underwent pretreatment FDG-PET/CT, and reported that FDG-PET/CT had sensitivity, specificity, and accuracy of 100%, 95%, and 98%, respectively, for differentiating MPM from benign pleural disease. Yildirim and colleagues[154] prospectively evaluated 31 patients with asbestos exposure and pleural disease, and showed that FDG-PET/CT could identify malignant from benign pleural disease with sensitivity and specificity of 94% and 100%, respectively when using a threshold SUV_{max} of greater than 2.2. In a retrospective study of 55 patients with suspected MPM, Mavi and colleagues[155] reported that the RI (from 1 to 2 hours) of tumor on DTP FDG-PET was significantly higher in both newly diagnosed and recurrent MPM in comparison with benign pleural disease.

Accurate staging of disease is critical for the proper selection of patients for aggressive surgical procedures and multimodality therapy. Identification of both nodal disease and distant metastatic disease in patients with MPM is improved through the use of FDG-PET/CT. For example, in a prospective study of 29 patients with MPM, Erasmus and colleagues[156] reported that FDG-PET/CT precluded surgery in 38% of patients by identification of locally advanced tumor and extrathoracic metastatic disease not visualized on conventional imaging. FDG-PET/CT has also been shown to have superior accuracy (94%) relative to mediastinoscopy (75%) for assessment of T4 and N2/N3 disease in a prospective study of 42 patients with MPM by Sorensen and colleagues,[157] preventing noncurative surgery in 29%.

FDG-PET is also useful in prognosticating patient outcome before therapy. In a prospective study of 21 patients with MPM, Kaira and colleagues[158] reported that tumor FDG uptake was significantly correlated with immunohistochemical markers of glucose uptake and phosphorylation, hypoxia, angiogenesis, and cell proliferation, and that high tumor FDG uptake on PET was significantly associated with a worse OS. Flores and colleagues[159] prospectively evaluated 137 patients with MPM, and reported that tumor SUV_{max} greater than 10 on pretreatment FDG-PET was associated with a

1.9-fold greater risk of death on multivariate analysis. Similarly, Abakay and colleagues[160] retrospectively studied 177 patients with MPM, and reported that tumor SUV_{max} greater than 5 was a poor prognostic factor. Nowak and colleagues[161] prospectively evaluated 89 patients with MPM who underwent pretreatment FDG-PET, reporting that sarcomatoid histology was the strongest prognostic factor and that tumor TLG was a better prognosticator of survival than CT-based disease stage on multivariate analysis in patients with nonsarcomatoid MPM. Klabatsa and colleagues[162] retrospectively analyzed 60 patients with MPM, and reported that a high TLG on pretreatment FDG-PET/CT was associated with decreased OS at borderline statistical significance. Lee and colleagues[163] retrospectively evaluated 13 patients with MPM who underwent pretreatment FDG-PET/CT, and reported that total MTV and TLG were independent factors associated with tumor progression on multivariate analysis. Moreover, time to progression was significantly shorter in patients with a high total MTV or TLG than in those with a low total MTV or TLG.

FDG-PET also plays a role in response assessment of patients with MPM (**Fig. 6**). Tsutani and colleagues[164] prospectively studied 50 patients with resectable MPM who underwent FDG-PET/CT before and after neoadjuvant platinum-based chemotherapy followed by extrapleural pneumonectomy without or with RT, and reported that a metabolic response to neoadjuvant therapy (defined as a decrease in tumor SUV_{max} of $\geq$30%) was an independent factor for improved OS, and was more useful than response by modified RECIST to predict patient outcome. As such, FDG-PET/CT may be useful for the selection of patients most likely to benefit from extrapleural pneumonectomy after neoadjuvant chemotherapy. Francis and colleagues[165] prospectively evaluated 23 patients with MPM who underwent CT and FDG-PET before and after 1 cycle of chemotherapy, and reported a significant correlation between a decrease in tumor TLG and improved survival. Neither a reduction in tumor SUV_{max} nor CT demonstrated a statistically significant association with patient survival. Veit-Haibach and colleagues[166] prospectively studied 41 patients with MPM who underwent CT and FDG-PET/CT before and after 3 cycles of chemotherapy. Baseline CT parameters, baseline PET/CT parameters, and change in tumor SUV following therapy were reported not to be significantly associated with patient survival, whereas decreases in tumor MTV and TLG on PET/CT in addition to CT-based response were significantly associated with OS.

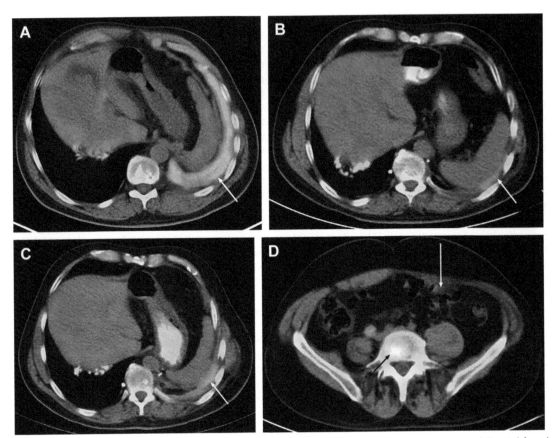

Fig. 6. A 51-year-old man with malignant pleural mesothelioma undergoing staging assessment. (*A*) Axial fused baseline FDG-PET/CT image shows avid FDG uptake (SUV$_{max}$ 13) in markedly thickened left pleura (*arrow*) resulting from locally advanced stage III malignant pleural mesothelioma. No regional lymphadenopathy or distant metastatic disease was seen. (*B*) Axial fused FDG-PET/CT image after radical pleurectomy, intraoperative photodynamic therapy, and adjuvant chemoradiation therapy shows interval decrease in thickness and FDG uptake (SUV$_{max}$ 3.7) of left pleura (*arrow*), indicating partial metabolic response. (*C*) Axial fused FDG-PET/CT image obtained 5 months later for restaging reveals interval increase in thickness and FDG uptake (SUV$_{max}$ 6.5) of left pleura (*arrow*). (*D*) Axial fused FDG-PET/CT image through pelvis from same study shows new FDG-avid bone marrow metastasis in L5 vertebra (*short black arrow*) along with new FDG-avid peritoneal spread of tumor (*long white arrow*). These findings on restaging examination indicate progressive metabolic disease.

Lastly, FDG-PET is accurate for detecting recurrent disease and estimating the extent of locoregional and distant metastatic disease (see **Fig. 6**). Gerbaudo and colleagues[167] prospectively evaluated 50 patients with MPM who underwent FDG-PET/CT for restaging on average 11 months after surgical therapy, and reported sensitivity, specificity, PPV, NPV, and accuracy for restaging FDG-PET/CT of 98%, 75%, 95%, 86%, and 94%, respectively. In addition, PET/CT helped in the selection of 29% of patients who benefited from additional previously unplanned treatment at the time of failure. Survival after relapse was independently predicted by the pattern of FDG uptake and PET nodal status on multivariate analysis, whereas OS was only predicted by tumor SUV$_{max}$ measured from pretreatment FDG-PET/CT. Bille and colleagues[168] retrospectively assessed 32 patients with MPM

who were treated with multimodality therapy and who underwent posttreatment FDG-PET/CT imaging every 6 months after treatment, and reported a statistically significant correlation between the SUV$_{max}$ and TLG of recurrent MPM with OS.

At present, current guidelines suggest the use of FDG-PET/CT for the staging of patients with MPM who are being considered for surgery, preferably before talc pleurodesis, which can induce increased FDG uptake caused by inflammation, and for RT planning.[169,170] The use of FDG-PET for other clinical applications in patients with MPM requires further investigation.

Esophageal Cancer

FDG-PET is useful in improving the staging of esophageal cancer (**Fig. 7**). In a meta-analysis of

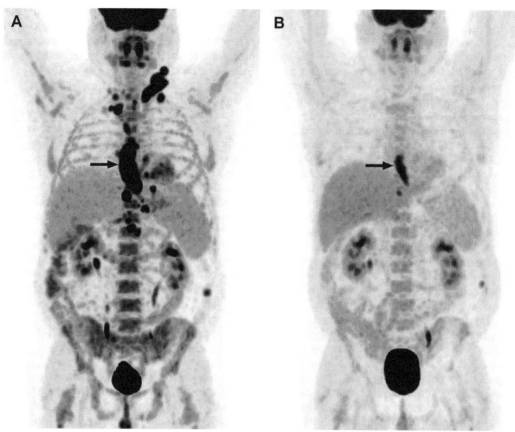

Fig. 7. A 52-year-old man with esophageal adenocarcinoma undergoing staging assessment. (*A*) Coronal PET MIP image from baseline FDG-PET/CT shows FDG-avid (SUV_{max} 45.1) tumor in mid and distal esophagus (*arrow*) along with extensive FDG-avid supraclavicular, mediastinal, and upper retroperitoneal lymphadenopathy. (*B*) Coronal PET MIP image from FDG-PET/CT after chemotherapy shows interval improvement in FDG uptake (SUV_{max} 9.8) of esophageal mass (*arrow*) and near complete resolution of regional lymphadenopathy, consistent with partial metabolic response.

7 studies of patients with esophageal cancer, Shi and colleagues[171] reported a nodal station level pooled sensitivity, specificity, and accuracy of 62% (95% CI 40%–79%), 96% (95% CI 93%–98%), and 95% (95% CI 92%–96%), respectively, and a patient-level pooled sensitivity, specificity, and accuracy of 55% (95% CI 34%–74%), 76% (95% CI 66%–83%), and 75% (95% CI 71%–79%), respectively, for pretreatment FDG-PET/CT. Yamada and colleagues[172] retrospectively evaluated 258 patients with esophageal squamous cell carcinoma who underwent pretreatment FDG-PET/CT followed by esophagectomy and radical lymphadenectomy, to investigate the diagnostic accuracy of FDG-PET/CT for lymph node staging of esophageal cancer. The sensitivity, specificity, PPV, NPV, and accuracy of FDG-PET/CT were 26%, 98%, 82%, 77%, and 82%, respectively, where 39% of the metastatic nodes were less than 8 mm in size and difficult to detect

by FDG-PET/CT. Kato and colleagues[173] prospectively studied 167 patients with esophageal squamous cell carcinoma who underwent pretreatment FDG-PET/CT, and reported that for individual nodal group evaluation, PET/CT compared with PET alone had a significantly higher sensitivity (46% vs 33%) and accuracy (95% vs 93%), with comparable specificities of 99%. Similarly, Yuan and colleagues[174] reported that FDG-PET/CT significantly improved the sensitivity, NPV, and accuracy of locoregional lymph node assessment in patients with esophageal squamous cell carcinoma.

The DTP technique may improve the diagnostic performance of FDG-PET for the staging of esophageal cancer. For example, Hu and colleagues[175] prospectively studied 34 patients with esophageal squamous cell carcinoma, and reported sensitivity, specificity, PPV, NPV, and accuracy of 89%, 92%, 73%, 97%, and 91%, respectively, for DTP FDG-PET in detecting regional lymph node metastases, compared with 76%, 85%, 56%, 93%, and 83% for STP FDG-PET.

Studies have shown that the use of FDG-PET for staging significantly affects management in patients with esophageal cancer. Barber and colleagues[176] prospectively assessed 139 patients with esophageal cancer, and reported that pretreatment FDG-PET/CT changed the stage group in 40% of patients and changed management in 34%. Similarly, Gillies and colleagues[177] retrospectively evaluated 200 patients with esophageal cancer, and reported that pretreatment FDG-PET/CT changed management in 17% of patients. In a multicenter study, Chatterton and colleagues[178] prospectively evaluated 129 patients with esophageal cancer without definite distant metastatic disease. Pretreatment FDG-PET detected additional sites of disease in 41% of patients, leading to significant management changes in 38%, primarily as a result of identification of additional sites of disease or confirming previously equivocal sites of regional and distant metastases. PFS was significantly shorter in patients who were found to have additional lesions on FDG-PET. Blencowe and colleagues[179] retrospectively studied 238 patients with esophageal or esophagogastric cancer without evidence of distant metastatic disease on CT, and reported that staging FDG-PET/CT changed management in 38% by either detecting unsuspected distant metastases or confirming a lack of distant metastases, leading to improved patient selection for radical treatment.

FDG-PET is also useful for prognostication of clinical outcome in patients with esophageal cancer. Yasuda and colleagues[180] retrospectively assessed 76 patients with esophageal squamous cell carcinoma who underwent pretreatment FDG-PET followed by curative resection. PET-positive lymph nodes involved a significantly larger size of metastatic nests than PET-negative lymph nodes. Furthermore, patients with PET-negative lymph nodes had a significantly higher frequency of having 2 or fewer lymph node metastases (92% vs 15%), a higher 5-year RFS (75% vs 30%), a higher 5-year OS (70% vs 30%), and a lower postoperative recurrence rate (24% vs 69%), where PET nodal status was the most significant pretreatment risk factor for postoperative recurrence on multivariate analysis. Gillies and colleagues[181] prospectively assessed 121 patients with esophageal adenocarcinoma who underwent pretreatment FDG-PET/CT before neoadjuvant chemotherapy and surgical resection, and reported that the presence of FDG-avid regional lymph nodes was significantly associated with a worse DFS and OS. Sun and colleagues[182] retrospectively evaluated 72 patients with early esophageal adenocarcinoma who underwent pretreatment FDG-PET/CT before endoscopic mucosal resection, and reported that a high SUV_{max} ratio (SUV_{max} primary tumor/SUV_{max} liver) of 1.5 or greater was associated with tumor invasion depth and decreased OS.

Global measures of disease burden on FDG-PET are also useful biomarkers of clinical outcome. Chen and colleagues[183] retrospectively assessed 90 patients with locally advanced squamous cell carcinoma of the esophagus, and reported that MTV greater than 40 cm^3 on pretreatment FDG-PET/CT was significantly associated with decreased 1-year OS and decreased 1-year DFS. Similarly, I and colleagues[184] retrospectively evaluated 54 patients with esophageal squamous cell carcinoma, and reported that high primary tumor MTV on pretreatment FDG-PET/CT was significantly associated with the presence of regional lymph node metastatic disease on multivariate analysis. Hyun and colleagues[185] retrospectively assessed 151 patients with esophageal cancer (mostly squamous cell subtype) who underwent pretreatment FDG-PET, and reported that a high primary tumor MTV was significantly associated with decreased OS on multivariate analysis, whereas tumor SUV_{max} was not. Shum and colleagues[186] retrospectively studied 26 patients with esophageal squamous cell carcinoma, and reported that high primary tumor MTV on pretreatment FDG-PET/CT was significantly associated with decreased 1-year OS. Hatt and colleagues[187] retrospectively assessed 45 patients with esophageal cancer who underwent pretreatment FDG-PET/CT, and reported that high primary tumor MTV and functional tumor length were significantly associated with decreased OS on multivariate analysis.

FDG-PET has been shown to be useful for response assessment of esophageal cancer in many studies (see **Fig. 7**), some of which are presented here. In a prospective study of 62 patients with esophageal cancer who underwent FDG-PET before and after neoadjuvant chemoradiation therapy followed by surgical resection, Kim and colleagues[188] reported that compared with endoscopic biopsy and CT, CMR by FDG-PET showed the highest correlation with histopathologic complete response (with 71% concordance) and was significantly associated with improved DFS and OS. False-positive results for residual tumor on FDG-PET were related to radiation esophagitis and reactive mediastinal lymphadenopathy, whereas false-negative results were related to the presence of small residual disease. Miyata and colleagues[189] prospectively evaluated 211 patients with esophageal squamous cell carcinoma who underwent FDG-PET/CT before and after neoadjuvant chemotherapy followed by surgery. Multivariate analysis identified posttreatment tumor SUV_{max} as an independent prognostic factor of OS, with 5-year OS of 62.2% versus 35.1% for patients with posttreatment SUV_{max} of less than 3.5 versus 3.5 or greater, respectively. Furthermore, Miyata and colleagues[190] also reported from this same study group that patients with posttreatment PET-positive lymph nodes on FDG-PET/CT had a shorter OS than those without PET-positive nodes (5-year OS 25.0% vs 62.6%), and that posttreatment nodal status on FDG-PET/CT is an independent prognostic factor of clinical outcome.

In a prospective study (the Metabolic response evalUatioN for Individualization of neoadjuvant Chemotherapy in esOphageal and esophagogastric adeNocarcinoma [MUNICON] trial) of 110 evaluable patients with locally advanced adenocarcinoma of the gastroesophageal junction or gastric cardia who underwent FDG-PET before and after 2 weeks of neoadjuvant chemotherapy followed by surgical resection, Lordick and colleagues[191] reported that metabolic responders had a significantly improved median event-free survival and median OS compared with metabolic nonresponders. Furthermore, metabolic response ($\geq$35% decrease in primary tumor SUV_{max}) was associated with complete or subtotal histologic response in 58% of patients. In a meta-analysis of 10 studies of patients with localized esophageal junctional cancer (predominantly adenocarcinoma) receiving neoadjuvant chemotherapy/chemoradiation, Zhu and colleagues[192] reported that an early metabolic response (ie, $\geq$35% decrease in primary tumor SUV_{max}) based on FDG-PET obtained before and 2 weeks after initiation of neoadjuvant therapy was associated with a significantly better OS and DFS. Cuenca and colleagues[193] prospectively evaluated 59 patients with locally advanced esophageal cancer who underwent FDG-PET/CT before and after 2 cycles of chemoradiation therapy, and reported that only a PET-based metabolic response was significantly associated with an improved 2-year OS on multivariate analysis. In a prospective study of 51 patients with esophageal adenocarcinoma who underwent FDG-PET/CT before and after neoadjuvant chemotherapy, Roedl and colleagues[194] reported that the decrease in MTV was a better predictor of histopathologic response, DFS, and OS than a decrease of tumor SUV or CT response based on RECIST or World Health Organization (WHO) criteria. In addition, they observed that the highest accuracy was achieved through use of tumor TLG to identify treatment responders, whereby a decrease of TLG of 78% or more predicted histopathologic response with sensitivity, specificity, and accuracy of 91%, 93%, and 92%, respectively.

Lastly, FDG-PET may play a role in the restaging of patients with esophageal cancer. In a prospective study of 56 patients with previously treated esophageal squamous cell carcinoma and suspected recurrence, Guo and colleagues[195] reported that FDG-PET/CT had sensitivity, specificity, and accuracy of 93%, 76%, and 87%, respectively, for the detection of recurrent disease. In multivariate analysis, high tumor SUV and the presence of systemic disease on PET/CT were significantly associated with a decreased OS. In another prospective study of 20 patients with locoregionally recurrent esophageal cancer following surgery who underwent FDG-PET before and less than 1 week after chemoradiation therapy, Jingu and colleagues[196] reported that cause-specific survival and local control rates were significantly better for patients with SUV_{max} 2.4 or less after chemotherapy, and that a decrease in FDG uptake greater than 68.5% was significantly correlated with an improved local control rate.

Current guidelines suggest the use of FDG-PET/CT for staging evaluation if there is no prior evidence of distant metastatic disease, and for response assessment 5 to 6 weeks or more following preoperative chemoradiation therapy or definitive chemoradiation therapy.[197] However, the guidelines emphasize that FDG-PET should not be used to select patients for surgery following preoperative chemoradiation, as RT-induced ulceration may be associated with FDG-avid false-positive results, precluding accurate detection of residual esophageal tumor. Nevertheless, FDG-PET/CT in combination with endoscopy is useful for identifying patients with a high risk of residual tumor following preoperative chemoradiation therapy.[198] The use of FDG-PET for other clinical applications in patients with esophageal cancer requires further investigation.

Thymic Epithelial Tumors

Thymic epithelial tumors are rare, and range from relatively benign thymomas to highly aggressive thymic carcinomas. The Masaoka-Koga stage classification is most commonly used for staging thymic epithelial tumors, with the TNM staging system less commonly used.[199,200] The WHO histologic classification system may be used to distinguish between low-risk thymomas (types A, AB, and B1), high-risk thymomas (types B2 and

B3), and thymic carcinomas including neuroendocrine epithelial tumors (type C), and generally has independent prognostic value in addition to tumor staging.[201,202]

FDG-PET/CT is useful for staging of thymic epithelial tumors, differentiating thymic carcinoma from thymoma, and distinguishing thymic tumors from thymic hyperplasia (**Fig. 8**). El-Bawab and colleagues[203] prospectively studied 25 patients with thymic abnormality, and reported that FDG-PET was useful in differentiating thymic hyperplasia and thymoma in patients with myasthenia gravis. Kaira and colleagues[204] prospectively assessed 49 patients with thymic epithelial tumors who underwent pretreatment FDG-PET, and reported that FDG uptake with significantly correlated with tumor GLUT-1, HIF-1α, VEGF, and p53, which were significantly associated with tumor grade and poor clinical outcome. Sung and colleagues[205] retrospectively assessed 33 patients with thymic epithelial tumors who underwent pretreatment FDG-PET/CT, and reported that the SUV_{max} of thymomas was significantly lower than that of thymic carcinomas. Moreover, FDG-PET/CT improved the detection of lymph node and pleural metastatic disease in comparison with CT alone. Other studies have similarly found that the degree of FDG uptake in thymomas is typically lower than that of thymic carcinomas, although there is generally overlap in the degree of FDG uptake within low-risk and high-risk thymomas, limiting the ability of FDG-PET to differentiate them.[206–209]

Inoue and colleagues[210] retrospectively evaluated 46 patients with thymic epithelial tumors who underwent pretreatment DTP FDG-PET (from 1 to 3 hours), and reported that a high early time-point SUV_{max} suggests the presence of high-risk thymoma or thymic carcinoma, and that a very high early time-point SUV_{max} is useful to differentiate thymic carcinomas from other thymic tumors. However, delayed time-point SUV_{max} was higher than early time-point SUV_{max} for all types of thymic epithelial tumors, and tumor RI was not useful for differentiating tumor subtypes.

FDG-PET may also be useful for response assessment and restaging. Thomas and colleagues[211] prospectively evaluated 56 patients with unresectable Masaoka stage III to IV thymic epithelial tumors with FDG-PET/CT before and after 6 weeks of treatment. A close correlation between early metabolic response and subsequent best response by RECIST was reported, with sensitivity and specificity for prediction of best response of 95% and 100%, respectively. In addition, metabolic responders had significantly longer

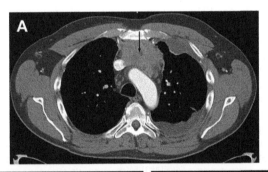

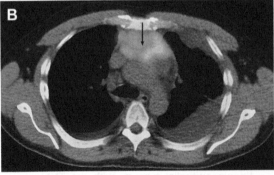
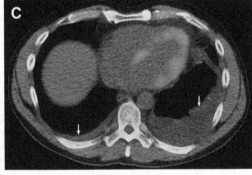

Fig. 8. A 54-year-old man with thymic carcinoma undergoing staging assessment. (*A*) Axial CT image shows 8.5-cm heterogeneously enhancing infiltrative soft-tissue mass (*arrow*) in anterior mediastinum obliterating left brachiocephalic vein, along with loculated left pleural effusion. (*B, C*) Axial fused baseline FDG-PET/CT images show avid FDG uptake (SUV_{max} 8.6) in mass (*arrow*) along with mild FDG uptake in pleural effusions (*short white arrows*), consistent with stage IV disease.

PFS (median 11.5 vs 4.6 months) and a trend toward longer OS (median 31.8 vs 18.4 months) than nonresponders. FDG uptake was again noted to be significantly higher in thymic carcinoma than in thymoma, although no significant difference in SUV_{max} was observed between low-risk and high-risk thymomas. Kaira and colleagues[212] prospectively studied 12 patients with unresectable thymic epithelial tumors who underwent FDG-PET before and after chemotherapy or RT. In the 6 patients with any response, the tumor to mediastinal (T/M) ratio after therapy was significantly lower than at baseline, and in the other 6 patients with SD no significant change in the T/M ratio was noted after therapy. Furthermore, a statistically significant difference in OS was observed in a subset of patients with PMR, compared with those with non-PMR. El-Bawab and colleagues[213] retrospectively assessed 37 thymoma patients who were treated with surgical excision, and reported that follow-up FDG-PET/CT was superior to CT for detection and localization of mediastinal recurrence. Moreover, FDG-PET/CT had sensitivity and specificity of 82% and 95%, respectively, compared with 71% and 85% for CT for recurrent thymoma.

Current guidelines suggest that FDG-PET/CT may be useful to stage disease, but do not presently recommend its use for other clinical applications in patients with thymic epithelial tumors.[214] More prospective research will be necessary to determine the role of FDG-PET for these additional applications.

SUMMARY

FDG-PET is a robust quantitative molecular imaging technique that complements structural imaging techniques for the evaluation of patients with thoracic malignancy. This article highlights many of the applications of FDG-PET in the thoracic oncologic setting. It is important for clinicians and scientists to be aware of these applications so as to optimize patient management and outcome, and to pursue additional prospective study of those applications involving the use of FDG-PET for which the current evidence base is limited.

REFERENCES

1. Hansell DM, Bankier AA, MacMahon H, et al. Fleischner Society: glossary of terms for thoracic imaging. Radiology 2008;246(3):697–722.
2. Kanne JP, Jensen LE, Mohammed TL, et al. ACR Appropriateness Criteria(R) radiographically detected solitary pulmonary nodule. J Thorac Imaging 2013;28(1):W1–3.
3. Gould MK, Maclean CC, Kuschner WG, et al. Accuracy of positron emission tomography for diagnosis of pulmonary nodules and mass lesions: a meta-analysis. JAMA 2001;285(7):914–24.
4. Cronin P, Dwamena BA, Kelly AM, et al. Solitary pulmonary nodules: meta-analytic comparison of cross-sectional imaging modalities for diagnosis of malignancy. Radiology 2008;246(3):772–82.
5. Fletcher JW, Kymes SM, Gould M, et al. A comparison of the diagnostic accuracy of ^{18}F-FDG PET and CT in the characterization of solitary pulmonary nodules. J Nucl Med 2008;49(2):179–85.
6. Kubota K, Murakami K, Inoue T, et al. Additional effects of FDG-PET to thin-section CT for the differential diagnosis of lung nodules: a Japanese multicenter clinical study. Ann Nucl Med 2011;25(10):787–95.
7. Jeong SY, Lee KS, Shin KM, et al. Efficacy of PET/CT in the characterization of solid or partly solid solitary pulmonary nodules. Lung Cancer 2008;61(2):186–94.
8. Yi CA, Lee KS, Kim BT, et al. Tissue characterization of solitary pulmonary nodule: comparative study between helical dynamic CT and integrated PET/CT. J Nucl Med 2006;47(3):443–50.
9. Bar-Shalom R, Kagna O, Israel O, et al. Noninvasive diagnosis of solitary pulmonary lesions in cancer patients based on 2-fluoro-2-deoxy-D-glucose avidity on positron emission tomography/computed tomography. Cancer 2008;113(11):3213–21.
10. Kagna O, Solomonov A, Keidar Z, et al. The value of FDG-PET/CT in assessing single pulmonary nodules in patients at high risk of lung cancer. Eur J Nucl Med Mol Imaging 2009;36(6):997–1004.
11. Kim SK, Allen-Auerbach M, Goldin J, et al. Accuracy of PET/CT in characterization of solitary pulmonary lesions. J Nucl Med 2007;48(2):214–20.
12. Nomori H, Watanabe K, Ohtsuka T, et al. Evaluation of F-18 fluorodeoxyglucose (FDG) PET scanning for pulmonary nodules less than 3 cm in diameter, with special reference to the CT images. Lung Cancer 2004;45(1):19–27.
13. Chun EJ, Lee HJ, Kang WJ, et al. Differentiation between malignancy and inflammation in pulmonary ground-glass nodules: the feasibility of integrated (18)F-FDG PET/CT. Lung Cancer 2009;65(2):180–6.
14. Heyneman LE, Patz EF. PET imaging in patients with bronchioloalveolar cell carcinoma. Lung Cancer 2002;38(3):261–6.
15. Yap CS, Schiepers C, Fishbein MC, et al. FDG-PET imaging in lung cancer: how sensitive is it for bronchioloalveolar carcinoma? Eur J Nucl Med Mol Imaging 2002;29(9):1166–73.
16. Lee HY, Lee KS, Han J, et al. Mucinous versus nonmucinous solitary pulmonary nodular bronchioloalveolar carcinoma: CT and FDG PET

findings and pathologic comparisons. Lung Cancer 2009;65(2):170–5.

17. Shim SS, Han J. FDG-PET/CT imaging in assessing mucin-producing non-small cell lung cancer with pathologic correlation. Ann Nucl Med 2010;24(5):357–62.

18. Sawada E, Nambu A, Motosugi U, et al. Localized mucinous bronchioloalveolar carcinoma of the lung: thin-section computed tomography and fluorodeoxyglucose positron emission tomography findings: Jpn J Radiol 2010;28(4):251–8.

19. Chong S, Lee KS, Kim BT, et al. Integrated PET/CT of pulmonary neuroendocrine tumors: diagnostic and prognostic implications. AJR Am J Roentgenol 2007;188(5):1223–31.

20. Daniels CE, Lowe VJ, Aubry MC, et al. The utility of fluorodeoxyglucose positron emission tomography in the evaluation of carcinoid tumors presenting as pulmonary nodules. Chest 2007;131(1):255–60.

21. Raz DJ, Odisho AY, Franc BL, et al. Tumor fluoro-2-deoxy-D-glucose avidity on positron emission tomographic scan predicts mortality in patients with early-stage pure and mixed bronchioloalveolar carcinoma. J Thorac Cardiovasc Surg 2006;132(5):1189–95.

22. Okada M, Tauchi S, Iwanaga K, et al. Associations among bronchioloalveolar carcinoma components, positron emission tomographic and computed tomographic findings, and malignant behavior in small lung adenocarcinomas. J Thorac Cardiovasc Surg 2007;133(6):1448–54.

23. Lee HY, Han J, Lee KS, et al. Lung adenocarcinoma as a solitary pulmonary nodule: prognostic determinants of CT, PET, and histopathologic findings. Lung Cancer 2009;66(3):379–85.

24. Watanabe K, Nomori H, Ohtsuka T, et al. [F-18]Fluorodeoxyglucose positron emission tomography can predict pathological tumor stage and proliferative activity determined by Ki-67 in clinical stage IA lung adenocarcinomas. Jpn J Clin Oncol 2006;36(7):403–9.

25. Maeda R, Isowa N, Onuma H, et al. The maximum standardized uptake values on positron emission tomography to predict the Noguchi classification and invasiveness in clinical stage IA adenocarcinoma measuring 2 cm or less in size. Interact Cardiovasc Thorac Surg 2009;9(1):70–3.

26. Sathekge MM, Maes A, Pottel H, et al. Dual time-point FDG PET-CT for differentiating benign from malignant solitary pulmonary nodules in a TB endemic area. S Afr Med J 2010;100(9):598–601.

27. Kwee TC, Torigian DA, Alavi A. Nononcological applications of positron emission tomography for evaluation of the thorax. J Thorac Imaging 2013;28(1):25–39.

28. Gould MK, Sanders GD, Barnett PG, et al. Cost-effectiveness of alternative management strategies for patients with solitary pulmonary nodules. Ann Intern Med 2003;138(9):724–35.

29. Gould MK, Donington J, Lynch WR, et al. Evaluation of individuals with pulmonary nodules: when is it lung cancer? Diagnosis and management of lung cancer, 3rd ed: American College of Chest Physicians evidence-based clinical practice guidelines. Chest 2013;143(Suppl 5):e93S–120S.

30. MacMahon H, Austin JH, Gamsu G, et al. Guidelines for management of small pulmonary nodules detected on CT scans: a statement from the Fleischner Society. Radiology 2005;237(2):395–400.

31. Naidich DP, Bankier AA, MacMahon H, et al. Recommendations for the management of subsolid pulmonary nodules detected at CT: a statement from the Fleischner Society. Radiology 2013;266(1):304–17.

32. Fletcher JW, Djulbegovic B, Soares HP, et al. Recommendations on the use of ^{18}F-FDG PET in oncology. J Nucl Med 2008;49(3):480–508.

33. Ravenel JG, Mohammed TL, Movsas B, et al. ACR Appropriateness Criteria(R) noninvasive clinical staging of bronchogenic carcinoma. J Thorac Imaging 2010;25(4):W107–11.

34. Ettinger DS, Akerley W, Borghaei H, et al. Non-small cell lung cancer, version 2.2013. J Natl Compr Canc Netw 2013;11(6):645–53 [quiz: 53].

35. Silvestri GA, Gonzalez AV, Jantz MA, et al. Methods for staging non-small cell lung cancer: diagnosis and management of lung cancer, 3rd ed: American College of Chest Physicians evidence-based clinical practice guidelines. Chest 2013;143(Suppl 5):e211S–50S.

36. The diagnosis and treatment of lung cancer (update). NICE clinical guideline. 121,2011;1–173. Available at: www.nice.org.uk/guidance/cg121.

37. Langer A. A systematic review of PET and PET/CT in oncology: a way to personalize cancer treatment in a cost-effective manner? BMC Health Serv Res 2010;10:283.

38. Gould MK, Kuschner WG, Rydzak CE, et al. Test performance of positron emission tomography and computed tomography for mediastinal staging in patients with non-small-cell lung cancer: a meta-analysis. Ann Intern Med 2003;139(11):879–92.

39. Wu Y, Li P, Zhang H, et al. Diagnostic value of fluorine 18 fluorodeoxyglucose positron emission tomography/computed tomography for the detection of metastases in non-small-cell lung cancer patients. Int J Cancer 2013;132(2):E37–47.

40. Lv YL, Yuan DM, Wang K, et al. Diagnostic performance of integrated positron emission tomography/computed tomography for mediastinal lymph node staging in non-small cell lung cancer: a bivariate systematic review and meta-analysis. J Thorac Oncol 2011;6(8):1350–8.

41. Toloza EM, Harpole L, McCrory DC. Noninvasive staging of non-small cell lung cancer: a review of

the current evidence. Chest 2003;123(Suppl 1): 137S–46S.

42. Kubota K, Murakami K, Inoue T, et al. Additional value of FDG-PET to contrast enhanced-computed tomography (CT) for the diagnosis of mediastinal lymph node metastasis in non-small cell lung cancer: a Japanese multicenter clinical study. Ann Nucl Med 2011;25(10):777–86.

43. Ose N, Sawabata N, Minami M, et al. Lymph node metastasis diagnosis using positron emission tomography with 2-[^{18}F] fluoro-2-deoxy-D-glucose as a tracer and computed tomography in surgical cases of non-small cell lung cancer. Eur J Cardiothorac Surg 2012;42(1):89–92.

44. Lee PC, Port JL, Korst RJ, et al. Risk factors for occult mediastinal metastases in clinical stage I non-small cell lung cancer. Ann Thorac Surg 2007;84(1):177–81.

45. Li L, Ren S, Zhang Y, et al. Risk factors for predicting the occult nodal metastasis in T1-2N0M0 NSCLC patients staged by PET/CT: potential value in the clinic. Lung Cancer 2013;81(2):213–7.

46. Trister AD, Pryma DA, Xanthopoulos E, et al. Prognostic value of primary tumor FDG uptake for occult mediastinal lymph node involvement in clinically N2/N3 Node-negative non-small cell lung cancer. Am J Clin Oncol 2012. [Epub ahead of print].

47. Li Y, Su M, Li F, et al. The value of (1)(8)F-FDG-PET/CT in the differential diagnosis of solitary pulmonary nodules in areas with a high incidence of tuberculosis. Ann Nucl Med 2011;25(10):804–11.

48. de Langen AJ, Raijmakers P, Riphagen I, et al. The size of mediastinal lymph nodes and its relation with metastatic involvement: a meta-analysis. Eur J Cardiothorac Surg 2006;29(1):26–9.

49. Pieterman RM, van Putten JW, Meuzelaar JJ, et al. Preoperative staging of non-small-cell lung cancer with positron-emission tomography. N Engl J Med 2000;343(4):254–61.

50. Hillner BE, Siegel BA, Shields AF, et al. Relationship between cancer type and impact of PET and PET/CT on intended management: findings of the national oncologic PET registry. J Nucl Med 2008; 49(12):1928–35.

51. Zeliadt SB, Loggers ET, Slatore CG, et al. Preoperative PET and the reduction of unnecessary surgery among newly diagnosed lung cancer patients in a community setting. J Nucl Med 2014;55(3):379–85.

52. Takeuchi S, Khiewvan B, Fox PS, et al. Impact of initial PET/CT staging in terms of clinical stage, management plan, and prognosis in 592 patients with non-small-cell lung cancer. Eur J Nucl Med Mol Imaging 2014;41(5):906–14.

53. Li J, Xu W, Kong F, et al. Meta-analysis: accuracy of ^{18}FDG PET-CT for distant metastasis staging in lung cancer patients. Surg Oncol 2013;22(3): 151–5.

54. Lu Y, Xie D, Huang W, et al. ^{18}F-FDG PET/CT in the evaluation of adrenal masses in lung cancer patients. Neoplasma 2010;57(2):129–34.

55. Kumar R, Xiu Y, Yu JQ, et al. ^{18}F-FDG PET in evaluation of adrenal lesions in patients with lung cancer. J Nucl Med 2004;45(12):2058–62.

56. Liu T, Xu JY, Xu W, et al. Fluorine-18 deoxyglucose positron emission tomography, magnetic resonance imaging and bone scintigraphy for the diagnosis of bone metastases in patients with lung cancer: which one is the best?–a meta-analysis. Clin Oncol (R Coll Radiol) 2011;23(5):350–8.

57. Qu X, Huang X, Yan W, et al. A meta-analysis of (1)(8)FDG-PET-CT, (1)(8)FDG-PET, MRI and bone scintigraphy for diagnosis of bone metastases in patients with lung cancer. Eur J Radiol 2012; 81(5):1007–15.

58. Kruger S, Mottaghy FM, Buck AK, et al. Brain metastasis in lung cancer. Comparison of cerebral MRI and ^{18}F-FDG-PET/CT for diagnosis in the initial staging. Nuklearmedizin 2011;50(3):101–6.

59. Lee HY, Lee KS, Kim BT, et al. Diagnostic efficacy of PET/CT plus brain MR imaging for detection of extrathoracic metastases in patients with lung adenocarcinoma. J Korean Med Sci 2009;24(6): 1132–8.

60. Torigian DA, Zaidi H, Kwee TC, et al. PET/MR imaging: technical aspects and potential clinical applications. Radiology 2013;267(1):26–44.

61. Heusch P, Buchbender C, Kohler J, et al. Thoracic staging in lung cancer: prospective comparison of ^{18}F-FDG PET/MRI and ^{18}F-FDG PET/CT. J Nucl Med 2014;55(3):373–8.

62. Usuda K, Sagawa M, Motono N, et al. Advantages of diffusion-weighted imaging over positron emission tomography-computed tomography in assessment of hilar and mediastinal lymph node in lung cancer. Ann Surg Oncol 2013;20(5):1676–83.

63. Kim YN, Yi CA, Lee KS, et al. A proposal for combined MRI and PET/CT interpretation criteria for preoperative nodal staging in non-small-cell lung cancer. Eur Radiol 2012;22(7):1537–46.

64. Kohan AA, Kolthammer JA, Vercher-Conejero JL, et al. N staging of lung cancer patients with PET/MRI using a three-segment model attenuation correction algorithm: initial experience. Eur Radiol 2013;23(11):3161–9.

65. Yildirim D, Tamam M, Sanli Y, et al. Virtual bronchoscopy using FDG-PET/CT images for the evaluation of lung cancer. Eur Rev Med Pharmacol Sci 2012;16(14):1951–60.

66. Paesmans M, Berghmans T, Dusart M, et al. Primary tumor standardized uptake value measured on fluorodeoxyglucose positron emission tomography is of prognostic value for survival in non-small

cell lung cancer: update of a systematic review and meta-analysis by the European Lung Cancer Working Party for the International Association for the Study of Lung Cancer Staging Project. J Thorac Oncol 2010;5(5):612–9.

67. Uehara H, Tsutani Y, Okumura S, et al. Prognostic role of positron emission tomography and high-resolution computed tomography in clinical stage IA lung adenocarcinoma. Ann Thorac Surg 2013; 96(6):1958–65.

68. Kadota K, Colovos C, Suzuki K, et al. FDG-PET SUVmax combined with IASLC/ATS/ERS histologic classification improves the prognostic stratification of patients with stage I lung adenocarcinoma. Ann Surg Oncol 2012;19(11):3598–605.

69. Ulger S, Demirci NY, Eroglu FN, et al. High FDG uptake predicts poorer survival in locally advanced nonsmall cell lung cancer patients undergoing curative radiotherapy, independently of tumor size. J Cancer Res Clin Oncol 2014;140(3):495–502.

70. Muto J, Hida Y, Kaga K, et al. Use of maximum standardized uptake value on fluorodeoxyglucose positron-emission tomography in predicting lymph node involvement in patients with primary non-small cell lung cancer. Anticancer Res 2014; 34(2):805–10.

71. Ishibashi T, Kaji M, Kato T, et al. ^{18}F-FDG uptake in primary lung cancer as a predictor of intratumoral vessel invasion. Ann Nucl Med 2011;25(8):547–53.

72. Chung HW, Lee KY, Kim HJ, et al. FDG PET/CT metabolic tumor volume and total lesion glycolysis predict prognosis in patients with advanced lung adenocarcinoma. J Cancer Res Clin Oncol 2014; 140(1):89–98.

73. Zhang H, Wroblewski K, Liao S, et al. Prognostic value of metabolic tumor burden from (18)F-FDG PET in surgical patients with non-small-cell lung cancer. Acad Radiol 2013;20(1):32–40.

74. Lee P, Bazan JG, Lavori PW, et al. Metabolic tumor volume is an independent prognostic factor in patients treated definitively for non-small-cell lung cancer. Clin Lung Cancer 2012;13(1):52–8.

75. Chen HH, Chiu NT, Su WC, et al. Prognostic value of whole-body total lesion glycolysis at pretreatment FDG PET/CT in non-small cell lung cancer. Radiology 2012;264(2):559–66.

76. Hamberg LM, Hunter GJ, Alpert NM, et al. The dose uptake ratio as an index of glucose metabolism: useful parameter or oversimplification? J Nucl Med 1994;35(8):1308–12.

77. Zhuang H, Pourdehnad M, Lambright ES, et al. Dual time point ^{18}F-FDG PET imaging for differentiating malignant from inflammatory processes. J Nucl Med 2001;42(9):1412–7.

78. Basu S, Kung J, Houseni M, et al. Temporal profile of fluorodeoxyglucose uptake in malignant lesions and normal organs over extended time periods in patients with lung carcinoma: implications for its utilization in assessing malignant lesions. Q J Nucl Med Mol Imaging 2009;53(1):9–19.

79. Cheng G, Alavi A, Werner TJ, et al. Serial changes of FDG uptake and diagnosis of suspected lung malignancy: a lesion-based analysis. Clin Nucl Med 2014;39(2):147–55.

80. Kaneko K, Sadashima E, Irie K, et al. Assessment of FDG retention differences between the FDG-avid benign pulmonary lesion and primary lung cancer using dual-time-point FDG-PET imaging. Ann Nucl Med 2013;27(4):392–9.

81. Kadaria D, Archie DS, SultanAli I, et al. Dual time point positron emission tomography/computed tomography scan in evaluation of intrathoracic lesions in an area endemic for histoplasmosis and with high prevalence of sarcoidosis. Am J Med Sci 2013;346(5):358–62.

82. Lin YY, Chen JH, Ding HJ, et al. Potential value of dual-time-point (1)(8)F-FDG PET compared with initial single-time-point imaging in differentiating malignant from benign pulmonary nodules: a systematic review and meta-analysis. Nucl Med Commun 2012;33(10):1011–8.

83. Barger RL Jr, Nandalur KR. Diagnostic performance of dual-time ^{18}F-FDG PET in the diagnosis of pulmonary nodules: a meta-analysis. Acad Radiol 2012;19(2):153–8.

84. Zhang L, Wang Y, Lei J, et al. Dual time point [18]FDG-PET/CT versus single time point ^{18}F-FDG-PET/CT for the differential diagnosis of pulmonary nodules: a meta-analysis. Acta Radiol 2013;54(7):770–7.

85. Hu M, Han A, Xing L, et al. Value of dual-time-point FDG PET/CT for mediastinal nodal staging in non-small-cell lung cancer patients with lung comorbidity. Clin Nucl Med 2011;36(6):429–33.

86. Alkhawaldeh K, Biersack HJ, Henke A, et al. Impact of dual-time-point F-18 FDG PET/CT in the assessment of pleural effusion in patients with non-small-cell lung cancer. Clin Nucl Med 2011; 36(6):423–8.

87. Demura Y, Tsuchida T, Ishizaki T, et al. ^{18}F-FDG accumulation with PET for differentiation between benign and malignant lesions in the thorax. J Nucl Med 2003;44(4):540–8.

88. Uesaka D, Demura Y, Ishizaki T, et al. Evaluation of dual-time-point ^{18}F-FDG PET for staging in patients with lung cancer. J Nucl Med 2008;49(10):1606–12.

89. Kim SJ, Kim YK, Kim IJ, et al. Limited predictive value of dual-time-point F-18 FDG PET/CT for evaluation of pathologic N1 status in NSCLC patients. Clin Nucl Med 2011;36(6):434–9.

90. Yen RF, Chen KC, Lee JM, et al. ^{18}F-FDG PET for the lymph node staging of non-small cell lung cancer in a tuberculosis-endemic country: is dual time point imaging worth the effort? Eur J Nucl Med Mol Imaging 2008;35(7):1305–15.

91. Li M, Wu N, Liu Y, et al. Regional nodal staging with ^{18}F-FDG PET-CT in non-small cell lung cancer: additional diagnostic value of CT attenuation and dual-time-point imaging. Eur J Radiol 2012;81(8): 1886–90.

92. Kasai T, Motoori K, Horikoshi T, et al. Dual-time point scanning of integrated FDG PET/CT for the evaluation of mediastinal and hilar lymph nodes in non-small cell lung cancer diagnosed as operable by contrast-enhanced CT. Eur J Radiol 2010; 75(2):143–6.

93. Tsuchida T, Demura Y, Sasaki M, et al. Differentiation of histological subtypes in lung cancer with ^{18}F-FDG-PET 3-point imaging and kinetic analysis. Hell J Nucl Med 2011;14(3):224–7.

94. Chen HH, Lee BF, Su WC, et al. The increment in standardized uptake value determined using dual-phase ^{18}F-FDG PET is a promising prognostic factor in non-small-cell lung cancer. Eur J Nucl Med Mol Imaging 2013;40(10):1478–85.

95. Houseni M, Chamroonrat W, Zhuang J, et al. Prognostic implication of dual-phase PET in adenocarcinoma of the lung. J Nucl Med 2010;51(4):535–42.

96. Satoh Y, Nambu A, Onishi H, et al. Value of dual time point F-18 FDG-PET/CT imaging for the evaluation of prognosis and risk factors for recurrence in patients with stage I non-small cell lung cancer treated with stereotactic body radiation therapy. Eur J Radiol 2012;81(11):3530–4.

97. Kim SJ, Kim YK, Kim IJ, et al. Limited prognostic value of dual time point F-18 FDG PET/CT in patients with early stage (stage I & II) non-small cell lung cancer (NSCLC). Radiother Oncol 2011; 98(1):105–8.

98. Mac Manus MP, Hicks RJ, Ball DL, et al. F-18 fluorodeoxyglucose positron emission tomography staging in radical radiotherapy candidates with nonsmall cell lung carcinoma: powerful correlation with survival and high impact on treatment. Cancer 2001;92(4):886–95.

99. Kolodziejczyk M, Kepka L, Dziuk M, et al. Impact of [18F]fluorodeoxyglucose PET-CT staging on treatment planning in radiotherapy incorporating elective nodal irradiation for non-small-cell lung cancer: a prospective study. Int J Radiat Oncol Biol Phys 2011;80(4):1008–14.

100. Bradley J, Bae K, Choi N, et al. A phase II comparative study of gross tumor volume definition with or without PET/CT fusion in dosimetric planning for non-small-cell lung cancer (NSCLC): primary analysis of Radiation Therapy Oncology Group (RTOG) 0515. Int J Radiat Oncol Biol Phys 2012;82(1):435–41.e1.

101. Nawara C, Rendl G, Wurstbauer K, et al. The impact of PET and PET/CT on treatment planning and prognosis of patients with NSCLC treated with radiation therapy. Q J Nucl Med Mol Imaging 2012;56(2):191–201.

102. Satoh Y, Onishi H, Nambu A, et al. Volume-based parameters measured by using FDG PET/CT in patients with stage I NSCLC treated with stereotactic body radiation therapy: prognostic value. Radiology 2014;270(1):275–81.

103. Vu CC, Matthews R, Kim B, et al. Prognostic value of metabolic tumor volume and total lesion glycolysis from (1)(8)F-FDG PET/CT in patients undergoing stereotactic body radiation therapy for stage I non-small-cell lung cancer. Nucl Med Commun 2013;34(10):959–63.

104. Takeda A, Yokosuka N, Ohashi T, et al. The maximum standardized uptake value (SUVmax) on FDG-PET is a strong predictor of local recurrence for localized non-small-cell lung cancer after stereotactic body radiotherapy (SBRT). Radiother Oncol 2011;101(2):291–7.

105. Nair VJ, Macrae R, Sirisegaram A, et al. Pretreatment [(18)F]-fluoro-2-deoxy-glucose positron emission tomography maximum standardized uptake value as predictor of distant metastasis in early-stage non-small cell lung cancer treated with definitive radiation therapy: rethinking the role of positron emission tomography in personalizing treatment based on risk status. Int J Radiat Oncol Biol Phys 2014;88(2):312–8.

106. Mac Manus MP, Hicks RJ, Matthews JP, et al. Positron emission tomography is superior to computed tomography scanning for response-assessment after radical radiotherapy or chemoradiotherapy in patients with non-small-cell lung cancer. J Clin Oncol 2003;21(7):1285–92.

107. Hicks RJ. Role of ^{18}F-FDG PET in assessment of response in non-small cell lung cancer. J Nucl Med 2009;50(Suppl 1):31S–42S.

108. Mac Manus MP, Ding Z, Hogg A, et al. Association between pulmonary uptake of fluorodeoxyglucose detected by positron emission tomography scanning after radiation therapy for non-small-cell lung cancer and radiation pneumonitis. Int J Radiat Oncol Biol Phys 2011;80(5):1365–71.

109. Guerrero T, Johnson V, Hart J, et al. Radiation pneumonitis: local dose versus [(18)F]-fluorodeoxyglucose uptake response in irradiated lung. Int J Radiat Oncol Biol Phys 2007;68(4):1030–5.

110. Petit SF, van Elmpt WJ, Oberije CJ, et al. [(18)F]fluorodeoxyglucose uptake patterns in lung before radiotherapy identify areas more susceptible to radiation-induced lung toxicity in non-small-cell lung cancer patients. Int J Radiat Oncol Biol Phys 2011;81(3):698–705.

111. Clarke K, Taremi M, Dahele M, et al. Stereotactic body radiotherapy (SBRT) for non-small cell lung cancer (NSCLC): is FDG-PET a predictor of outcome? Radiother Oncol 2012;104(1):62–6.

112. Coon D, Gokhale AS, Burton SA, et al. Fractionated stereotactic body radiation therapy in the treatment

of primary, recurrent, and metastatic lung tumors: the role of positron emission tomography/computed tomography-based treatment planning. Clin Lung Cancer 2008;9(4):217–21.

113. Mac Manus MP, Hicks RJ, Matthews JP, et al. Metabolic (FDG-PET) response after radical radiotherapy/chemoradiotherapy for non-small cell lung cancer correlates with patterns of failure. Lung Cancer 2005;49(1):95–108.

114. Machtay M, Duan F, Siegel BA, et al. Prediction of survival by [18F]fluorodeoxyglucose positron emission tomography in patients with locally advanced non-small-cell lung cancer undergoing definitive chemoradiation therapy: results of the ACRIN 6668/RTOG 0235 trial. J Clin Oncol 2013;31(30):3823–30.

115. van Loon J, Grutters J, Wanders R, et al. Follow-up with 18FDG-PET-CT after radical radiotherapy with or without chemotherapy allows the detection of potentially curable progressive disease in non-small cell lung cancer patients: a prospective study. Eur J Cancer 2009;45(4):588–95.

116. van Loon J, Grutters JP, Wanders R, et al. 18FDG-PET-CT in the follow-up of non-small cell lung cancer patients after radical radiotherapy with or without chemotherapy: an economic evaluation. Eur J Cancer 2010;46(1):110–9.

117. Tiseo M, Ippolito M, Scarlattei M, et al. Predictive and prognostic value of early response assessment using 18FDG-PET in advanced non-small cell lung cancer patients treated with erlotinib. Cancer Chemother Pharmacol 2014;73(2):299–307.

118. Zander T, Scheffler M, Nogova L, et al. Early prediction of nonprogression in advanced non-small-cell lung cancer treated with erlotinib by using [(18)F]fluorodeoxyglucose and [(18)F]fluorothymidine positron emission tomography. J Clin Oncol 2011;29(13):1701–8.

119. Bengtsson T, Hicks RJ, Peterson A, et al. 18F-FDG PET as a surrogate biomarker in non-small cell lung cancer treated with erlotinib: newly identified lesions are more informative than standardized uptake value. J Nucl Med 2012;53(4):530–7.

120. Zhang C, Liu J, Tong J, et al. 18F-FDG-PET evaluation of pathological tumour response to neoadjuvant therapy in patients with NSCLC. Nucl Med Commun 2013;34(1):71–7.

121. Hellwig D, Groschel A, Graeter TP, et al. Diagnostic performance and prognostic impact of FDG-PET in suspected recurrence of surgically treated non-small cell lung cancer. Eur J Nucl Med Mol Imaging 2006;33(1):13–21.

122. Keidar Z, Haim N, Guralnik L, et al. PET/CT using 18F-FDG in suspected lung cancer recurrence: diagnostic value and impact on patient management. J Nucl Med 2004;45(10):1640–6.

123. Dane B, Grechushkin V, Plank A, et al. PET/CT vs. non-contrast CT alone for surveillance 1-year post

lobectomy for stage I non-small-cell lung cancer. Am J Nucl Med Mol Imaging 2013;3(5):408–16.

124. Toba H, Sakiyama S, Otsuka H, et al. 18F-fluorodeoxyglucose positron emission tomography/computed tomography is useful in postoperative follow-up of asymptomatic non-small-cell lung cancer patients. Interact Cardiovasc Thorac Surg 2012;15(5):859–64.

125. He YQ, Gong HL, Deng YF, et al. Diagnostic efficacy of PET and PET/CT for recurrent lung cancer: a meta-analysis. Acta Radiol 2014;55(3):309–17.

126. Colt HG, Murgu SD, Korst RJ, et al. Follow-up and surveillance of the patient with lung cancer after curative-intent therapy: diagnosis and management of lung cancer, 3rd ed: American College of Chest Physicians evidence-based clinical practice guidelines. Chest 2013;143(Suppl 5):e437S–54S.

127. Kalemkerian GP, Akerley W, Bogner P, et al. Small cell lung cancer. J Natl Compr Canc Netw 2013;11(1):78–98.

128. Kalemkerian GP, Gadgeel SM. Modern staging of small cell lung cancer. J Natl Compr Canc Netw 2013;11(1):99–104.

129. Jett JR, Schild SE, Kesler KA, et al. Treatment of small cell lung cancer: diagnosis and management of lung cancer, 3rd ed: American College of Chest Physicians evidence-based clinical practice guidelines. Chest 2013;143(Suppl 5):e400S–19S.

130. Bradley JD, Dehdashti F, Mintun MA, et al. Positron emission tomography in limited-stage small-cell lung cancer: a prospective study. J Clin Oncol 2004;22(16):3248–54.

131. Brink I, Schumacher T, Mix M, et al. Impact of [18F]FDG-PET on the primary staging of small-cell lung cancer. Eur J Nucl Med Mol Imaging 2004;31(12):1614–20.

132. Chin R Jr, McCain TW, Miller AA, et al. Whole body FDG-PET for the evaluation and staging of small cell lung cancer: a preliminary study. Lung Cancer 2002;37(1):1–6.

133. Kut V, Spies W, Spies S, et al. Staging and monitoring of small cell lung cancer using [18F]fluoro-2-deoxy-D-glucose-positron emission tomography (FDG-PET). Am J Clin Oncol 2007;30(1):45–50.

134. Fischer BM, Mortensen J, Langer SW, et al. A prospective study of PET/CT in initial staging of small-cell lung cancer: comparison with CT, bone scintigraphy and bone marrow analysis. Ann Oncol 2007;18(2):338–45.

135. Sohn BS, Lee DH, Kim EK, et al. The role of integrated 18F-FDG PET-CT as a staging tool for limited-stage small cell lung cancer: a retrospective study. Onkologie 2012;35(7–8):432–8.

136. Vinjamuri M, Craig M, Campbell-Fontaine A, et al. Can positron emission tomography be used as a staging tool for small-cell lung cancer? Clin Lung Cancer 2008;9(1):30–4.

137. Azad A, Chionh F, Scott AM, et al. High impact of 18F-FDG-PET on management and prognostic stratification of newly diagnosed small cell lung cancer. Mol Imaging Biol 2010;12(4):443–51.

138. Schumacher T, Brink I, Mix M, et al. FDG-PET imaging for the staging and follow-up of small cell lung cancer. Eur J Nucl Med 2001;28(4):483–8.

139. Shen YY, Shiau YC, Wang JJ, et al. Whole-body 18F-2-deoxyglucose positron emission tomography in primary staging small cell lung cancer. Anticancer Res 2002;22(2B):1257–64.

140. Blum R, MacManus MP, Rischin D, et al. Impact of positron emission tomography on the management of patients with small-cell lung cancer: preliminary experience. Am J Clin Oncol 2004;27(2):164–71.

141. Hauber HP, Bohuslavizki KH, Lund CH, et al. Positron emission tomography in the staging of small-cell lung cancer: a preliminary study. Chest 2001; 119(3):950–4.

142. Niho S, Fujii H, Murakami K, et al. Detection of unsuspected distant metastases and/or regional nodes by FDG-PET [corrected] scan in apparent limited-disease small-cell lung cancer. Lung Cancer 2007;57(3):328–33.

143. Kamel EM, Zwahlen D, Wyss MT, et al. Whole-body (18)F-FDG PET improves the management of patients with small cell lung cancer. J Nucl Med 2003;44(12):1911–7.

144. Pandit N, Gonen M, Krug L, et al. Prognostic value of [18F]FDG-PET imaging in small cell lung cancer. Eur J Nucl Med Mol Imaging 2003;30(1):78–84.

145. Reymen B, Van Loon J, van Baardwijk A, et al. Total gross tumor volume is an independent prognostic factor in patients treated with selective nodal irradiation for stage I to III small cell lung cancer. Int J Radiat Oncol Biol Phys 2013;85(5):1319–24.

146. Oh JR, Seo JH, Chong A, et al. Whole-body metabolic tumour volume of 18F-FDG PET/CT improves the prediction of prognosis in small cell lung cancer. Eur J Nucl Med Mol Imaging 2012;39(6):925–35.

147. Zhu D, Ma T, Niu Z, et al. Prognostic significance of metabolic parameters measured by (18)F-fluorodeoxyglucose positron emission tomography/computed tomography in patients with small cell lung cancer. Lung Cancer 2011;73(3):332–7.

148. van Loon J, Offermann C, Bosmans G, et al. 18FDG-PET based radiation planning of mediastinal lymph nodes in limited disease small cell lung cancer changes radiotherapy fields: a planning study. Radiother Oncol 2008;87(1):49–54.

149. van Loon J, De Ruysscher D, Wanders R, et al. Selective nodal irradiation on basis of (18)FDG-PET scans in limited-disease small-cell lung cancer: a prospective study. Int J Radiat Oncol Biol Phys 2010;77(2):329–36.

150. Yamamoto Y, Kameyama R, Murota M, et al. Early assessment of therapeutic response using FDG PET in small cell lung cancer. Mol Imaging Biol 2009;11(6):467–72.

151. Onitilo AA, Engel JM, Demos JM, et al. Prognostic significance of 18 F-fluorodeoxyglucose - positron emission tomography after treatment in patients with limited stage small cell lung cancer. Clin Med Res 2008;6(2):72–7.

152. van Loon J, Offermann C, Ollers M, et al. Early CT and FDG-metabolic tumour volume changes show a significant correlation with survival in stage I-III small cell lung cancer: a hypothesis generating study. Radiother Oncol 2011;99(2):172–5.

153. Orki A, Akin O, Tasci AE, et al. The role of positron emission tomography/computed tomography in the diagnosis of pleural diseases. Thorac Cardiovasc Surg 2009;57(4):217–21.

154. Yildirim H, Metintas M, Entok E, et al. Clinical value of fluorodeoxyglucose-positron emission tomography/computed tomography in differentiation of malignant mesothelioma from asbestos-related benign pleural disease: an observational pilot study. J Thorac Oncol 2009;4(12):1480–4.

155. Mavi A, Basu S, Cermik TF, et al. Potential of dual time point FDG-PET imaging in differentiating malignant from benign pleural disease. Mol Imaging Biol 2009;11(5):369–78.

156. Erasmus JJ, Truong MT, Smythe WR, et al. Integrated computed tomography-positron emission tomography in patients with potentially resectable malignant pleural mesothelioma: staging implications. J Thorac Cardiovasc Surg 2005;129(6):1364–70.

157. Sorensen JB, Ravn J, Loft A, et al. Preoperative staging of mesothelioma by 18F-fluoro-2-deoxy-D-glucose positron emission tomography/computed tomography fused imaging and mediastinoscopy compared to pathological findings after extrapleural pneumonectomy. Eur J Cardiothorac Surg 2008;34(5):1090–6.

158. Kaira K, Serizawa M, Koh Y, et al. Relationship between 18F-FDG uptake on positron emission tomography and molecular biology in malignant pleural mesothelioma. Eur J Cancer 2012;48(8): 1244–54.

159. Flores RM, Akhurst T, Gonen M, et al. Positron emission tomography predicts survival in malignant pleural mesothelioma. J Thorac Cardiovasc Surg 2006;132(4):763–8.

160. Abakay A, Komek H, Abakay O, et al. Relationship between 18 FDG PET-CT findings and the survival of 177 patients with malignant pleural mesothelioma. Eur Rev Med Pharmacol Sci 2013;17(9): 1233–41.

161. Nowak AK, Francis RJ, Phillips MJ, et al. A novel prognostic model for malignant mesothelioma incorporating quantitative FDG-PET imaging with clinical parameters. Clin Cancer Res 2010;16(8): 2409–17.

162. Klabatsa A, Chicklore S, Barrington SF, et al. The association of (18)F-FDG PET/CT parameters with survival in malignant pleural mesothelioma. Eur J Nucl Med Mol Imaging 2014;41(2):276–82.

163. Lee HY, Hyun SH, Lee KS, et al. Volume-based parameter of (18)F-FDG PET/CT in malignant pleural mesothelioma: prediction of therapeutic response and prognostic implications. Ann Surg Oncol 2010;17(10):2787–94.

164. Tsutani Y, Takuwa T, Miyata Y, et al. Prognostic significance of metabolic response by positron emission tomography after neoadjuvant chemotherapy for resectable malignant pleural mesothelioma. Ann Oncol 2013;24(4):1005–10.

165. Francis RJ, Byrne MJ, van der Schaaf AA, et al. Early prediction of response to chemotherapy and survival in malignant pleural mesothelioma using a novel semiautomated 3-dimensional volume-based analysis of serial ^{18}F-FDG PET scans. J Nucl Med 2007;48(9):1449–58.

166. Veit-Haibach P, Schaefer NG, Steinert HC, et al. Combined FDG-PET/CT in response evaluation of malignant pleural mesothelioma. Lung Cancer 2010;67(3):311–7.

167. Gerbaudo VH, Mamede M, Trotman-Dickenson B, et al. FDG PET/CT patterns of treatment failure of malignant pleural mesothelioma: relationship to histologic type, treatment algorithm, and survival. Eur J Nucl Med Mol Imaging 2011;38(5):810–21.

168. Bille A, Chicklore S, Okiror L, et al. Patterns of disease progression on ^{18}F-fluorodeoxyglucose positron emission tomography-computed tomography in patients with malignant pleural mesothelioma undergoing multimodality therapy with pleurectomy/decortication. Nucl Med Commun 2013;34(11): 1075–83.

169. Ettinger DS, Krug LM, Akerley W, et al. NCCN Guidelines Version 1.2014 Malignant Pleural Mesothelioma. 2014. NCCN.org.

170. Varghese TK Jr, Hofstetter WL, Rizk NP, et al. The society of thoracic surgeons guidelines on the diagnosis and staging of patients with esophageal cancer. Ann Thorac Surg 2013;96(1):346–56.

171. Shi W, Wang W, Wang J, et al. Meta-analysis of [18]FDG PET-CT for nodal staging in patients with esophageal cancer. Surg Oncol 2013;22(2): 112–6.

172. Yamada H, Hosokawa M, Itoh K, et al. Diagnostic value of (18)F-FDG PET/CT for lymph node metastasis of esophageal squamous cell carcinoma. Surg Today 2013. [Epub ahead of print].

173. Kato H, Kimura H, Nakajima M, et al. The additional value of integrated PET/CT over PET in initial lymph node staging of esophageal cancer. Oncol Rep 2008;20(4):857–62.

174. Yuan S, Yu Y, Chao KS, et al. Additional value of PET/CT over PET in assessment of locoregional lymph nodes in thoracic esophageal squamous cell cancer. J Nucl Med 2006;47(8):1255–9.

175. Hu Q, Wang W, Zhong X, et al. Dual-time-point FDG PET for the evaluation of locoregional lymph nodes in thoracic esophageal squamous cell cancer. Eur J Radiol 2009;70(2):320–4.

176. Barber TW, Duong CP, Leong T, et al. ^{18}F-FDG PET/CT has a high impact on patient management and provides powerful prognostic stratification in the primary staging of esophageal cancer: a prospective study with mature survival data. J Nucl Med 2012;53(6):864–71.

177. Gillies RS, Middleton MR, Maynard ND, et al. Additional benefit of (1)(8)F-fluorodeoxyglucose integrated positron emission tomography/computed tomography in the staging of oesophageal cancer. Eur Radiol 2011;21(2):274–80.

178. Chatterton BE, Ho Shon I, Baldey A, et al. Positron emission tomography changes management and prognostic stratification in patients with oesophageal cancer: results of a multicentre prospective study. Eur J Nucl Med Mol Imaging 2009;36(3): 354–61.

179. Blencowe NS, Whistance RN, Strong S, et al. Evaluating the role of fluorodeoxyglucose positron emission tomography-computed tomography in multi-disciplinary team recommendations for oesophago-gastric cancer. Br J Cancer 2013; 109(6):1445–50.

180. Yasuda T, Higuchi I, Yano M, et al. The impact of (1)(8)F-fluorodeoxyglucose positron emission tomography positive lymph nodes on postoperative recurrence and survival in resectable thoracic esophageal squamous cell carcinoma. Ann Surg Oncol 2012;19(2):652–60.

181. Gillies RS, Middleton MR, Han C, et al. Role of positron emission tomography-computed tomography in predicting survival after neoadjuvant chemotherapy and surgery for oesophageal adenocarcinoma. Br J Surg 2012;99(2):239–45.

182. Sun G, Tian J, Gorospe EC, et al. Utility of baseline positron emission tomography with computed tomography for predicting endoscopic resectability and survival outcomes in patients with early esophageal adenocarcinoma. J Gastroenterol Hepatol 2013;28(6):975–81.

183. Chen SW, Hsieh TC, Ding HJ, et al. Pretreatment metabolic tumor volumes to predict the short-term outcome of unresectable locally advanced squamous cell carcinoma of the esophagus treated with definitive chemoradiotherapy. Nucl Med Commun 2014;35(3):291–7.

184. I HS, Kim SJ, Kim IJ, et al. Predictive value of metabolic tumor volume measured by ^{18}F-FDG PET for regional lymph node status in patients with esophageal cancer. Clin Nucl Med 2012; 37(5):442–6.

185. Hyun SH, Choi JY, Shim YM, et al. Prognostic value of metabolic tumor volume measured by ^{18}F-fluorodeoxyglucose positron emission tomography in patients with esophageal carcinoma. Ann Surg Oncol 2010;17(1):115–22.

186. Shum WY, Ding HJ, Liang JA, et al. Use of pretreatment metabolic tumor volumes on PET-CT to predict the survival of patients with squamous cell carcinoma of esophagus treated by curative surgery. Anticancer Res 2012;32(9):4163–8.

187. Hatt M, Visvikis D, Albarghach NM, et al. Prognostic value of ^{18}F-FDG PET image-based parameters in oesophageal cancer and impact of tumour delineation methodology. Eur J Nucl Med Mol Imaging 2011;38(7):1191–202.

188. Kim MK, Ryu JS, Kim SB, et al. Value of complete metabolic response by (18)F-fluorodeoxyglucose-positron emission tomography in oesophageal cancer for prediction of pathologic response and survival after preoperative chemoradiotherapy. Eur J Cancer 2007;43(9):1385–91.

189. Miyata H, Yamasaki M, Takahashi T, et al. Determinants of response to neoadjuvant chemotherapy for esophageal cancer using ^{18}F-fluorodeoxyglucose positron emission tomography (^{18}F-FDG-PET). Ann Surg Oncol 2014;21(2):575–82.

190. Miyata H, Yamasaki M, Takahashi T, et al. Relevance of [^{18}F]fluorodeoxyglucose positron emission tomography-positive lymph nodes after neoadjuvant chemotherapy for squamous cell oesophageal cancer. Br J Surg 2013;100(11):1490–7.

191. Lordick F, Ott K, Krause BJ, et al. PET to assess early metabolic response and to guide treatment of adenocarcinoma of the oesophagogastric junction: the MUNICON phase II trial. Lancet Oncol 2007;8(9):797–805.

192. Zhu W, Xing L, Yue J, et al. Prognostic significance of SUV on PET/CT in patients with localised oesophagogastric junction cancer receiving neoadjuvant chemotherapy/chemoradiation: a systematic review and meta-analysis. Br J Radiol 2012; 85(1017):e694–701.

193. Cuenca X, Hennequin C, Hindie E, et al. Evaluation of early response to concomitant chemoradiotherapy by interim ^{18}F-FDG PET/CT imaging in patients with locally advanced oesophageal carcinomas. Eur J Nucl Med Mol Imaging 2013; 40(4):477–85.

194. Roedl JB, Colen RR, Holalkere NS, et al. Adenocarcinomas of the esophagus: response to chemoradiotherapy is associated with decrease of metabolic tumor volume as measured on PET-CT. Comparison to histopathologic and clinical response evaluation. Radiother Oncol 2008; 89(3):278–86.

195. Guo H, Zhu H, Xi Y, et al. Diagnostic and prognostic value of ^{18}F-FDG PET/CT for patients with suspected recurrence from squamous cell carcinoma of the esophagus. J Nucl Med 2007;48(8):1251–8.

196. Jingu K, Kaneta T, Nemoto K, et al. (18)F-fluorodeoxyglucose positron emission tomography immediately after chemoradiotherapy predicts prognosis in patients with locoregional postoperative recurrent esophageal cancer. Int J Clin Oncol 2010;15(2):184–90.

197. Ajani JA, Bentrem DJ, Besh S, et al. NCCN guidelines version 2.2013. Esophageal and esophagogastric junction cancers. 2013. NCCN.org.

198. Erasmus JJ, Munden RF, Truong MT, et al. Preoperative chemo-radiation-induced ulceration in patients with esophageal cancer: a confounding factor in tumor response assessment in integrated computed tomographic-positron emission tomographic imaging. J Thorac Oncol 2006;1(5): 478–86.

199. Detterbeck FC, Nicholson AG, Kondo K, et al. The Masaoka-Koga stage classification for thymic malignancies: clarification and definition of terms. J Thorac Oncol 2011;6(7 Suppl 3):S1710–6.

200. Masaoka A. Staging system of thymoma. J Thorac Oncol 2010;5(10 Suppl 4):S304–12.

201. Kondo K, Yoshizawa K, Tsuyuguchi M, et al. WHO histologic classification is a prognostic indicator in thymoma. Ann Thorac Surg 2004;77(4):1183–8.

202. Moran CA, Weissferdt A, Kalhor N, et al. Thymomas I: a clinicopathologic correlation of 250 cases with emphasis on the World Health Organization schema. Am J Clin Pathol 2012;137(3):444–50.

203. El-Bawab H, Al-Sugair AA, Rafay M, et al. Role of fluorine-18 fluorodeoxyglucose positron emission tomography in thymic pathology. Eur J Cardiothorac Surg 2007;31(4):731–6.

204. Kaira K, Endo M, Abe M, et al. Biologic correlation of 2-[^{18}F]-fluoro-2-deoxy-D-glucose uptake on positron emission tomography in thymic epithelial tumors. J Clin Oncol 2010;28(23):3746–53.

205. Sung YM, Lee KS, Kim BT, et al. ^{18}F-FDG PET/CT of thymic epithelial tumors: usefulness for distinguishing and staging tumor subgroups. J Nucl Med 2006;47(10):1628–34.

206. Seki N, Sakamoto S, Karube Y, et al. ^{18}F-fluorodeoxyglucose positron emission tomography for evaluation of thymic epithelial tumors: utility for World Health Organization classification and predicting recurrence-free survival. Ann Nucl Med 2014;28(3):257–62.

207. Toba H, Kondo K, Sadohara Y, et al. ^{18}F-fluorodeoxyglucose positron emission tomography/computed tomography and the relationship between fluorodeoxyglucose uptake and the expression of hypoxia-inducible factor-1alpha, glucose transporter-1 and vascular endothelial growth factor in thymic epithelial tumours. Eur J Cardiothorac Surg 2013;44(2):e105–12.

208. Lococo F, Cesario A, Okami J, et al. Role of combined ^{18}F-FDG-PET/CT for predicting the WHO malignancy grade of thymic epithelial tumors: a multicenter analysis. Lung Cancer 2013;82(2):245–51.

209. Otsuka H. The utility of FDG-PET in the diagnosis of thymic epithelial tumors. J Med Invest 2012; 59(3–4):225–34.

210. Inoue A, Tomiyama N, Tatsumi M, et al. (18)F-FDG PET for the evaluation of thymic epithelial tumors: correlation with the World Health Organization classification in addition to dual-time-point imaging. Eur J Nucl Med Mol Imaging 2009;36(8):1219–25.

211. Thomas A, Mena E, Kurdziel K, et al. ^{18}F-fluorodeoxyglucose positron emission tomography in the management of patients with thymic epithelial tumors. Clin Cancer Res 2013;19(6):1487–93.

212. Kaira K, Murakami H, Miura S, et al. ^{18}F-FDG uptake on PET helps predict outcome and response after treatment in unresectable thymic epithelial tumors. Ann Nucl Med 2011;25(4):247–53.

213. El-Bawab HY, Abouzied MM, Rafay MA, et al. Clinical use of combined positron emission tomography and computed tomography in thymoma recurrence. Interact Cardiovasc Thorac Surg 2010;11(4):395–9.

214. Ettinger DS, Riely GJ, Akerley W, et al. NCCN guidelines version 1.2014. Thymomas and thymic carcinomas. 2014. NCCN.org.

[¹⁸F]Fluorodeoxyglucose PET/Computed Tomography in Gastrointestinal Malignancies

CrossMark

Maarten L. Donswijk, MD[a,b], Søren Hess, MD[c],
Ties Mulders, MD, PhD[a,b], Marnix G.E.H. Lam, MD, PhD[a,b],*

KEYWORDS

• Gastrointestinal • GI • Malignancy • [¹⁸F]Fluorodeoxyglucose • PET/CT

KEY POINTS

• The major strength of 2-deoxy-2-[¹⁸F]fluoro-ᴅ-glucose (FDG)-PET/computed tomography (CT) lies in detecting distant metastases in patients with gastrointestinal malignancy who are at high risk for metastasized disease, and in patients with undetermined results on conventional imaging modalities.
• Opportunities for FDG-PET/CT lie in the area of prognostication and response assessment, as metabolic changes precede morphologic changes and offer valuable supplemental information on tumor biology.
• Further solidification of FDG-PET/CT in clinical practice may be achieved by addressing issues on quantification, standardization, and cost-effectiveness, and by aiming at new indications, to improve management particularly in patients with gastrointestinal malignancies.

INTRODUCTION

The widespread use of 2-deoxy-2-[¹⁸F]fluoro-ᴅ-glucose (FDG)-PET does not need an introduction. This article discusses the current state-of-the-art application of FDG-PET in the management of patients with gastrointestinal malignancies. The last decade has seen a steep increase in the use of FDG-PET in conjunction with computed tomography (CT), namely low-dose CT or contrast-enhanced CT (ceCT), as a hybrid imaging modality. Most recent studies concern hybrid PET/CT scanners. When relevant, distinction is made in this article between PET as a stand-alone imaging modality or PET combined with low-dose CT or ceCT. Furthermore, when used here PET and PET/CT apply to FDG-PET and FDG-PET/CT, respectively.

Gastrointestinal malignancies include many different cell types, several common malignancies of which may be imaged by PET/CT. This article focuses on gastric carcinoma, pancreatic carcinoma, hepatocellular carcinoma, cholangiocarcinoma, colorectal carcinoma, and stroma cell tumors. The role of PET/CT in staging these malignancies is discussed, in addition to (re)staging, detection of recurrent disease, patient selection/prognostication, and response assessment, with reference to the currently available literature.

The authors have nothing to disclose.
[a] Department of Radiology, University Medical Center Utrecht, Heidelberglaan 100, Utrecht 3584 CX, The Netherlands; [b] Department of Nuclear Medicine, University Medical Center Utrecht, Heidelberglaan 100, Utrecht 3584 CX, The Netherlands; [c] Department of Nuclear Medicine, Odense University Hospital, Sdr. Boulevard 29, 5000 Odense, Denmark
* Corresponding author. Departments of Radiology and Nuclear Medicine, University Medical Center Utrecht, Utrecht 3584 CX, The Netherlands.
E-mail address: m.lam@umcutrecht.nl

PET Clin 9 (2014) 421–441
http://dx.doi.org/10.1016/j.cpet.2014.07.001
1556-8598/14/$ – see front matter © 2014 Elsevier Inc. All rights reserved.

GASTRIC CANCER
Introduction

Gastric cancer is a serious health issue worldwide. In Europe it remains the sixth most commonly diagnosed cancer, but the fourth commonest cause of cancer-related mortality. There are marked geographic variations in the worldwide distribution, with the highest incidence in Asia, South America, and Eastern Europe, and the lowest incidence in Western Europe and the United States. Although there has been a general decline in incidence, there has been a relative increase in adenocarcinomas of the gastric cardia and the gastroesophageal junction.[1] Despite improved surgical procedures the overall prognosis remains austere, and the goal of curative treatment is microscopic radical resection. However, this is achievable in only 30% of patients; moreover, a large number of patients experience relapse within the first 2 years after radical resection. Most recurrences are discovered late, when they give rise to clinical symptoms; the disease is usually disseminated at this point in time, and very rarely is salvage resection or curative oncologic treatment an option. Thus the overall 5-year survival rate is less than 20%, and because of the high incidence of recurrent disease and the overall poor prognosis, improved staging, along with better and earlier detection of recurrence, is in high demand.

PET and PET/CT have been proposed and proved to be valuable in some settings, but there are several important issues with the use of FDG for gastric cancer that impede its use to some extent. First, there is some physiologic uptake in the gastric mucosa, both focally and diffusely, in patients without malignancies. There tends to be increased gastric uptake in the more proximal fundus. One might therefore advocate a higher index of suspicion regarding high FDG uptake in the lower distal third of the stomach (antrum). Studies have shown that the common, though controversial, maximum standardized uptake value (SUV_{max}) of 2.5 indicating malignancy can be measured in the nonmalignant gastric mucosa as well. The physiologic FDG uptake may be mitigated by additional consumption of water or milk, but this approach has not gained widespread use.[2] Furthermore, several benign conditions can exhibit focally or diffusely increased FDG uptake (eg, *Helicobacter pylori* infections, gastritis or other inflammatory conditions).[3] Thus, Heusner and colleagues[4] concluded from their examination of 546 patients with nonspecific FDG uptake in the esophageal or gastric mucosa, and no evidence of malignancies, that this finding does not predict cancer development and should not be investigated further if there are no corresponding features on CT images.

Another important caveat is different accumulation patterns depending on histologic type of malignant cells in the stomach. FDG uptake depends on the expression of glucose transporter 1 (GLUT1), which is overexpressed in many cancers. However, in gastric carcinoma overexpression of GLUT1 is not so straightforward; it generally occurs at a late stage in carcinogenesis, and is a marker of disease progression and poor outcome. In an analysis of GLUT1 expression in tubular adenomas and gastric carcinomas, Kawamura and colleagues[5] found that none of the adenomas and only 30% of carcinomas overall expressed GLUT1, with papillary adenocarcinomas being the histologic type with the highest abundance of GLUT1 (44% of cases), followed by tubular and poorly differentiated adenocarcinomas (32% and 28%, respectively), while GLUT1 was virtually nonexistent in signet-ring cell carcinomas (**Fig. 1**) and mucinous adenocarcinomas (6% and 2%, respectively). Similarly, Yamada and colleagues[6] found FDG uptake in only 48% of gastric carcinomas, with cohesive carcinomas (ie, papillary, tubular, and solid-type poorly differentiated adenocarcinomas) being significantly more FDG-avid than noncohesive carcinomas (ie, signet-ring cell and nonsolid-type poorly differentiated carcinomas), that is, in 67% versus 14%, respectively. Thus, early and noncohesive gastric carcinoma may not be sufficiently FDG-avid to be detectable.

Staging

The National Comprehensive Cancer Network has established the accuracy of PET/CT staging in a variety of malignancies.[7] Regarding gastric cancer, combined PET/CT was found to have a higher overall accuracy than stand-alone PET and CT, 84% compared with 63% and 64%, respectively, leading to a change in management in approximately one-third of patients. This accuracy was especially true for detecting distant metastases and stage IV disease, whereas sensitivity was generally low for locally advanced disease including local lymph nodes. In the latter, PET and PET/CT has shown consistently poorer accuracy than ceCT and endoscopic ultrasonography (EUS) (48%–72% vs 69%) owing to a lack of sensitivity (22%–40% vs 83%), whereas PET has higher accuracy for distant metastases (86% vs 62%). Specificity, on the other hand, was consistently high, with overall values greater than 95%. PET/CT has to some extent alleviated these numbers, but is still outperformed by ceCT on sensitivity

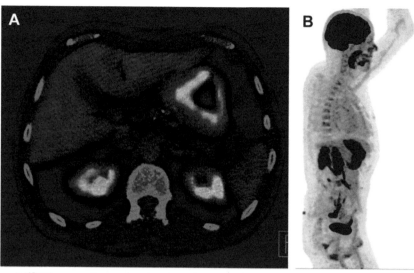

Fig. 1. 2-Deoxy-2-[^{18}F]fluoro-D-glucose (FDG)-PET/computed tomography (CT) in a patient with signet cell adeno-carcinoma of the stomach. (*A*) Transaxial slice through the antrum shows marked FDG uptake and a thick tumorous stomach wall. Maximum-intensity projection from oblique (*B*) shows intense FDG uptake in the stomach.

and accuracy, whereas specificity remains equal and/or higher. Compared with ceCT the sensitivity, specificity, positive predictive value (PPV), negative predictive value (NPV), and accuracy were 41% versus 75%, 100% versus 92%, 100% versus 98%, 26% versus 42%, and 51% versus 72%, respectively.[2,7] However, with regard to distant metastases, PET/CT is second to none, especially for peritoneal metastases, as shown by Yang and colleagues,[8] who found sensitivity, specificity, accuracy, PPV, and NPV of 74%, 93%, 88%, 81%, and 93%, respectively. These results were significantly better than those for ceCT (ie, 39%, 94%, 78%, 72%, and 79%, respectively).

Recurrence Detection

Several studies have assessed the efficacy of PET/CT for the detection of recurrence in various settings of gastric cancer. The earliest studies used stand-alone PET and were retrospective, but the results were promising. Jadvar and colleagues[9] examined 18 patients and found PET and ceCT to be discordant in 4. PET was true positive in 3 where other imaging was negative, and false negative in one patient with a true positive ceCT. De Potter and colleagues[10] found similar results in 33 patients with mediocre sensitivity and specificity for recurrence of 70% and 69%, respectively. However, another important finding of this study was a significantly poorer prognosis in PET-positive patients with proven recurrence in comparison with PET-negative ones; mean survival was 18.5 ± 12.5 months versus 6.9 ± 6.5 months, respectively.

In the last decade, PET/CT has gained widespread use and has surpassed stand-alone PET in many clinical settings. However, in one of the first studies, Sim and colleagues[11] found comparable values with sensitivity and specificity of 68% and 71%, respectively, which was inferior to ceCT especially in detecting peritoneal seeding. Thus these investigators found no additional value from PET/CT when compared with ceCT. On the other hand, another early study by Sun[12] found overall accuracy of PET/CT of 83% with NPV of 78% and PPV of 86%. As an important additional result, PET/CT was true positive in half of the patients (11 patients) in whom CT was negative or equivocal, and treatment was changed in 30% of patients based on PET/CT. Similar results were described by Park and colleagues[13] in 105 patients. Again the key feature was an excellent PPV of 89% both on a per-patient and a per-lesion basis. Nakamoto and colleagues[14] evaluated PET/CT for recurrence detection in different clinical settings, looking at 3 different subgroups of patients suspected of recurrence: patients suspected based on other imaging modalities (group A, recurrence incidence 67%), patients suspected based on elevated tumor markers without definitive findings (group B, recurrence incidence 58%), and patients with no evidence of recurrence (group C, recurrence incidence 7%). PET/CT showed decreasing sensitivity from group A through C at 81%, 73%, and 50%, respectively, with consistent specificities of 87% to 88%. Treatment strategy was influenced by PET/CT findings in 42% to 48% in groups A and B, and 7% in group

C. The investigators concluded that PET/CT was most influential when recurrence was suspected based on actual findings. In a retrospective head-to-head comparison of PET/CT and ceCT, Kim and colleagues[15] found no overall statistically significant differences between the 2 modalities on a per-patient basis, but PET/CT had a sensitivity comparable with or better than ceCT in most settings, including locoregional recurrence (43% vs 43%), regional lymph nodes (28% vs 28%), liver (75% vs 50%), and distant metastases (100% vs 71%), with comparable specificity and accuracy. Only with regard to detection of peritoneal carcinomatosis was PET/CT far less sensitive than ceCT (18% vs 64%), although with comparable specificity and accuracy. In addition, PET/CT detected 15 clinically relevant additional lesions including secondary cancers in 8 patients. In a recent prospective head-to-head comparison of PET/CT and ceCT, Bilici and colleagues[16] found even more striking results, with PET/CT being significantly superior to ceCT with regard to overall sensitivity (96% vs 63%), specificity (100% vs 10%), accuracy (97% vs 47%), PPV (100% vs 63%), and NPV (91% vs 10%). Furthermore, PET/CT changed patient management in 53% of patients; 9 patients had additional, previously unplanned therapy while 9 other patients had previously planned therapy discontinued. Finally, a recent retrospective study by Sharma and colleagues[17] in nonoriental Asians also substantiated the efficacy of PET/CT with good overall per-study sensitivity, specificity, and accuracy of 96%, 80%, and 88%, respectively, and very high accuracy greater than 95% in most locations on a per-region based analysis of lymph nodes, liver, lung, bone, and other sites. Lowest accuracy (89%) was found for local recurrence. This problem was also assessed by Choi and colleagues,[18] who retrospectively reviewed PET/CT and measured SUV_{max} at the anastomotic site in sequential scans in 19 patients operated on for gastric cancer. The investigators found consistently elevated SUV_{max} at the site of anastomosis, and concluded that SUV_{max} was unable to definitively differentiate physiologic uptake or postoperative inflammatory changes from actual recurrence.

Response Evaluation, Prognosis, and Impact on Management

In one of the earliest studies on PET for response assessment was in gastric cancer, Couper and colleagues[19] examined 14 patients in a feasibility study, with a visual response in all patients, whereas only 4 demonstrated measurable response on ceCT. However, data on this topic are still relatively sparse. In general, chemotherapy induces a measurable tumor response in nearly half of the patients with metastatic disease, but one-third of the patients experience progression. Neoadjuvant chemotherapy has now become a mainstay strategy in locally advanced stages, improving overall prognosis in responders. However, nonresponders experience inferior prognosis owing to toxicity from chemotherapy and because ineffective chemotherapy promotes progression in the preoperative period.[20] Thus, an important challenge regarding preoperative chemotherapy is to distinguish responders from nonresponders beforehand. Two groups have provided valuable insight into PET in this clinical setting, with PET response defined as a decrease in SUV of greater than 35% compared with baseline. In an early 2003 article, Ott and colleagues[21] presented data elaborated on in their 2008 article, partly including the same patient base. Metabolic responders were shown to have much higher histopathologic response rates (69% vs 17% response rates). Median survival was not reached in the former group, whereas it was 24 months in the latter group.

Lordick[22] assessed response in 2 so-called MUNICON studies. Reliable response assessment was shown to be possible as early as 14 days after the first series of neoadjuvant chemotherapy, allowing for nonresponders to proceed directly to surgery (MUNICON-I), and progression-free survival was significantly higher in responders than in nonresponders (29.7 vs 14.1 months). In the ensuing MUNICON-II study, nonresponders were switched to salvage neoadjuvant chemotherapy before surgery, increasing the rate of histopathologic response (26% vs 0% in MUNICON-I), but the primary end point of increasing the number of R0 resection from 74% to 94% was not reached. There was also no prognostic benefit for nonresponders, and although progression-free survival was slightly higher compared with MUNICON-I (15.3% vs 14.1%), overall survival was less (18.3 vs 24.3 months). Overall, there is a clear potential for using PET/CT to evaluate response to treatment by tailoring the strategy in accordance with tumor biology, but larger and, preferably, multicenter studies are warranted to firmly establish both the clinical benefit and more standardized approaches to the quantification of metabolic response.

Summary

Early studies of PET/CT in gastric cancer have shown considerable promise, although inherent features related to tumor biology may impede its use in some histopathologic subgroups. At present, National Comprehensive Cancer Network (NCCN) practice guidelines on gastric cancer only give limited mention of PET/CT as an adjunctive modality for the detection of distant metastases in the preoperative setting.[23] In general only few studies are available for analysis, and further and larger prospective studies are required to more firmly establish the role of PET/CT in gastric cancer with regard to improving preoperative staging and response assessment, and earlier detection of recurrence.

PANCREATIC CANCER
Introduction

Pancreatic cancer is the third most common cancer of the gastrointestinal tract and the fifth leading cause of cancer deaths in the United States, while it is the tenth most common cancer and the eighth leading cause of cancer-related mortality in Europe. Pancreatic cancer comprises different histologic types, with ductal adenocarcinomas accounting for more than 90% of cases, with the remainder divided into acinar cell carcinoma, cystic neoplasms, and islet cell tumors and other neuroendocrine tumors. The latter types are not addressed herein.

Despite developments in diagnostic procedures, imaging, and treatment, pancreatic cancer still harbors one of the poorest prognoses; 5-year survival rates remain low at only a few percent, and median survival is approximately 18 months for patients with resectable disease, 6 to 9 months for patients with locally advanced, nonresectable disease, and 3 to 6 months for patients with metastatic disease at diagnosis. Overall more than 95% of patients will eventually die from their disease, primarily because of the high incidence of patients with metastatic disease at diagnosis; only approximately 20% present initially with potentially resectable disease.

Various conventional imaging modalities are used in the initial diagnostic workup: ultrasonography, CT, and magnetic resonance (MR) imaging. However, several diagnostic issues remain for the initial diagnostic workup (eg, early detection), staging purposes (eg, lesion localization, proximity to vessels, invasion of adjacent structures, regional and distant metastases), response evaluation, and detection of recurrent disease. In recent years, EUS has been increasingly implemented, especially for local staging, while PET/CT is being investigated in all of the afore mentioned areas.

Initial Diagnosis and Staging

After its introduction, stand-alone PET was used for differentiating benign pancreatic lesions from malignant ones. For example, differentiating carcinoma with focal uptake from the diffuse uptake of pancreatitis. The pivotal 2001 tabulated summary by Gambhir and colleagues[24] identified 26 studies on pancreatic cancer and found a weighted average sensitivity and specificity of 94% and 90%, respectively, compared with 82% and 75%, respectively, for ceCT. Furthermore, there was a change of management in 50% of patients. A recent meta-analysis[25] substantiated these results comparing PET, PET/CT, and EUS, finding overall pooled sensitivities of 88%, 90%, and 81%, respectively, and specificities of 83%, 80%, and 93%, respectively. However, only few prospective studies on PET/CT for the initial diagnosis of pancreatic cancer have been published to date, and there are some issues with comparison arising from the different reported data on CT protocols; sensitivities and specificities range from 85% to 89% and 56% to 94%, respectively. A separate clinical entity is cystic lesions including intrapapillary mucinous neoplasms, and also in this respect, PET/CT has been shown to be superior to ceCT in discriminating benign cysts from malignant neoplasms (**Fig. 2**).

Preoperative staging is of paramount importance in avoiding futile surgery because 25% to 30% of patients considered resectable present with nondetected metastases on laparotomy. At present, ceCT is the most validated method and is considered the reference standard regarding locoregional spread and lymph node involvement, supplemented by EUS, whereas PET is considered inferior in the evaluation of resectability (involvement of vessels and adjacent structures), even when coregistered with ceCT, probably because of high metabolic activity in the primary tumor, which may obscure peripancreatic structures. Moreover, studies on PET for lymph node involvement have been disappointing, with sensitivities below 50%.[26,27] This lack in sensitivity may in some patients relate to hyperglycemia, which may decrease FDG uptake in malignant lesions. However, PET is considered superior to ceCT for detecting distant metastases and leads to a change of management in a considerable portion of patients. In a study by Heinrich and colleagues,[28] 16 of 59 patients had distant metastases; 13 were detected by PET, and in 5 cases they were detected only by PET, which led to a change of management in 16% of patients. Another study by Bang and colleagues[29] found a higher accuracy for PET compared with ceCT with regard to liver metastases. PET changed the initial stage in approximately 27% and changed the resectability status in 22% of cases. However, controversies remain, especially regarding liver metastases, and several studies have failed to

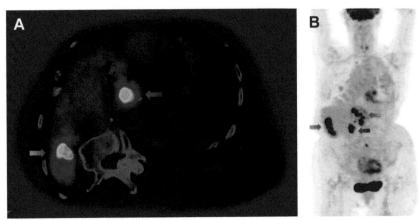

Fig. 2. FDG-PET/CT in a patient with adenocarcinoma of the pancreas. Transaxial slice through the pancreas (*A*) and maximum-intensity projection (*B*) show marked focal FDG uptake in the pancreatic head (*red arrow*). Blue arrows denote physiologic renal FDG excretion.

corroborate these results. The sensitivity of PET has been found to be only about 50% for sub-centimeter liver lesions, which is considered inferior to ceCT. Further studies are needed because most studies hitherto used stand-alone PET or early-generation PET/CT with only low-dose CT and no contrast enhancement. The first study on PET/ceCT clearly showed superiority compared with stand-alone PET and PET/CT without contrast enhancement: sensitivity of PET and PET/CT was 100%, with specificities of 44% and 56%, respectively. For PET/ceCT the corresponding values were 96%, and 82%, respectively.[30] It is conceivable that this approach, combined with further technical developments, multiple-time-point imaging, and quantification will alleviate these caveats.

Recurrence Detection

With some 40% of the patients having recurrence within the first year after resection, recurrence detection is of great importance in instituting palliative chemotherapy in a timely fashion. ceCT may have difficulty in distinguishing malignant cells from benign, post-therapy changes such as radiation-induced or surgery-induced necrosis or fibrosis. PET/CT may be particularly helpful in this setting, and for patients with rising tumor markers and negative conventional workup. Ruf and colleagues[31] compared PET and CT or MR imaging in 31 patients suspected of tumor recurrence. PET detected 96% of patients with recurrence compared with 39% with ceCT or MR imaging. The latter did detect more hepatic lesions than PET, but PET detected all extrahepatic recurrences and 2 extra-abdominal recurrences, neither of which were demonstrated by ceCT or MR imaging. Three earlier studies have found PET to be particularly sensitive in patients with elevated tumor markers and indeterminate ceCT results. Rose and colleagues[32] identified all patients with recurrence, 4 in the surgical bed, and 4 new liver lesions. Franke and colleagues[33] found PET to provide added value in half of the patients, resulting in subsequent change of management. In the study by Jadvar and Fischman,[34] PET identified recurrence in 15% of patients with nondiagnostic ceCT findings, and altered management in two-thirds of patients (ie, earlier initiation of chemotherapy). In a more recent study, Sperti and colleagues[35] found recurrence in 63 of 72 patients (87.5%); ceCT detected the recurrence in 35 patients, PET in 61 patients, and additionally 2 patients had a secondary cancer resected because of findings on PET/CT. Only a few studies have assessed PET/CT in this setting: Kitajima and colleagues[36] compared PET/CT and PET/ceCT in 45 patients with suspected recurrence. Sensitivity, specificity, and accuracy of PET/CT were 83%, 91%, and 87%, respectively, while corresponding numbers for PET/ceCT were 92%, 95%, and 93%, respectively. Casneuf and colleagues[37] found similar values in a comparison between PET, ceCT, and PET/CT, with sensitivity and accuracy of PET/CT of 90% and 92%, respectively, whereas sensitivity for ceCT alone was 80%. Similarly, in a recent study by Asagi and colleagues,[27] PET/ceCT found all cases of recurrence (11 of 11 patients), compared with 7 of 11 by ceCT alone.

Response Evaluation, Prognosis, and Impact on Management

As with many other cancers, PET has been found to be more accurate than ceCT for response evaluation by reflecting tumor viability instead of only changes in morphologic dimensions. Moreover, as mentioned earlier, ceCT may have difficulty in distinguishing malignant tissue from the necrotic or fibrotic changes accompanying radiotherapy. Bang and colleagues[29] found significantly longer progression-free survival in PET responders than in PET nonresponders: 399 versus 233 days. Similarly, Heinrich and colleagues[28] found that patients with higher baseline metabolic activity responded better to neoadjuvant chemotherapy. The value of SUV has also been assessed, and Maemura and colleagues[38] found metastatic pancreatic cancer to have higher baseline SUV than localized tumors. Sperti and colleagues[35] found SUV greater than 4 to be associated with shorter survival. Kittaka and colleagues[39] recently showed a better pathologic response to preoperative chemoradiotherapy in patients with high baseline SUV and a large change in SUV_{max} following therapy compared with patients with no or lesser metabolic response. Similarly, Topkan and colleagues[40] found a positive correlation between changes in SUV_{max} measured at baseline and after concurrent chemoradiotherapy in 19 patients with unresectable locally advanced pancreatic cancer; there was significantly higher overall survival (17 vs 9.8 months, respectively) and progression-free survival (8.4 vs 3.8 months, respectively) when comparing patients with greater SUV_{max} changes with patients with lesser SUV_{max} changes. Several studies have assessed the impact of PET/CT on clinical management and have found a positive impact in 16% to 41% on the initial staging,[26,28,41,42] whereas one study by Javery and colleagues[43] found negligible impact on management with regard to staging and restaging, and even a negative impact on biopsy planning, but a positive impact in half of the patients when assessing response to therapy.

Summary

Early studies of PET in pancreatic cancer have shown promise, and it is likely that PET/ceCT will further positively affect patient management by improved preoperative staging and response assessment, and earlier recurrence detection. Only few investigators have assessed the potential cost-effectiveness, but preliminary results were positive, with patient benefit because of avoidance of futile surgeries.[44] However, in general only few studies are available for analysis, and further and larger prospective studies are required to more firmly establish the role of PET/CT in pancreatic cancer. Accordingly, NCCN practice guidelines state that the role of PET/CT in pancreatic cancer

remains unclear and, at present, should be considered an adjunct to conventional imaging and be reserved for the detection of distant metastases in high-risk patients.[45]

PRIMARY LIVER MALIGNANCIES
Introduction

Primary liver malignancies are the sixth most common type of cancer worldwide.[46] The most common form, which accounts for 90% of cases, is hepatocellular carcinoma. Others include cholangiocarcinoma and more rare types of cancers. The prognosis of primary liver malignancies is very poor, with a 5-year survival rate ranging from 5% to 20%.[47] Accurate diagnosis and staging may lead to a more appropriate treatment and improved clinical outcomes. Surgical resection is the primary curative option for most of these cancers, and earlier and more accurate detection may increase the likelihood of a timely intervention. However, despite a plethora of clinically available imaging techniques, the disease seems to be overlooked most of the time, only to be discovered at surgical exploration. Conventional imaging such as ceCT and MR imaging capitalize on anatomic changes to detect disease. By contrast, PET is based on the identification of molecular biological changes. The metabolic difference between cancer and normal tissue is the hallmark of PET. Detectability on PET may be independent of the structural changes seen on conventional imaging.[48]

Initial Diagnosis and Staging

The cornerstone of oncologic staging of primary liver malignancies is MR imaging and ceCT. To date the additional value of PET has been limited, confirmed by the NCCN guidelines, which state that "PET is not considered adequate" for staging. Despite this limitation, several investigators have explored the diagnostic value of PET in the staging of primary liver malignancies. Normally, malignancies are characterized by high FDG uptake, which differentiates them from normal tissue. Well-differentiated hepatocellular carcinomas have low expression of GLUT1 and very high expression of glucose-6-phosphatase, comparable with normal liver tissue, which hampers the diagnosis and staging with PET even more.[49] This aspect is exemplified by the work of Kahn and colleagues,[50] who found sensitivity of 55% for PET, compared with 90% for ceCT, in identifying hepatocellular carcinoma. In line with this, Bohm and colleagues[51] found sensitivity of only 52% for PET in comparison with ultrasonography (61%), ceCT (81%) and MR imaging (89%).

The most promising use of PET is the detection of extrahepatic lesions or metastases, which makes extensive surgery or toxic chemotherapies redundant. These lesions may be overlooked on ceCT. In the same article that showed inferior results of PET on detecting primary malignancies, Bohm and colleagues[51] found sensitivity for detecting metastasis of 63% for PET, compared with 47% for ceCT and 40% for MR imaging. In fact, the findings on PET had a direct impact on operative management in 9 patients (18%). This result is supported by a prospective study that found PET to have a clinically significant impact in 26 of 91 (28%) patients with hepatocellular carcinoma.[52] These studies were all small but showed consistent results. A recently conducted meta-analysis of 3 studies, not including the 2 studies mentioned earlier, and 239 patients by Lin and colleagues[53] on the accuracy of PET in detecting extrahepatic metastasis, showed pooled estimates of sensitivity, specificity, positive likelihood ratio, and negative likelihood ratio of 76.6%, 98.0%, 14.7, and 0.3, respectively.

The differentiation of the tumor is also an interesting characteristic to detect on imaging. Several studies have evaluated FDG uptake on PET for differentiation of the cancer. For instance, one study found that a significant difference existed in the SUV between well and moderately differentiated hepatocellular carcinomas, and between well and poorly differentiated hepatocellular carcinomas.[54] In a similar study regarding SUV, Seo and colleagues[55] found a correlation between SUV and survival in a study of 70 patients who underwent curative resection. Besides a statistically higher SUV between poorly differentiated and well-differentiated hepatocellular carcinomas, disease-free survival was much lower among the poorly differentiated or higher-SUV lesions.

The detection of cholangiocarcinoma by PET is hampered by the same limitations as the detection of hepatocellular carcinoma. The resectability rate is low, because at the time of diagnosis this disease is frequently beyond the limits of surgical therapy, which is the only possibility for long-term survival.[56] Therefore, early tumor detection is of major importance. PET may assist in this matter (**Fig. 3**). Although most biliary tract cancers are FDG-avid, only a limited number of studies have been performed on the use of PET in the staging of cholangiocarcinoma, and its role is still controversial, although the NCCN guidelines state that "PET scanning might be useful for detecting lymph node involvement and distant metastatic disease."

In one study, PET/CT and ceCT provided a comparable accuracy for cholangiocarcinomas (n = 47), with sensitivity of 93% and 78% and specificity of 80% and 80%. All distant metastases (n = 12) were detected by PET/CT, but only 3 of 12 by CT (P<.001). Regional lymph node metastases were detected by PET/CT and ceCT in only 12% versus 24%.[57] It was reported in a consecutive series of 50 patients that the specificity of cancer detection is higher for the nodular type than for the infiltrating type; sensitivity was 85% for the nodular morphology, whereas it was only 18% for the infiltrating type.[58]

These promising results were confirmed by a study comparing PET/CT, ceCT, and MR imaging in 123 patients.[59] The overall values of PET/CT in

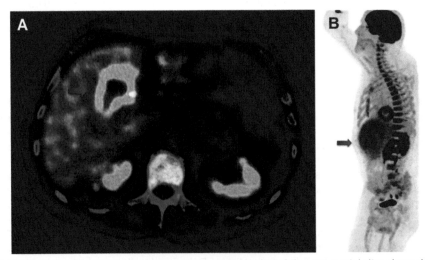

Fig. 3. FDG-PET/CT in a patient with cholangiocarcinoma in the liver hilus. Transaxial slice through the liver (*A*) and maximum-intensity projection from oblique (*B*) show marked circular FDG uptake and a cold central area in the liver hilus (*arrow*), compatible with a Klatskin tumor.

primary tumor detection for sensitivity, specificity, PPV, NPV, and accuracy were 84.0%, 79.3%, 92.9%, 60.5%, and 82.9%, respectively. PET/CT demonstrated no statistically significant advantage over ceCT and MR cholangiopancreatography in the diagnosis of primary tumor. Furthermore, PET/CT revealed significantly higher accuracy over CT in the diagnosis of regional lymph node metastases (75.9% vs 60.9%, P = .004) and distant metastases (88.3% vs 78.7%, P = .004). This finding is important, as patients with distant metastases have an extremely poor prognosis and are excluded from curative surgery.

Recurrence Detection

Little is reported on the detection of recurrent malignant disease in primary liver malignancies. In a series of 93 patients with hepatocellular carcinomas who underwent curative resection, 26 patients (27.9%) had recurrences. In these patients, the SUV of the tumor and the SUV ratio between the tumor and nontumor were strongly correlated with tumor differentiation ($P<.01$). In a univariate analysis, predictors of early tumor recurrence were tumor/nontumor ratio and a high SUV of the cancer. However, in a multivariate analysis, none of these retained statistical significance.[60]

It was shown in a systematic review comprising 109 patients and 4 studies that the pooled estimates of sensitivity and specificity of PET in the detection of recurrent hepatocellular carcinoma were 81.7% and 88.9%.[53]

Response Evaluation, Prognosis, and Impact on Management

Because primary liver malignancies are characterized by an aggressive course, monitoring of the disease is extremely important. Identified prognostic factors may lead to improved patient selection and identification of high-risk groups, which may lead to prognostic advantage in selected patient groups. For hepatocellular carcinoma, the most identified prognostic factor is the SUV. Indeed, it was found in 135 patients with locally advanced disease, who were treated with localized concurrent chemoradiotherapy, that patients with low tumor SUVs had a higher disease control rate than those with high tumor SUVs (86.8% vs 68.5%; $P<.05$). Both the progression-free survival (8.4 vs 5.2 months; $P<.01$) and overall survival (17.9 vs 11.3 months; $P<.05$) were significantly longer in the low SUV group than in the high SUV group.[61] This finding was supported in some smaller series, which found that the overall survival was significantly longer in the lower tumor/nontumor SUV ratio group than in the higher SUV ratio

group (5-year survival rate 63% vs 29%; $P<.01$).[62] Another study found in 29 patients that the SUV of the tumor was an independent prognostic factor for progression-free survival in multivariate analysis.[63] Moreover, it was found in 63 patients that the tumor to nontumor ratio was an independent predictive factor, even after correction of confounding factors. The ratios in the groups with late recurrence (after 1 year) and no recurrence were significantly lower than that in the early recurrence (within 1 year) group. The tumor to nontumor ratio was an independent predictive factor of the time to initial recurrence by multivariate analysis,[64] although this was not found by others.[60]

Some investigators laboriously tried to identify prognostic factors, whereas others have tried to characterize patients to evaluate response of treatment. Ahn and colleagues[65] investigated 189 patients with hepatocellular carcinoma who underwent curative resection and analyzed prognostic factors and surgery type. Major hepatectomy minimizes tumor recurrence, but is harmful because of decreased hepatic functional reserve. It was tested as to whether the characteristics of PET were capable of selecting a proper patient group suitable for major hepatectomy. The overall survival and recurrence-free survival were significantly better following major hepatectomy rather than minor hepatectomy in patients whose preoperative PET indicated that the maximum SUV of the tumor was 4 or greater and the tumor to nontumor SUV ratio was 1.5 or greater. More interesting is that the median overall survival did not differ significantly between the major and minor hepatectomy groups. Therefore, PET proved to be suitable in selecting which cases to apply for a major surgical procedure. Another study in 35 patients with unresectable malignancies, who underwent radiotherapy, tested whether SUV could select patients who would respond favorably to radiotherapy. In patients with a high SUV there was a response rate of 46%, versus 17% in patients with a low SUV for the tumor.[59] This interesting finding in a small study needs further confirmation, but indicates that especially aggressive tumors might benefit from external radiotherapy.

For cholangiocarcinomas, there is little literature on prognosis and response evaluation. Two studies have assessed the SUV to assist in the prognostic evaluation of patients. In 69 patients, Furukawa and colleagues[66] found that the 3-year survival rate in patients with an SUV of 6.3 or less was 74.3%, whereas it was only 44.1% for those with values greater than 6.3. Univariate analysis showed that the SUV_{max} was one of the significant prognostic factors for overall survival ($P = .0119$), whereas it retained no statistical significance in a multivariate model. Another study included 19 patients who underwent radioembolization for a cholangiocarcinoma.[67] The SUV_{max} and the SUV_{mean} significantly predicted survival by Kaplan-Meier analysis. Responders were identified by a high ΔSUV_{max} and ΔSUV_{mean}, which were defined as the difference between SUV before and after treatment. These responders had a median survival of 114 weeks, versus 19 weeks (nonresponders) and 69 weeks in patients with stable disease ($P<.05$).

Summary

Although the literature on the use of PET in hepatocellular carcinoma and cholangiocarcinoma is scarce, it has been shown that PET has limited sensitivity for diagnosing hepatocellular carcinoma in comparison with ceCT and MR imaging. The accuracy of PET in detecting cholangiocarcinoma is higher, and almost comparable with conventional imaging techniques. The most valuable feature of PET is the detection of distant metastases.

The strongest prognostic factor in patients with primary liver malignancies remains the SUV, with multiple studies showing significant associations in both hepatocellular carcinoma and cholangiocarcinoma. As the evidence is limited, and most studies are conducted retrospectively and with limited power, more research is needed in this field.

COLORECTAL MALIGNANCIES AND LIVER METASTASES
Introduction

Malignancies of the colon and rectum (colorectal carcinoma [CRC]) are the third most common malignancy and the third leading cause of cancer death in both men and women in the United States and many other Western countries.[68] About 100 new cases per 100,000 population are diagnosed every year with a 55% to 60% predominance in men. Major risk factors for developing CRC are a positive family history and inflammatory bowel disease; lifestyle factors are of less influence. Mortality rates are declining because of early detection of (pre-)cancerous lesions by screening programs and increasingly effective treatments. Nevertheless, about one-third of patients will die from CRC, and survival rates are greatly influenced by the stage of the disease. Furthermore, different treatment regimens have their own side effects. Therefore, adequate staging and selection of treatment is of vital importance.

Initial Diagnosis and Staging

Colonoscopy is the gold standard for detection of CRC, owing to its high sensitivity and high specificity (histopathology). CT-colonoscopy is a good alternative, especially if (complete) colonoscopy is not possible, or in cases where the exact tumor location cannot be determined, with sensitivity of 96% (95% confidence interval [CI] 94%–98%), which is comparable with that of colonoscopy (95%; 95% CI 90%–97%).[69] PET has no role in primary tumor detection. However, incidental focal bowel uptake on PET is regularly encountered and warrants further investigations. Peng and colleagues[70] found focal colonic uptake in 1.35% of the scans in a prospective study with greater than 10,000 PET scans, yielding cancerous and precancerous lesions in 20.5% and 23.5% of cases, respectively, confirmed by colonoscopy and pathology.

Primary tumor and lymph node staging

In daily practice, ceCT is used to determine primary tumor extent of CRC and lymph node status, with additional MR imaging or ultrasonography in rectal carcinomas. However, Buijsen and colleagues[71] demonstrated that PET/CT improves tumor delineation in radiotherapy planning of rectal cancer. In a study by Mori and Oguchi,[72] potential secondary malignancies proximal to a nonpassable tumor on colonoscopy were evaluated by PET/CT. In a total of 52 retrospectively analyzed patients who underwent PET before surgical resection, 16 of 17 additional tumors 8 mm or larger and proximal to the nonpassable tumor were correctly identified by PET. Smaller tumors, however, could not be detected, and distinction between adenoma and carcinoma could not reliably be made. Mainenti and colleagues[73] used PET/CT in identifying the primary tumor and defining local extent, correctly classifying the T stage in 33 of 35 patients, showing an accuracy of 94.3% (95% CI 87%–100%). These data show that PET may be an accurate modality for identifying primary tumor and defining local extent of CRC, especially in cases where specific questions need complementary imaging (treatment planning, nondiagnostic colonoscopy, and so forth). Further studies are needed for confirmation and definition of clinical value.

N staging with PET was the subject of a recent meta-analysis performed by Lu and colleagues.[74] A total of 409 patients from 10 studies were analyzed. The pooled estimates of sensitivity, specificity, positive likelihood ratio, and negative likelihood ratio of PET(/CT) in the detection of pretherapeutic lymph node involvement in patients with CRC were 42.9%, 87.9%, 2.82, and 0.69, respectively. Although specificity was found to be high, overall diagnostic accuracy was low (0.707). Low sensitivity for lymph node metastases might be due to insufficient spatial resolution of the PET scanner for small-sized lymph nodes, and obscuring of nodes by physiologic activity in the intestine and urinary bladder, or by the nearby primary tumor. The investigators concluded that there is no solid evidence to support the routine clinical application of PET(/CT) in the pretherapeutic evaluation of lymph node status in patients with CRC.

Detection of liver metastases

Detection of liver metastases has an important role in staging CRC, owing to the common dissemination route of hematologic metastases via the portal vein to the liver, and because liver metastases still hold potential for curative treatment. Another important factor related to treatment is the detection of extrahepatic metastases, which severely limit the potential for curative treatment. Prognosis and treatment options, however, are variable and depend on the number and site of extrahepatic metastases.[75] In the staging of CRC, noninvasive imaging plays an important role in: (1) detection of metastases at the time of initial diagnosis (synchronous metastases); (2) evaluation of resectability of liver metastases, or indications for other local therapies; (3) detection of recurring malignancy or metachronous metastases; and (4) follow-up during or after therapy for liver metastases.

Points mentioned under (1) and (2) depend on good per-patient detection and, to a somewhat lesser extent, per-lesion detection of liver metastases by various imaging techniques (discussed next); topics (3) and (4) are addressed under "Recurrence Detection."

In a meta-analysis, Niekel and colleagues[76] searched the literature between 1990 and 2010 for prospective studies comparing ceCT, MR imaging, and PET(/ceCT) in initial staging of CRC. Thirty-nine eligible studies were found, reporting on a total of 3391 patients. The pooled sensitivity estimates of ceCT, MR imaging, and PET on a per-lesion basis were 74.4%, 80.3%, and 81.4%, respectively (no statistical differences between groups). On a per-patient basis, the sensitivities of ceCT, MR imaging, and PET were 83.6%, 88.2%, and 94.1%, respectively (sensitivity of ceCT significantly lower than that of PET, $P = .025$). Per-patient specificity estimates were comparably high (>90%) for all modalities. There was no indication that different scanning protocols performed differently (ie, portal, arterial, and portal

phase imaging in ceCT, or different protocols and contrast materials in MR imaging). Data on PET combined with ceCT were too limited to compare with the other modalities. In an earlier meta-analysis by the same research group, lower sensitivities were found for ceCT and MR imaging.[77] Niekel and colleagues therefore argued that MR imaging has caught up with PET. However, data comparing MR imaging with PET/ceCT are limited. Another recent meta-analysis by Floriani and colleagues[78] yielded comparable results, although in this meta-analysis retrospective studies were also included.

Regarding the size of liver lesions, sensitivity of MR imaging for lesions smaller than 10 mm was significantly higher than that of ceCT ($P = .006$),[76] but data were limited for PET. In a study comparing 131 patients, selected for hepatic surgery of CRC liver metastases, ceCT and PET performed comparably, with detection of only 16% of lesions smaller than 10 mm, 72% to 75% of lesions between 10 and 20 mm, and 95% to 97% of lesions larger than 20 mm.[79] However, finding unexpected smaller hepatic metastases during hepatic surgery by intraoperative ultrasonography and palpation did not impose major changes in surgical management, as during surgery only 9 of 131 patients (6.8%) in this study appeared to have too extensive hepatic involvement to achieve curative resection. When it comes to evaluation of hepatic involvement, PET is not so superior over ceCT and MR imaging that it should inevitably be used as a first-line investigation. However, when ceCT or MR imaging is doubtful, PET should be used as a second-line investigation for evaluation of hepatic involvement.

Detection of extrahepatic metastases and impact on surgical management

Usually, ceCT is used to stage the liver and the rest of the abdomen plus chest. No randomized trials have been undertaken to determine the additional value of abdominal CT for detection of extrahepatic disease, and neither is the exact value of thoracic CT over chest radiography known. Serum carcinoembryonic antigen (CEA) is a specific, though not very sensitive, test to detect metastases of CRC at primary staging or during follow-up.[80]

The major advantage of PET in CRC is its ability to detect extrahepatic metastases. In a meta-analysis by Patel and colleagues,[81] 3 studies comprising a total of 178 patients were included that evaluated the diagnostic accuracy of PET/CT for the detection of extrahepatic lesions. In these studies PET was combined with non–contrast-enhanced, low-dose CT.[82–84] Given the heterogeneity in this small number of studies, no pooled estimates could be derived. The results of these studies suggest that PET/CT is more sensitive than ceCT for determining the presence of extrahepatic metastases (75%–89% vs 58%–64%, patient-based analysis), although specificities were in the same range (95%–96 vs 87%–97%).

Chan and colleagues[85] performed a systematic review to provide evidence-based guideline recommendations. Six studies were identified assessing the role of PET in the staging of CRC. Some studies showed no significant change in staging of distant metastases,[86–88] but others showed that PET had better performance than ceCT in detecting distant metastases,[89,90] and correctly changed management in 24% of cases.[90] Chan and colleagues pointed out that the studies which showed changes in M status and change of management included a large proportion of patients with advanced-stage CRC. In such a setting, differences in diagnostic performance between PET and ceCT are enhanced and more often significant. PET seems to have a higher detection rate than ceCT for extrahepatic metastases on a per-lesion basis, but in many cases this will not change M status (as this only denotes presence or absence of distant metastases, not number and site of metastases). Furthermore, finding additional extrahepatic metastases does not necessarily change management. However, in a select group of patients with solitary metastasis or oligometastases, the higher sensitivity of PET for extrahepatic metastases can play an important role. This group of patients comprises mainly those with hepatic metastases who are regarded as eligible for surgery.

Ruers and colleagues[91] performed a randomized controlled trial including 150 patients selected for surgical treatment of liver metastases from CRC. The primary outcome measure was futile laparotomy, defined as any laparotomy that did not result in complete tumor treatment, revealed benign disease, or did not result in a disease-free survival period longer than 6 months. Seventy-five patients in the control arm had conventional preoperative workup including ceCT of chest and abdomen, and 75 patients in the experimental arm had PET in addition to this. Patient and tumor characteristics were similar for both groups. The number of futile laparotomies was 34 (45%) in the control arm without PET and 21 (28%) in the experimental arm with PET; the relative risk reduction was 38% ($P = .042$). These results are in line with a change of management in 8% to 20% of patients reported in studies mentioned in the meta-analysis by Patel and colleagues.[81] The

multidisciplinary treatment team in the study by Ruers and colleagues had the freedom to disregard the additional findings of the PET. If all PET findings would have been accepted, the number of futile laparotomies could have been reduced even further by more than 65%. Ruers and colleagues[91] concluded that addition of PET to the workup for surgical resection of colorectal liver metastases prevented unnecessary surgery in 1 of 6 patients, and that PET should be implemented in the standard workup of such patients.

Recurrence Detection

Recurrent disease (local recurrence or metastases) may be detected by PET, even when conventional workup (including ceCT) fails to do so. Maas and colleagues[92] performed a meta-analysis to compare the diagnostic performance of PET(/CT), ceCT, and MR imaging as whole-body imaging modalities for the detection of local and/or distant recurrent disease in CRC patients who had a (high) suspicion of recurrent disease, based on clinical findings or increase in CEA. Data on MR imaging as whole-body imaging modality were limited (only 1 study). Other included studies, both prospective and retrospective, reported on PET (n = 12), PET/CT (n = 5), and ceCT (n = 5). Pooled data were used to calculate areas under the receiver-operating characteristic curve (AUC). AUCs for PET, PET/CT, and CT were 0.94 (95% CI 0.90–0.97), 0.94 (95% CI 0.87–0.98), and 0.83 (95% CI 0.72–0.90), respectively. In patient-based analyses, PET/CT had a slightly higher diagnostic performance than PET, with an AUC of 0.95 (95% CI 0.89–0.97) for PET/CT versus 0.92 (95% CI 0.86–0.96) for PET. It should be mentioned that in the PET/CT studies, various protocols were used for the CT part of PET/CT (with or without oral contrast and/or intravenous contrast).

Lu and colleagues[93] assessed the diagnostic performance of PET or PET/CT in the detection of recurrent CRC in patients with elevated CEA. In this meta-analysis, 11 studies with a total of 510 patients were included. The pooled estimates of sensitivity and specificity and positive and negative likelihood ratios of PET in the detection of tumor recurrence in CRC patients with elevated CEA were 90.3% (95% CI 85.5%–94.0%), 80.0% (95% CI 67.0%–89.6%), 2.88 (95% CI 1.37–6.07), and 0.12 (95% CI 0.07–0.20), respectively. The pooled estimates of sensitivity of PET/CT tended to be somewhat higher than PET without CT, and the specificity tended to be somewhat lower, but both were not significantly different from PET. Again, various CT protocols were used in the CT part of PET/CT.

In both meta-analyses discussed, PET(/CT) was regarded as a valuable diagnostic tool. Its superior accuracy over ceCT suggests that in clinical practice PET(/CT) should be the modality of choice for evaluation of patients suspected of recurring CRC. Additional studies are needed to confirm this finding.

Response Assessment and Prognosis

In multiple studies PET has been used to characterize CRC and predict prognosis regarding treatment stratification and early assessment of tumor response to therapy. PET may be used in evaluation of preoperative chemoradiotherapy in primary rectal cancer, chemotherapy in advanced CRC, and evaluation of effects of local therapies for liver metastases (**Fig. 4**).

Janssen and colleagues[94] predicted treatment response in the primary tumor in 30 patients with rectal cancer as early as 2 weeks after start of a 3-month neoadjuvant chemoradiotherapy scheme. Subsequently this model was evaluated to predict the pathology-based response in a second group of 21 patients. A cutoff value of 48% SUV_{max} reduction was selected to differentiate

responders from nonresponders (specificity of 100%, sensitivity of 64%). Applying this cutoff value to the second patient group resulted in specificity and sensitivity of 93% and 83%, respectively This PET-based prediction may be used to adjust timing and extent of surgery.

Byström and colleagues[95] used PET for early evaluation of response to palliative chemotherapy and for prediction of long-term outcome after 2 cycles of chemotherapy in a clinical trial including 51 patients with metastatic CRC. Response was assessed by ceCT after every 4 cycles of chemotherapy. The mean baseline SUV for all tumor lesions per patient was higher in nonresponders than in responders (mean 7.4 vs 5.6, $P = .02$). There was a strong correlation between metabolic response (changes in SUV) and objective response ($r = 0.57$, $P = .00001$), with sensitivity of 77% and specificity of 76%. No significant correlation between metabolic response and time to progression or overall survival was found. Byström and colleagues concluded that although metabolic response assessed by FDG-PET reflects radiologic tumor volume changes, the sensitivity and specificity are too low to support the routine use of PET in metastatic CRC. Furthermore, PET failed

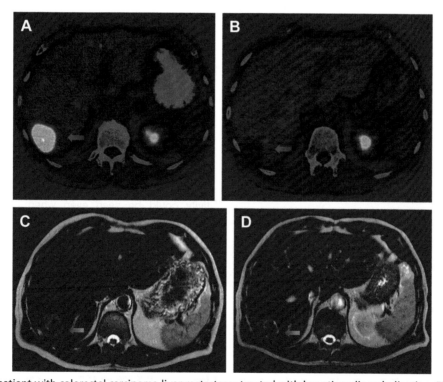

Fig. 4. A patient with colorectal carcinoma liver metastases treated with hepatic radioembolization. FDG-PET/CT pretreatment (*A*) and 6 weeks posttreatment (*B*) show a marked complete metabolic response (*red arrows*), whereas magnetic resonance imaging pretreatment (*C*) and 6 weeks posttreatment (*D*) show only a partial anatomic response (*blue arrows*).

to reflect long-term outcome and should not be used as surrogate end point for hard end-point benefit.

de Geus-Oei and colleagues[96] performed a systematic review including 15 studies assessing PET in early preoperative therapy evaluation and 5 studies determining the predictive value of PET in early response monitoring in metastatic CRC. The investigators concluded that, although the studies included showed large heterogeneity, by and large they indicated that PET is a significant predictor of therapy outcome in both situations.

Reasons for somewhat conflicting conclusions may be the heterogeneity and small size of studies on these topics. Furthermore, significant findings on a group level may not translate into adequate accuracy on a patient level to justify deviation from standard of care in therapeutic management. However, the potential of FDG-PET in early therapy response assessment in CRC appeals and further randomized trials may determine the position of FDG-PET in treatment schemes.

Summary

In CRC, PET(/CT) already has proved its additional value to conventional diagnostic modalities. Patients considered for hepatic surgery may especially benefit from PET, as PET may change management in up to 50% of cases in selected patient groups. Furthermore, care for patients with equivocal findings on conventional diagnostic imaging, patients suspected of recurrent disease, and patients with neoadjuvant treatment may be substantially optimized by PET. Implementation in standard clinical practice should be aimed for if not already accomplished. Current NCNN practice guidelines endorse the role of PET in patients with potentially resectable synchronous or metachronous disease, and to a lesser extent in patients with suspected recurrence and negative conventional workup.[97]

STROMA CELL TUMORS
Introduction

Gastrointestinal stroma cell tumors (GISTs) are soft-tissue tumors arising from the gastrointestinal tract. Although they share features with other soft-tissue tumors, and in the past frequently have been classified under several different entities, GISTs have specific features that set them apart from other soft-tissue tumors. Discovery of the C-kit proto-oncogene mutation, a feature of nearly all GISTs,[98] led to better ability to detect and correctly classify GISTs. Incidence rates were estimated at 150 new cases per year in the United States in the late 1990s,[99] but are now estimated

at 4000 to 5000 new cases each year (1.5 per 100,000).[68] GISTs can arise in every part of the gastrointestinal tract, but are most frequently found in the stomach (50%–60%) and small bowel (20%–30%), with the remainder of cases in esophagus, colon, and rectum. About two-thirds of GISTs are malignant, but most GISTs in the esophagus are benign and can be incidentally found at endoscopy.[99] Being resistant to radiotherapy and cytotoxic chemotherapy, treatment options were few for advanced GISTs in which curative resection could not be reached until the introduction of targeted therapies 10 years ago, with imatinib being the first.[100] Nevertheless, mortality rates are high, with only 53% 2-year survival in advanced-stage GIST.[68]

Response Assessment and Prognosis

The primary role of PET in GIST is in therapy response assessment and prognostication. In the early evaluation of imatinib, a tyrosine kinase inhibitor, as a potential therapy for metastatic GIST, PET was already used in a small series of patients as an early response assessment tool using the criteria of the European Organization for Research and Treatment of Cancer (EORTC),[101] and showed good correlation with clinical improvement and response objectified by ceCT after therapy (Fig. 5).[102]

Demetri and colleagues[103] assessed the efficacy and safety of imatinib in advanced GIST, and used PET complementary to ceCT in 64 patients to assess metabolic changes of the tumors. Histopathologic and molecular changes during treatment were evaluated in selected patients by means of serial biopsies of the tumor. In all responders, tumor-related glycolytic activity assessed by PET decreased markedly from baseline as early as 24 hours after a single dose of imatinib. Significant reduction of glycolytic activity could be seen even when biopsies still showed large numbers of viable residual tumor cells. Increases in tumor-related metabolic activity, activity at new sites, or both were seen in all patients with disease progression. PET results correlated with subsequent evidence of response or progression on ceCT or MR imaging.

In a small series of 21 patients (of whom 17 had GIST), Stroobants and colleagues[104] found that PET at baseline and day 8 of imatinib therapy predicted ceCT response at 8 weeks. Moreover, PET response was associated with longer progression-free survival (92% vs 12% at 1 year, $P<.01$).

Choi and colleagues[105] addressed the issue of CT being inadequate for early response monitoring of imatinib therapy in GIST when using standard

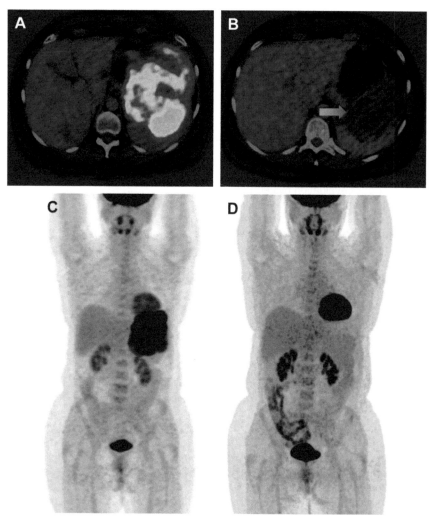

Fig. 5. FDG-PET/CT in a patient with GIST treated with imatinib. Transaxial slice through the stomach (*A*) and maximum-intensity projection (*C*) show intense FDG uptake in a large gastric stroma cell tumor before treatment, and complete metabolic response after 3 months of treatment (*B, D*), while CT shows a residual mass (*blue arrow*).

response criteria (RECIST), which are purely based on tumor size. In a series of 36 patients, the investigators reported both decreasing tumor density (reflecting tumor necrosis or decrease in tumor vessels) and decrease in FDG uptake in response to imatinib as good indicators and quantification of tumor response. About 20% of GISTs do not show elevated FDG uptake and cannot be monitored by PET.[105] Choi and colleagues concluded that monitoring tumor density on ceCT, either visually or quantitatively, provides a good alternative and is preferred over standard CT response criteria.

Despite the success of imatinib, about 14% of patients show primary imatinib resistance, and half of the patients with a good initial response will develop secondary resistance.[100] Newer tyrosine kinase inhibitors have become available to

address this issue. Prior and colleagues[106] evaluated response with PET after 4 weeks of therapy in 23 patients with GIST who had aborted previous imatinib therapy because of recent tumor progression or unacceptable imatinib toxicity. A decrease in SUV_{max} greater than 25% between baseline and after 1 therapeutic cycle of 4 weeks was strongly predictive of progression-free survival. The investigators stated that even a single PET scan at 4 weeks is able to predict progression-free survival and to discriminate responders from nonresponders.

In a multicenter study, Benjamin and colleagues[107] evaluated the efficacy and safety of motesanib in 138 patients with imatinib-resistant GIST. Response evaluation after 8 weeks was performed in 102 patients by ceCT according to RECIST and using the Choi criteria, and in 91 patients by PET according to EORTC. Patients were treated and evaluated by serial ceCTs up to 48 weeks. The tumor response rate based on EORTC criteria after 8 weeks of treatment was 30%, compared with a 3% response rate based on RECIST criteria. Based on the Choi response criteria, 41% had a tumor response after 8 weeks of treatment. However, Choi criteria for progression did not correlate well with real disease progression, as some patients marked as "progressive" in fact reached "stable disease" or "durable stable disease" (ie, ≥24 weeks). In conclusion, early response evaluation by ceCT according to Choi criteria and PET showed higher response rates than standard CT response criteria, and seemed to correlate better with objective antitumor activity.

Treglia and colleagues[100] conducted a literature review that included 19 original studies with a total of 628 GIST patients determining the role of PET in treatment response evaluation, of which some have already been discussed. From this literature review it was concluded that PET(/CT) has significant value in assessing treatment response to imatinib or other drugs in GIST patients, and that PET(/CT) allows an early assessment of treatment response and is a strong predictor of clinical outcome.

Summary

PET(/CT) is a valuable tool to monitor response in patients with GIST treated by tyrosine kinase inhibitors. Tumor response may be assessed as early as within 24 hours after the start of therapy, and metabolic changes precede structural changes on ceCT by weeks to months. However, about 20% of GISTs cannot be monitored by PET, and cost-effectiveness has not been proved in this still fairly rare malignancy; this might hamper implementation in standard clinical practice. At present, NCNN practice guidelines confirm the advantages of PET, but state that it should be used in addition to CT when this yields ambiguous results, and should not replace CT.[108]

DISCUSSION

PET/CT has proved to be a valuable imaging modality in the management of patients with gastrointestinal malignancies, including many different cell types. The primary strength of PET/CT is the combination of a whole-body imaging modality and its high sensitivity to detect malignant lesions. Its primary weakness is the relatively high rate of false-positive results and limited spatial resolution (Fig. 6).

In general, PET/CT is most valuable in the evaluation of M status/distant metastases. It performs best in patients who are at high risk of having M1 disease, and in patients with undetermined results on conventional imaging modalities, such as CT and MR imaging. For the evaluation of T status, a modality with better spatial resolution is needed to evaluate size, local spread, and possible ingrowth in surrounding structures. In part this may be solved by combining PET with diagnostic ceCT. Furthermore, for radiotherapy treatment planning it has been shown in several gastrointestinal malignancies that PET/CT has a valuable role, not so much for evaluation of T status, but especially as a sensitive imaging tool for delineation of local tumor activity. Unfortunately, the evaluation of N status is difficult in all cases. Although PET/CT is known for its high sensitivity, this may not be enough to detect small clusters of malignant cells within otherwise normal lymph nodes. In many cases PET/CT does not outperform more conventional imaging modalities in regard of detection of lymph node involvement. In the latter case all modalities perform rather poorly.

Besides staging, opportunities for PET/CT lie in the area of prognostication and response assessment. The functional information of glycolytic metabolism that may be quantified on PET/CT

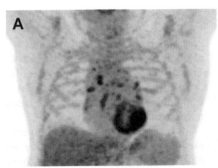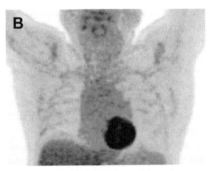

Fig. 6. A patient with colorectal carcinoma liver metastasis treated with hepatic radioembolization. A durable hepatic response was reported at 6 months after treatment (*A*), together with a sarcoid-like reaction with mediastinal lymphadenopathy. Follow-up at 9 months (*B*) with resolution of all abnormality confirmed this finding.

holds prognostic value in many cancer primaries, including gastrointestinal malignancies. This information may be used for improved patient selection before treatment. After treatment, conventional response monitoring using the well-known RE-CIST criteria may be supplemented by the evaluation of metabolic response using PET/CT, thus allowing one to monitor response early after treatment and possibly change treatment management accordingly.

The rapid development of hybrid imaging modalities and functional imaging tracers may be a threat to the widespread use of PET beyond staging alone. Besides new imaging strategies using new modalities and tracers, a focus should be placed on consolidation and further exploration of PET. There is a clear need for large prospective clinical trials on PET looking at quantification issues, standardization, cost-effectiveness, and new indications. It may be surmised that this will lead to improved patient management in general, and gastrointestinal malignancies in particular.

REFERENCES

1. Waddell T, Verheij M, Allum W, et al. Gastric cancer: ESMO-ESSO-ESTRO clinical practice guidelines for diagnosis, treatment and follow-up. Ann Oncol 2013;24(Suppl 6):vi57–63.

2. Shimada H, Okazumi S, Koyama M, et al. Japanese Gastric Cancer Association Task Force for Research Promotion: clinical utility of (1)(8)F-fluoro-2-deoxyglucose positron emission tomography in gastric cancer. A systematic review of the literature. Gastric Cancer 2011;14(1):13–21.

3. Takahashi H, Ukawa K, Ohkawa N, et al. Significance of (18)F-2-deoxy-2-fluoro-glucose accumulation in the stomach on positron emission tomography. Ann Nucl Med 2009;23(4):391–7.

4. Heusner TA, Hahn S, Hamami ME, et al. Gastrointestinal ^{18}F-FDG accumulation on PET without a corresponding CT abnormality is not an early indicator of cancer development. Eur Radiol 2009; 19(9):2171–9.

5. Kawamura T, Kusakabe T, Sugino T, et al. Expression of glucose transporter-1 in human gastric carcinoma: association with tumor aggressiveness, metastasis, and patient survival. Cancer 2001; 92(3):634–41.

6. Yamada A, Oguchi K, Fukushima M, et al. Evaluation of 2-deoxy-2-[^{18}F]fluoro-D-glucose positron emission tomography in gastric carcinoma: relation to histological subtypes, depth of tumor invasion, and glucose transporter-1 expression. Ann Nucl Med 2006;20(9):597–604.

7. Podoloff DA, Ball DW, Ben-Josef E, et al. NCCN Task Force: clinical utility of PET in a variety of tumor types. J Natl Compr Canc Netw 2009; 7(Suppl 2):S1–26.

8. Yang QM, Bando E, Kawamura T, et al. The diagnostic value of PET/CT for peritoneal dissemination of abdominal malignancies. Gan To Kagaku Ryoho 2006;33(12):1817–21.

9. Jadvar H, Tatlidil R, Garcia AA, et al. Evaluation of recurrent gastric malignancy with [F-18]-FDG positron emission tomography. Clin Radiol 2003;58(3): 215–21.

10. De Potter T, Flamen P, Van Cutsem E, et al. Whole-body PET with FDG for the diagnosis of recurrent gastric cancer. Eur J Nucl Med Mol Imaging 2002;29(4):525–9.

11. Sim SH, Kim YJ, Oh DY, et al. The role of PET/CT in detection of gastric cancer recurrence. BMC Cancer 2009;9:73.

12. Sun L. Clinical role of ^{18}F-fluorodeoxyglucose positron emission tomography/computed tomography in post-operative follow up of gastric cancer: initial results. World J Gastroenterol 2008;14(29):4627.

13. Park MJ, Lee WJ, Lim HK, et al. Detecting recurrence of gastric cancer: the value of FDG PET/CT. Abdom Imaging 2009;34(4):441–7.

14. Nakamoto Y, Togashi K, Kaneta T, et al. Clinical value of whole-body FDG-PET for recurrent gastric cancer: a multicenter study. Jpn J Clin Oncol 2009; 39(5):297–302.

15. Kim DW, Park SA, Kim CG. Detecting the recurrence of gastric cancer after curative resection: comparison of FDG PET/CT and contrast-enhanced abdominal CT. J Korean Med Sci 2011; 26(7):875–80.

16. Bilici A, Ustaalioglu BB, Seker M, et al. The role of (1)(8)F-FDG PET/CT in the assessment of suspected recurrent gastric cancer after initial surgical resection: can the results of FDG PET/CT influence patients' treatment decision making? Eur J Nucl Med Mol Imaging 2011;38(1):64–73.

17. Sharma P, Singh H, Suman SK, et al. ^{18}F-FDG PET/CT for detecting recurrent gastric adenocarcinoma: results from a non-Oriental Asian population. Nucl Med Commun 2012;33(9):960–6.

18. Choi BW, Zeon SK, Kim SH, et al. Significance of SUV on follow-up F-18 FDG PET at the anastomotic site of gastroduodenostomy after distal subtotal gastrectomy in patients with gastric cancer. Nucl Med Mol Imaging 2011;45(4):285–90.

19. Couper GW, McAteer D, Wallis F, et al. Detection of response to chemotherapy using positron emission tomography in patients with oesophageal and gastric cancer. Br J Surg 1998;85(10):1403–6.

20. de Geus-Oei LF, Vriens D, Arens AI, et al. FDG-PET/CT based response-adapted treatment. Cancer Imaging 2012;12:324–35.

21. Ott K, Herrmann K, Lordick F, et al. Early metabolic response evaluation by fluorine-18 fluorodeoxyglucose

positron emission tomography allows in vivo testing of chemosensitivity in gastric cancer: long-term results of a prospective study. Clin Cancer Res 2008; 14(7):2012–8.

22. Lordick F. Optimizing neoadjuvant chemotherapy through the use of early response evaluation by positron emission tomography. Recent Results Cancer Res 2012;196:201–11.

23. NCCN Clinical Practice Guidelines in Oncology (NCCN Guidelines®): gastric cancer, version 1.2014. Available at: http://www.nccn.org/profes sionals/physician_gls/PDF/gastric.pdf. Accessed June 17, 2014.

24. Gambhir SS, Czernin J, Schwimmer J, et al. A tabulated summary of the FDG PET literature. J Nucl Med 2001;42(Suppl 5):1S–93S.

25. Tang S, Huang G, Liu J, et al. Usefulness of ^{18}F-FDG PET, combined FDG-PET/CT and EUS in diagnosing primary pancreatic carcinoma: a meta-analysis. Eur J Radiol 2011;78(1):142–50.

26. Kauhanen SP, Komar G, Seppanen MP, et al. A prospective diagnostic accuracy study of ^{18}F-fluorodeoxyglucose positron emission tomography/computed tomography, multidetector row computed tomography, and magnetic resonance imaging in primary diagnosis and staging of pancreatic cancer. Ann Surg 2009;250(6):957–63.

27. Asagi A, Ohta K, Nasu J, et al. Utility of contrast-enhanced FDG-PET/CT in the clinical management of pancreatic cancer: impact on diagnosis, staging, evaluation of treatment response, and detection of recurrence. Pancreas 2013;42(1):11–9.

28. Heinrich S, Goerres GW, Schafer M, et al. Positron emission tomography/computed tomography influences on the management of resectable pancreatic cancer and its cost-effectiveness. Ann Surg 2005;242(2):235–43.

29. Bang S, Chung HW, Park SW, et al. The clinical usefulness of 18-fluorodeoxyglucose positron emission tomography in the differential diagnosis, staging, and response evaluation after concurrent chemoradiotherapy for pancreatic cancer. J Clin Gastroenterol 2006;40(10):923–9.

30. Strobel K, Heinrich S, Bhure U, et al. Contrast-enhanced ^{18}F-FDG PET/CT: 1-stop-shop imaging for assessing the resectability of pancreatic cancer. J Nucl Med 2008;49(9):1408–13.

31. Ruf J, Lopez Hanninen E, Oettle H, et al. Detection of recurrent pancreatic cancer: comparison of FDG-PET with CT/MRI. Pancreatology 2005;5(2–3):266–72.

32. Rose DM, Delbeke D, Beauchamp RD, et al. [18]Fluorodeoxyglucose-positron emission tomography in the management of patients with suspected pancreatic cancer. Ann Surg 1999;229(5):729–37 [discussion: 737–8].

33. Franke C, Klapdor R, Meyerhoff K, et al. 18-FDG positron emission tomography of the pancreas:

34. Jadvar H, Fischman AJ. Evaluation of pancreatic carcinoma with FDG PET. Abdom Imaging 2001; 26(3):254–9.

35. Sperti C, Pasquali C, Bissoli S, et al. Tumor relapse after pancreatic cancer resection is detected earlier by 18-FDG PET than by CT. J Gastrointest Surg 2010;14(1):131–40.

36. Kitajima K, Murakami K, Yamasaki E, et al. Performance of integrated FDG-PET/contrast-enhanced CT in the diagnosis of recurrent pancreatic cancer: comparison with integrated FDG-PET/non-contrast-enhanced CT and enhanced CT. Mol Imaging Biol 2010;12(4):452–9.

37. Casneuf V, Delrue L, Kelles A, et al. Is combined ^{18}F-fluorodeoxyglucose-positron emission tomography/computed tomography superior to positron emission tomography or computed tomography alone for diagnosis, staging and restaging of pancreatic lesions? Acta Gastroenterol Belg 2007;70(4):331–8.

38. Maemura K, Takao S, Shinchi H, et al. Role of positron emission tomography in decisions on treatment strategies for pancreatic cancer. J Hepatobiliary Pancreat Surg 2006;13(5):435–41.

39. Kittaka H, Takahashi H, Ohigashi H, et al. Role of (18) F-fluorodeoxyglucose positron emission tomography/computed tomography in predicting the pathologic response to preoperative chemoradiation therapy in patients with resectable T3 pancreatic cancer. World J Surg 2013;37(1):169–78.

40. Topkan E, Parlak C, Kotek A, et al. Predictive value of metabolic [18]FDG-PET response on outcomes in patients with locally advanced pancreatic carcinoma treated with definitive concurrent chemoradiotherapy. BMC Gastroenterol 2011;11:123.

41. Barber TW, Kalff V, Cherk MH, et al. ^{18}F-FDG PET/CT influences management in patients with known or suspected pancreatic cancer. Intern Med J 2011;41(11):776–83.

42. Yao J, Gan G, Farlow D, et al. Impact of F18-fluorodeoxyglycose positron emission tomography/computed tomography on the management of resectable pancreatic tumours. ANZ J Surg 2012;82(3):140–4.

43. Javery O, Shyn P, Mortele K. FDG PET or PET/CT in patients with pancreatic cancer: when does it add to diagnostic CT or MRI? Clin Imaging 2013;37(2): 295–301.

44. Dibble EH, Karantanis D, Mercier G, et al. PET/CT of cancer patients: part 1, pancreatic neoplasms. AJR Am J Roentgenol 2012;199(5):952–67.

45. NCCN Clinical Practice Guidelines in Oncology (NCCN Guidelines®): pancreatic adenocarcinoma, version 2.2014. Available at: http://www.nccn.org/professionals/physician_gls/PDF/pancreatic.pdf. Accessed June 17, 2014.

46. European Association for the Study of the Liver, European Organisation for Research and Treatment of Cancer. EASL-EORTC clinical practice guidelines: management of hepatocellular carcinoma. J Hepatol 2012;56(4):908–43.

47. National Cancer Institute, The SEER Cancer Statistics Review, 1975–2011. Available at: http://seer.cancer.gov/csr/1975_2011/results_merged/topic_survival.pdf. Accessed January 31, 2014.

48. Lan BY, Kwee SA, Wong LL. Positron emission tomography in hepatobiliary and pancreatic malignancies: a review. Am J Surg 2012;204(2):232–41.

49. Torizuka T, Tamaki N, Inokuma T, et al. In vivo assessment of glucose metabolism in hepatocellular carcinoma with FDG-PET. J Nucl Med 1995;36(10):1811–7.

50. Khan MA, Combs CS, Brunt EM, et al. Positron emission tomography scanning in the evaluation of hepatocellular carcinoma. J Hepatol 2000;32(5):792–7.

51. Bohm B, Voth M, Geoghegan J, et al. Impact of positron emission tomography on strategy in liver resection for primary and secondary liver tumors. J Cancer Res Clin Oncol 2004;130(5):266–72.

52. Wudel LJ Jr, Delbeke D, Morris D, et al. The role of [18F]fluorodeoxyglucose positron emission tomography imaging in the evaluation of hepatocellular carcinoma. Am Surg 2003;69(2):117–24 [discussion: 124–6].

53. Lin CY, Chen JH, Liang JA, et al. 18F-FDG PET or PET/CT for detecting extrahepatic metastases or recurrent hepatocellular carcinoma: a systematic review and meta-analysis. Eur J Radiol 2012;81(9):2417–22.

54. Paudyal B, Paudyal P, Oriuchi N, et al. Clinical implication of glucose transport and metabolism evaluated by 18F-FDG PET in hepatocellular carcinoma. Int J Oncol 2008;33(5):1047–54.

55. Seo S, Hatano E, Higashi T, et al. Fluorine-18 fluorodeoxyglucose positron emission tomography predicts tumor differentiation, P-glycoprotein expression, and outcome after resection in hepatocellular carcinoma. Clin Cancer Res 2007;13(2 Pt 1):427–33.

56. Jarnagin WR, Fong Y, DeMatteo RP, et al. Staging, resectability, and outcome in 225 patients with hilar cholangiocarcinoma. Ann Surg 2001;234(4):507–17 [discussion: 517–9].

57. Petrowsky H, Wildbrett P, Husarik DB, et al. Impact of integrated positron emission tomography and computed tomography on staging and management of gallbladder cancer and cholangiocarcinoma. J Hepatol 2006;45(1):43–50.

58. Anderson CD, Rice MH, Pinson CW, et al. Fluorodeoxyglucose PET imaging in the evaluation of gallbladder carcinoma and cholangiocarcinoma. J Gastrointest Surg 2004;8(1):90–7.

59. Kim JW, Seong J, Yun M, et al. Usefulness of positron emission tomography with fluorine-18-fluorodeoxyglucose in predicting treatment response in unresectable hepatocellular carcinoma patients treated with external beam radiotherapy. Int J Radiat Oncol Biol Phys 2012;82(3):1172–8.

60. Ahn SG, Kim SH, Jeon TJ, et al. The role of preoperative [18F]fluorodeoxyglucose positron emission tomography in predicting early recurrence after curative resection of hepatocellular carcinomas. J Gastrointest Surg 2011;15(11):2044–52.

61. Kim BK, Kang WJ, Kim JK, et al. 18F-fluorodeoxyglucose uptake on positron emission tomography as a prognostic predictor in locally advanced hepatocellular carcinoma. Cancer 2011;117(20):4779–87.

62. Hatano E, Ikai I, Higashi T, et al. Preoperative positron emission tomography with fluorine-18-fluorodeoxyglucose is predictive of prognosis in patients with hepatocellular carcinoma after resection. World J Surg 2006;30(9):1736–41.

63. Lee JH, Park JY, Kim do Y, et al. Prognostic value of 18F-FDG PET for hepatocellular carcinoma patients treated with sorafenib. Liver Int 2011;31(8):1144–9.

64. Kitamura K, Hatano E, Higashi T, et al. Preoperative FDG-PET predicts recurrence patterns in hepatocellular carcinoma. Ann Surg Oncol 2012;19(1):156–62.

65. Ahn SG, Jeon TJ, Lee SD, et al. A survival benefit of major hepatectomy for hepatocellular carcinoma identified by preoperative [18F] fluorodeoxyglucose positron emission tomography in patients with well-preserved hepatic function. Eur J Surg Oncol 2013;39(9):964–73.

66. Furukawa H, Ikuma H, Asakura-Yokoe K, et al. Preoperative staging of biliary carcinoma using 18F-fluorodeoxyglucose PET: prospective comparison with PET+CT, MDCT and histopathology. Eur Radiol 2008;18(12):2841–7.

67. Haug AR, Heinemann V, Bruns CJ, et al. 18F-FDG PET independently predicts survival in patients with cholangiocellular carcinoma treated with 90Y microspheres. Eur J Nucl Med Mol Imaging 2011;38(6):1037–45.

68. American Cancer Society, Colorectal Cancer Facts and Figures 2011–2013. Available at: http://www.cancer.org/acs/groups/content/@epidemiologysurveilance/documents/document/acspc-028323.pdffigures-2011-2013-page. Accessed November 19, 2013.

69. Pickhardt PJ, Hassan C, Halligan S, et al. Colorectal cancer: CT colonography and colonoscopy for detection–systematic review and meta-analysis. Radiology 2011;259(2):393–405.

70. Peng J, He Y, Xu J, et al. Detection of incidental colorectal tumours with 18F-labelled 2-fluoro-2-deoxyglucose positron emission tomography/computed tomography scans: results of a prospective study. Colorectal Dis 2011;13(11):e374–8.

71. Buijsen J, van den Bogaard J, van der Weide H, et al. FDG-PET/CT reduces the interobserver variability in rectal tumor delineation. Radiother Oncol 2012;102(3):371–6.

72. Mori S, Oguchi K. Application of (18)F-fluorodeoxyglucose positron emission tomography to detection of proximal lesions of obstructive colorectal cancer. Jpn J Radiol 2010;28(8):584–90.

73. Mainenti PP, Iodice D, Segreto S, et al. Colorectal cancer and 18FDG-PET/CT: what about adding the T to the N parameter in loco-regional staging? World J Gastroenterol 2011;17(11):1427–33.

74. Lu YY, Chen JH, Ding HJ, et al. A systematic review and meta-analysis of pretherapeutic lymph node staging of colorectal cancer by 18F-FDG PET or PET/CT. Nucl Med Commun 2012;33(11):1127–33.

75. Spolverato G, Ejaz A, Azad N, et al. Surgery for colorectal liver metastases: the evolution of determining prognosis. World J Gastrointest Oncol 2013;5(12):207–21.

76. Niekel MC, Bipat S, Stoker J. Diagnostic imaging of colorectal liver metastases with CT, MR imaging, FDG PET, and/or FDG PET/CT: a meta-analysis of prospective studies including patients who have not previously undergone treatment. Radiology 2010;257(3):674–84.

77. Bipat S, van Leeuwen MS, Comans EF, et al. Colorectal liver metastases: CT, MR imaging, and PET for diagnosis–meta-analysis. Radiology 2005; 237(1):123–31.

78. Floriani I, Torri V, Rulli E, et al. Performance of imaging modalities in diagnosis of liver metastases from colorectal cancer: a systematic review and meta-analysis. J Magn Reson Imaging 2010; 31(1):19–31.

79. Wiering B, Ruers TJ, Krabbe PF, et al. Comparison of multiphase CT, FDG-PET and intra-operative ultrasound in patients with colorectal liver metastases selected for surgery. Ann Surg Oncol 2007; 14(2):818–26.

80. Kievit J. Follow-up of patients with colorectal cancer: numbers needed to test and treat. Eur J Cancer 2002;38(7):986–99.

81. Patel S, McCall M, Ohinmaa A, et al. Positron emission tomography/computed tomographic scans compared to computed tomographic scans for detecting colorectal liver metastases: a systematic review. Ann Surg 2011;253(4):666–71.

82. Selzner M, Hany TF, Wildbrett P, et al. Does the novel PET/CT imaging modality impact on the treatment of patients with metastatic colorectal cancer of the liver? Ann Surg 2004;240(6):1027–34 [discussion: 1035–6].

83. Bellomi M, Rizzo S, Travaini LL, et al. Role of multidetector CT and FDG-PET/CT in the diagnosis of local and distant recurrence of resected rectal cancer. Radiol Med 2007;112(5):681–90 [in English, Italian].

84. Rappeport ED, Loft A, Berthelsen AK, et al. Contrast-enhanced FDG-PET/CT vs. SPIO-enhanced MRI vs. FDG-PET vs. CT in patients with liver metastases from colorectal cancer: a prospective study with intraoperative confirmation. Acta Radiol 2007;48(4):369–78.

85. Chan K, Welch S, Walker-Dilks C, et al. Evidence-based guideline recommendations on the use of positron emission tomography imaging in colorectal cancer. Clin Oncol (R Coll Radiol) 2012; 24(4):232–49.

86. Furukawa H, Ikuma H, Seki A, et al. Positron emission tomography scanning is not superior to whole body multidetector helical computed tomography in the preoperative staging of colorectal cancer. Gut 2006;55(7):1007–11.

87. Nahas CS, Akhurst T, Yeung H, et al. Positron emission tomography detection of distant metastatic or synchronous disease in patients with locally advanced rectal cancer receiving preoperative chemoradiation. Ann Surg Oncol 2008;15(3):704–11.

88. Kinner S, Antoch G, Bockisch A, et al. Whole-body PET/CT-colonography: a possible new concept for colorectal cancer staging. Abdom Imaging 2007; 32(5):606–12.

89. Kosugi C, Saito N, Murakami K, et al. Positron emission tomography for preoperative staging in patients with locally advanced or metastatic colorectal adenocarcinoma in lymph node metastasis. Hepatogastroenterol 2008;55(82–83):398–402.

90. Park IJ, Kim HC, Yu CS, et al. Efficacy of PET/CT in the accurate evaluation of primary colorectal carcinoma. Eur J Surg Oncol 2006;32(9):941–7.

91. Ruers TJ, Wiering B, van der Sijp JR, et al. Improved selection of patients for hepatic surgery of colorectal liver metastases with (18)F-FDG PET: a randomized study. J Nucl Med 2009;50(7):1036–41.

92. Maas M, Rutten IJ, Nelemans PJ, et al. What is the most accurate whole-body imaging modality for assessment of local and distant recurrent disease in colorectal cancer? A meta-analysis: imaging for recurrent colorectal cancer. Eur J Nucl Med Mol Imaging 2011;38(8):1560–71.

93. Lu YY, Chen JH, Chien CR, et al. Use of FDG-PET or PET/CT to detect recurrent colorectal cancer in patients with elevated CEA: a systematic review and meta-analysis. Int J Colorectal Dis 2013; 28(8):1039–47.

94. Janssen MH, Ollers MC, van Stiphout RG, et al. PET-based treatment response evaluation in rectal cancer: prediction and validation. Int J Radiat Oncol Biol Phys 2012;82(2):871–6.

95. Byström P, Berglund A, Garske U, et al. Early prediction of response to first-line chemotherapy by sequential [18F]-2-fluoro-2-deoxy-D-glucose positron emission tomography in patients with advanced colorectal cancer. Ann Oncol 2009;20(6):1057–61.

96. de Geus-Oei LF, Vriens D, van Laarhoven HW, et al. Monitoring and predicting response to therapy with ^{18}F-FDG PET in colorectal cancer: a systematic review. J Nucl Med 2009;50(Suppl 1):43S–54S.

97. NCCN Clinical Practice Guidelines in Oncology (NCCN Guidelines®): colon cancer, version 3.2014. Available at: http://www.nccn.org/profes sionals/physician_gls/PDF/colon.pdf.   Accessed June 30, 2014.

98. Isozaki K, Hirota S. Gain-of-function mutations of receptor tyrosine kinases in gastrointestinal stromal tumors. Curr Genomics 2006;7(8):469–75.

99. Pidhorecky I, Cheney RT, Kraybill WG, et al. Gastrointestinal stromal tumors: current diagnosis, biologic behavior, and management. Ann Surg Oncol 2000;7(9):705–12.

100. Treglia G, Mirk P, Stefanelli A, et al. ^{18}F-Fluorodeoxyglucose positron emission tomography in evaluating treatment response to imatinib or other drugs in gastrointestinal stromal tumors: a systematic review. Clin Imaging 2012;36(3):167–75.

101. Young H, Baum R, Cremerius U, et al. Measurement of clinical and subclinical tumour response using [^{18}F]-fluorodeoxyglucose and positron emission tomography: review and 1999 EORTC recommendations. European Organization for Research and Treatment of Cancer (EORTC) PET Study Group. Eur J Cancer 1999;35(13):1773–82.

102. van Oosterom AT, Judson I, Verweij J, et al. Safety and efficacy of imatinib (STI571) in metastatic gastrointestinal stromal tumours: a phase I study. Lancet 2001;358(9291):1421–3.

103. Demetri GD, von Mehren M, Blanke CD, et al. Efficacy and safety of imatinib mesylate in advanced gastrointestinal stromal tumors. N Engl J Med 2002;347(7):472–80.

104. Stroobants S, Goeminne J, Seegers M, et al. [18]FDG-Positron emission tomography for the early prediction of response in advanced soft tissue sarcoma treated with imatinib mesylate (Glivec). Eur J Cancer 2003;39(14):2012–20.

105. Choi H, Charnsangavej C, de Castro Faria S, et al. CT evaluation of the response of gastrointestinal stromal tumors after imatinib mesylate treatment: a quantitative analysis correlated with FDG PET findings. AJR Am J Roentgenol 2004;183(6):1619–28.

106. Prior JO, Montemurro M, Orcurto MV, et al. Early prediction of response to sunitinib after imatinib failure by ^{18}F-fluorodeoxyglucose positron emission tomography in patients with gastrointestinal stromal tumor. J Clin Oncol 2009;27(3):439–45.

107. Benjamin RS, Schoffski P, Hartmann JT, et al. Efficacy and safety of motesanib, an oral inhibitor of VEGF, PDGF, and Kit receptors, in patients with imatinib-resistant gastrointestinal stromal tumors. Cancer Chemother Pharmacol 2011;68(1):69–77.

108. NCCN Clinical Practice Guidelines in Oncology (NCCN Guidelines®): soft tissue sarcoma, version 2.2014. Available at: http://www.nccn.org/profes sionals/physician_gls/PDF/sarcoma.pdf. Accessed June 30, 2014.

Fluorine-18-fluorodeoxyglucose Positron Emission Tomography in Diffuse Large B-cell Lymphoma

Karen Juul Mylam, MD[a],*, Anne Lerberg Nielsen, MD[b],
Lars Møller Pedersen, MD[c], Martin Hutchings, MD, PhD[d]

KEYWORDS

• FDG-PET • Lymphoma • Staging • Response evaluation • Response criteria • Surveillance

KEY POINTS

- Fluorine-18-fluorodeoxyglucose positron emission tomography (FDG-PET)/computed tomography (CT) offers higher sensitivity and specificity for staging than CT alone.
- At present, there is insufficient evidence to change standard treatment based on the result of interim FDG-PET/CT scan.
- Tailored treatment trials according to the result of interim FDG-PET/CT are being conducted and results are awaited.
- FDG-PET is more accurate than CT to detect residual disease at the conclusion of therapy.
- FDG-PET/CT is recommended for staging and response evaluation after the completion of therapy.

INTRODUCTION

According to the World Health Organization (WHO) classification of lymphomas, non-Hodgkin lymphomas (NHLs) are subclassified according to their histologic lineage, immunophenotype, and maturation. Lymphomas are divided into aggressive and indolent lymphomas, and into B-cell and T-cell lymphomas.[1] The most common type of aggressive B-cell NHL is diffuse large B-cell lymphoma (DLBCL), which is generally very chemosensitive. However, even though most patients respond well to chemotherapy, 30% of patients with DLBCL still experience a relapse, most commonly within the first 2 years after therapy.

Most lymphomas are 18F-fluorodeoxyglucose (FDG) avid and the more aggressive the lymphoma, the higher the FDG avidity.[2] Weiler-Sagie and colleagues[3] performed a study among 766 patients with Hodgkin lymphoma (HL), DLBCL, and follicular lymphoma and found that 97% of patients with DLBCL had FDG-avid lesions, with an FDG uptake in DLBCL that was 3-fold higher than in indolent lymphomas.[4]

FDG–POSITRON EMISSION TOMOGRAPHY FOR INITIAL STAGING OF LYMPHOMA
FDG–Positron Emission Tomography Versus CT

Prognostication of patients with DLBCL currently consists of baseline standard laboratory

[a] Department of Hematology, Odense University Hospital, Sønder Boulevard 29, Odense 5000, Denmark;
[b] Department of Nuclear Medicine, Odense University Hospital, Sønder Boulevard 29, Odense 5000, Denmark;
[c] Department of Hematology, Roskilde Hospital, Køgevej 7-13, Roskilde 4000, Denmark; [d] Department of Hematology, Rigshospitalet, Copenhagen University Hospital, Blegdamsvej 9, Copenhagen 2100, Denmark
* Corresponding author.
E-mail address: karen.mylam@rsyd.dk

PET Clin 9 (2014) 443–455
http://dx.doi.org/10.1016/j.cpet.2014.06.001
1556-8598/14/$ – see front matter © 2014 Elsevier Inc. All rights reserved.

examinations, bone marrow biopsy, and FDG–positron emission tomography (PET)/CT. Ann Arbor staging is the currently most widely used staging classification for all types of lymphoma. Ann Arbor staging depends on both location of involved sites and on certain B symptoms likely to represent systemic dissemination of the lymphoma (**Table 1**).[5]

The Ann Arbor staging classification was designed to help in defining radiotherapy fields for patients with HL when this was the main treatment modality. It is still widely applied because patients are allocated to different treatment strategies according to their stage. The extension of the disease, as reflected by the stage, is one of the most important predictors of outcome for any type of lymphoma. However, to create a better prognostic model for aggressive NHL, the international prognostic index (IPI) was developed and incorporates additional adverse factors such as increased lactate dehydrogenase, more than 1 extranodal site, age above 60 years, performance status more than 1, and Ann Arbor stage 3 or 4.[6] A higher IPI allocates the patient to an adverse prognostic group.

The Cotswolds revision of the Ann Arbor staging system was published in 1990 and incorporated the use of CT into lymphoma staging.[7] An enhanced IPI (National Comprehensive Cancer Network [NCCN]-IPI) was recently devised to improve risk stratification in the rituximab era. This clinically based NCCN-IPI discriminates low-risk and high-risk patients with DLBCL better than the original IPI.[8]

Until 2000, CT was the standard imaging modality for staging; however, CT has several shortcomings, such as inability to identify malignancy in normal size lymph nodes or to differentiate between lymph nodes enlarged because of malignant and benign causes. FDG-PET depicts pathologic metabolism, which substantially adds information to morphologic imaging. Several studies have shown that FDG-PET/CT has higher staging accuracy than CT alone.[9,10] A meta-analysis by Isasi and colleagues[11] evaluated the diagnostic accuracy of FDG-PET in the staging of lymphoma and, out of a total of 14 patient-based studies, the median sensitivity was 90.3% and the median specificity was 91.1%. The impact of PET/CT on stage migration has mainly been studied in HL, and in DLBCL upstaging occurs more often than downstaging, although both situations occur.[12,13] Stage I disease is less frequently found and skeletal lesions are more frequently found in the PET era.[14] Although upstaging occurs in 11% to 41% of patients undergoing staging FDG-PET/CT, the frequency of therapy change as a result of FDG-PET/CT for staging is 8% to 25%,[10,12,13,15,16] even though no studies have shown an improved outcome for patients treated more aggressively because of this stage migration. Limited literature exists on staging performed with whole-body diffusion-weighted imaging (WB-DWI), but a smaller study comparing staging results of 12 patients with DLBCL undergoing both PET/CT and WB-DWI found that the two modalities performed equally well.[17] Both the NCCN guidelines and the new guidelines from the International Conference on Malignant Lymphomas imaging working group recommend performing FDG-PET scans in DLBCL at baseline because of the high staging accuracy and potential therapeutic impact (**Fig. 1**).[18]

FDG-PET in Detection of Bone Marrow Involvement

Routine bone marrow biopsy is performed in order to detect extranodal involvement in patients who have disease limited to the lymph nodes detected on the imaging. The ability of FDG-PET to detect bone marrow involvement has been a controversial issue. Early studies did not convincingly

Table 1
Ann Arbor staging

Ann Arbor Stage I	Ann Arbor Stage II	Ann Arbor Stage III	Ann Arbor Stage IV
Involvement of a single lymph node region (I) or of a single extralymphatic organ or site (IE)	Involvement of 2 or more lymph node regions or lymphatic structures on the same side of the diaphragm alone (II) or with involvement of limited, contiguous, extralymphatic organ or tissue (IIE)	Involvement of lymph node regions on both sides of the diaphragm (III), which may include the spleen (IIIS) or limited, contiguous, extralymphatic organ or site (IIIE), or both (IIIES)	Diffuse or disseminated foci of involvement of 1 or more extralymphatic organs or tissues, with or without associated lymphatic involvement

Liver, lung, and bone marrow involvement always indicates stage IV disease.

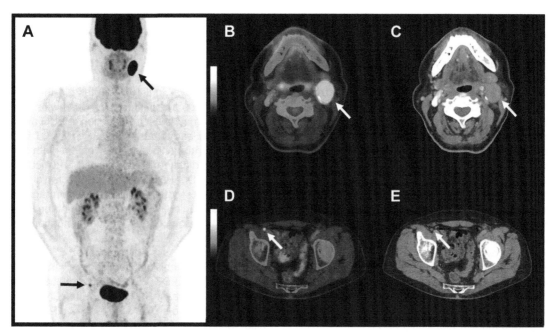

Fig. 1. Staging small parailiac lymph node. Baseline FDG PET/CT of patient with diffuse large cell B-cell lymphoma showing focal FDG-uptake on left side of neck and in pelvic region on the maximal intensity projection (*A, arrows*). A large lymph node in the left side of the neck is demonstrated on PET/CT and CT (*B and C, arrows*). PET/CT also reveals a small but intense FDG-avid lymph node in right parailiac region (*D, arrow*), not exceeding the size of pathologic lymph nodes on CT (*E, arrow*) and could be overlooked on CT alone.

show that FDG-PET can replace bone marrow biopsy. Present guidelines still recommend performing bone marrow biopsy in all patients with DLBCL who are eligible for curative treatment and in whom there is a possible therapeutic impact.[18] However, bone marrow biopsy has many false-negative results caused by sampling error.[19] Pakos and colleagues[19] performed a meta-analysis showing that FDG-PET had a pooled sensitivity and specificity of 43% and 88% respectively for the detection of bone marrow involvement in a mixed group of NHL. The low sensitivity was mainly explained by difficulties interpreting diffuse FDG uptake, leading to a high number of false-negative results. Adams and colleagues[20] performed a systematic review and meta-analysis including 7 studies with DLBCL and showed that FDG-PET/CT achieves pooled sensitivity and specificity estimates of 88.7% (range, 84.0%–95.8%) and 99.8% (range, 99.0%–100.0%) for the detection of bone marrow involvement. The investigators concluded that positive focal and diffuse FDG-PET findings of bone marrow could obviate subsequent bone marrow biopsy. Patients with PET-negative bone marrow should continue to have bone marrow biopsy taken if it has prognostic and/or therapeutic implications. This advice was confirmed in a recent retrospective study that found that 5 of 16

patients with a positive bone marrow biopsy were classified as negative for bone marrow involvement after FDG-PET/CT.[21] Khan and colleagues[22] also challenged the need to perform routine bone marrow biopsy in all patients with DLBCL. The investigators presented data on 130 patients with DLBCL and found that out of 44 stage IV patients none were allocated to this stage because of bone marrow biopsy alone. FDG-PET/CT had a much higher sensitivity of 94% in detecting bone marrow involvement than bone marrow biopsy (40%), whereas the specificity was 100% for both methods. There is currently no consensus as to whether diffuse bone marrow uptake should be regarded as positive or negative for bone marrow involvement. In a homogenous cohort of patients with DLBCL, Khan and colleagues did not face interpretation difficulties in patients with diffuse marrow FDG uptake by using strict criteria for the differentiation between diffuse infiltrating lymphoma and low-grade diffuse uptake caused by reactive conditions. Furthermore, patients with positive bone marrow biopsy had worse progression-free survival (PFS) than stage IV patients without bone marrow infiltration. The reason for this difference in outcome is highly speculative because of the low number of positive bone marrow biopsies in this particular study. A possible explanation might be that FDG-PET is capable of detecting limited infiltration compared with a bone marrow aspirate relying on blindly targeting a large area for disease that is known to have a focal character. When a biopsy is positive in this situation, extensive disease is likely. For staging purposes, bone marrow biopsy seems to add limited value to FDG-PET/CT alone, but the decision to omit bone marrow biopsy in patients with DLBCL still seems problematic. Sehn and colleagues[23] showed that bone marrow biopsy provides prognostic information that is independent of the IPI. A multivariate analysis was performed to assess the independent prognostic significance of bone marrow involvement after adjusting for IPI. Concordant bone marrow involvement remained a significant negative prognostic factor for both PFS and overall survival (OS). In contrast, discordant bone marrow involvement was not independent of the IPI score with regard to PFS and OS. This information is not currently exploited for clinical purposes, which limits the purpose of performing bone marrow biopsies (**Fig. 2**).

FDG-PET in Detecting Extranodal Lesions and Central Nervous System Lymphoma

Detection of extranodal involvement is important because a worse prognosis and a higher stage mean a different therapeutic approach. Extranodal involvement has been reported in 25% to 40% of all NHL cases, depending on geography.[24–26] Several studies specifically suggest the superiority of FDG-PET compared with CT for assessment of extranodal involvement.[27,28] Schaefer and colleagues[9] found the sensitivity and specificity for extranodal involvement to be 88% and 100%, respectively, for PET/CT, versus 50% and 90% for contrast-enhanced CT.

Primary central nervous system lymphoma (PCNSL) is a rare type of extranodal lymphoma confined to the brain, eyes, leptomeninges, and spinal cord. Using FDG-PET for the detection of intracranial lymphoma may be hampered by the presence of physiologic FDG uptake in the brain cortex. Steroids administered in cases with brain involvement may cause a reduction in FDG accumulation and lead to falsely negative PET/CT findings and leptomeningeal involvement with low volume and diffuse disease burden is difficult to assess with FDG-PET. Therefore, intracranial lymphoma is most often evaluated with magnetic resonance imaging, which is also part of the International Working Group recommendation for PCNSL.[29] As many as 8% of patients with PCNSL may have occult systemic disease.[30,31] A case report by Karantanis and colleagues[32] suggests that whole-body FDG-PET detected multiple sites of extranodal disease in patients with PCNSL that were not detected on CT. Mohile and colleagues[33] also found systemic FDG-PET/CT–positive disease in 7% of patients with suspected PCNSL, which would have been missed with CT; this finding supports using FDG-PET/CT as a useful tool for staging. The limitation of the PCNSL studies is low patient numbers caused by the low incidence of the disease. Only conventional CT is currently part of the International Working Group recommendation for the staging of patients with PCNSL.[29]

FDG-PET and the Use of Dual-time-point PET

Multiple studies have indicated that dual-time-point imaging with PET can differentiate between benign metabolic activity and malignant lesions. Dual-time-point PET imaging (DTPI) is the

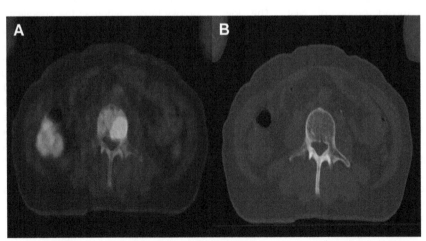

Fig. 2. (*A*) *Arrow* indicating diffuse large B-cell lymphoma located in the bone marrow of FDG-PET/CT scan. (*B*) *Arrow* indicating lesion not visible on CT.

acquisition of 2 PET scans: one scan after the routine time interval of 60 minutes followed by a delayed scan performed 120 to 180 minutes after the injection of FDG. Most FDG-avid malignancies have increased maximum standardized uptake value (SUV_{max}) on the delayed time point of imaging.[34–36] The biggest value of DTPI is probably the increased sensitivity caused by continued clearance of background activity and continued FDG accumulation in the malignant lesions. A longer distribution time allows improved blood pool and urinary tract clearance of FDG and thus lower background activity, leading to better imaging quality and better distinction between physiologic/benign FDG uptake and malignant uptake. Image quality is often poor in obese patients and background activity is often high in patients with renal failure and poorly controlled diabetes because of decreased clearance. In these cases DTPI may help detect lesions.

FDG-PET FOR EARLY RESPONSE EVALUATION

Ann Arbor staging and IPI are the most widely used tools for deciding first-line treatment strategy. However, they rely on pretherapeutic criteria without taking into account the individual patient's sensitivity to treatment. A prompt response to first-line therapy is associated with a longer PFS in patients with HL and DLBCL,[37] and is more strongly prognostic than any pretherapeutic marker. More than 20 studies have been conducted on interim FDG-PET in aggressive NHL/DLBCL in order to differentiate responders from nonresponders according to their early FDG-PET/CT results (**Fig. 3**). Hoping that this modality and strategy could be used as a prognostic marker that could allocate patients to more aggressive treatment strategies in high-risk patients or even de-escalation regimens in low-risk patients has initiated great interest.

The first emerging results were encouraging, showing that FDG-PET/CT could predict outcome after 2 to 4 cycles of chemotherapy[38–42] and even as early as after 1 course of treatment.[43,44] However, the later data questioned the usefulness of interim FDG-PET/CT, especially owing to low positive predictive values (PPV). Pregno and colleagues[45] showed that, among 66 prospectively enrolled patients who had FDG-PET/CT scans performed after 3 to 4 cycles of rituximab, cyclophosphamide, doxorubicin, vincristin, prednisolone (R-CHOP) therapy, interim FDG-PET/CT was not able to accurately predict outcome. According to Deauville visual interpretation, 2-year PFS was 85% in PET-negative patients and 72% in PET-positive patients ($P = .05$). Because of the high number of false-positive results of interim FDG-PET/CT among the recent studies (PPV 32%–83%),[45–59] Moskowitz[60] recommended that PET-positive results always be confirmed with a biopsy of the metabolically active site. One possible explanation for the lack of predictive ability of interim PET might be different timing of the PET acquisition (after 1, 2, 3, or 4 courses of chemotherapy). Most studies perform PET scan after 2 to 4 courses of chemotherapy, which is 2 time points at which PET has different meanings. PET after 2 cycles of chemotherapy probably provides early information on chemosensitivity and enables differentiation of responders from nonresponders, whereas FDG uptake after 4 courses might reflect tumor regrowth. Pooling patients with PET scans performed at different time points is problematic. Another

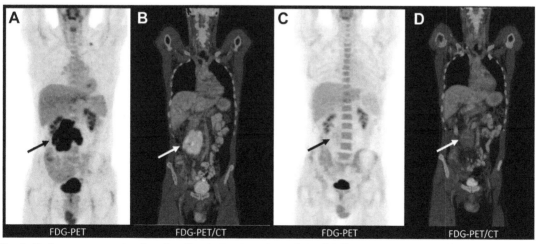

Fig. 3. Early response evaluation. Baseline FDG-PET/CT (*A* and *B*) of diffuse large cell B-cell lymphoma showing FDG-avid abdominal bulky tumor (*arrow*) and lymph node in left clavicular region. After 3 series of chemotherapy residual tissue is visible on CT (*D, arrow*) but without pathologic FDG-uptake (*C* and *D, arrow*).

possible reason might be the better prognosis in patients since the introduction of the standard use of rituximab and the reactive process that is associated with rituximab therapy generating more false-positive results.

Using imaging such as FDG-PET for early response evaluation can only be justified if the result of the scan can be used to alter treatment and this treatment change may translate into better outcome. As long as such evidence is absent, interim PET in patients with DLBCL is not strongly recommended outside clinical trials. The positron emission tomography guided therapy of aggressive non-hodgkin lymphomas (PETAL) study, from the Essen group, is one of the largest clinical trials on tailored treatment according to an interim PET result (www.clinicaltrials.gov identifier NCT00554164). Recruitment of the PETAL trial was stopped in December 2012 after registration of a total 1072 patients. After inclusion of 100, 200, and 300 patients, safety analyses were performed showing that interim PET with SUV-based evaluation was predictive of outcome. Relapse rate in poor responders to the first 2 cycles of R-CHOP was consistently 3 to 4 times higher than in good responders but the final outcome data are awaited (Dührsen U, personal communication, 2013).

Different interpretation criteria are used for lymphoma FDG-PET/CT imaging. These criteria are subdivided into visual assessment scales and quantitative measurements.

Interpretation of Interim PET Using International Harmonization Project Criteria

The consensus recommendation for FDG-PET/CT in response assessment in lymphoma according to the International Harmonization Project (IHP) was developed for the interpretation of FDG-PET/CT scans after the completion of therapy.[61] IHP uses the mediastinal blood pool activity to define a positive FDG-PET/CT study for residual lesions larger than 2 cm. In lesions smaller than 2 cm the surrounding background activity is used as reference background. The studies are assessed as either positive or negative. Despite IHP criteria being developed to determine remission status after conclusion of front-line therapy, some studies have applied these criteria to the evaluation of interim PET/CT scans. Cashen and colleagues[56] performed a study among 50 patients with advanced-stage DLBCL and applying IHP criteria to interim FDG-PET/CT was associated with low PPV of 42% and a slightly higher negative predictive value of 77% for the prediction of relapse, thus not supporting the use of IHP for

interim assessment. Uptake higher than the mediastinal blood pool is not necessarily associated with a poor prognosis in patients evaluated during therapy. Because IHP is a binary scoring system not allowing intensity grading of FDG uptake it does not allow interpretation according to the clinical context or timing in relation to numbers of courses of chemotherapy. Because of these limitations, the Deauville 5-point scale (5PS) was developed to reflect different degrees of FDG uptake and different therapeutic situations with different demands for a high NPV and a high PPV.

Interpretation of Interim PET Using Deauville 5PS

Similar to the study by Cashen and colleagues,[56] an earlier study by Itti and colleagues[62] also failed to predict outcome in patients with interim PET/CT using mediastinal blood pool as reference. In contrast, using liver as the background reference, PET-positive and PET-negative patients were clearly differentiated with 2-year PFS of 51.8% and 81.8%, respectively. An early PET/CT does not necessarily have to be negative in order to predict a superior outcome. Evaluation of PET/CT scans at midtherapy had to be redefined with a threshold lower than the IHP criteria to reflect a dynamic process, which takes place in early evaluation. The Deauville 5PS was recommended at the first international workshop on interim PET held in Deauville in 2009.[63] This set of criteria grades the intensity of the residual uptake relative to various background references in order to accommodate the dynamic behavior of tumor decrease during treatment. Baseline and interim PET/CT scans are scored according to uptake in sites initially involved by lymphoma as (1) no uptake, (2) uptake less than or equal to mediastinum blood pool, (3) uptake less than or equal to liver, (4) moderately increased uptake greater than liver, or (5) markedly increased uptake greater than liver and/or new lesions. The Deauville 5PS is now routinely used for the interpretation of interim FDG-PET/CT scans at many institutions. A score of 1 to 3 is regarded as negative and 4 or 5 as positive for midtherapy scans as proposed in the international validation study.[64] This cutoff between Deauville score 3 and 4 was chosen from the evaluation of patients with HL after 2 courses of ABVD. Reporting of interim PET/CT scans using this 5PS with a cutoff between score 3 and 4 has very good interobserver agreement. Barrington and colleagues[65] discovered this result in an assessment study between expert readers from 4 different European centers, which supports the strength of the Deauville 5PS as a robust tool for response evaluation. It is likely that the threshold defining a negative and positive FDG-PET/CT scan should be redefined according to the timing of PET (1–4 courses), the type of lymphoma, and the desired end point.

Visual interpretation is subjective and although the Deauville 5PS is the simplest and best interpretation tool to date it has its limitations. Deauville 5PS is subject to individual interpretation of contrast between lesion and background rather than pure intensity of the residual activity. If the background varies in a patient, the residual activity might also be interpreted differently in relation to the reference. Furthermore, Deauville scores of 4 and 5 rely on an individual interpretation of moderately and markedly increased uptake compared with liver, which also is highly subjective. A more objective cutoff is needed and it has been proposed that uptake 2 times or 3 times the activity of normal liver could be the solution.[66] This proposal led to the suggestion that quantification might help the visual definition of scores of 4 and 5, and studies are underway to improve the predictive values of Deauville 5PS by semiquantification.

Interpretation of Interim PET Using Quantitative Analysis

Great effort has been devoted to developing a semiquantitative method to determine whether an interim FDG-PET/CT scan should be considered positive or negative. SUV is often used in clinical PET imaging as a semiquantitative, functional measurement of radiotracer activity, normalized for dose and body weight (or lean body mass or body surface area). Using the change in SUV_{max} from baseline to the interim scan (ΔSUV_{max}) has been shown to be predictive of PFS and OS. However, the cutoff seems to vary according to the timing of imaging and therefore the results might be difficult to reproduce.

Lin and colleagues[50] presented the first large quantitative study in 2007. Analyzing 92 patients diagnosed with DLBCL, a ΔSUV_{max} of 66% was an optimal cutoff to predict 2-year event-free survival (EFS). Patients with ΔSUV_{max} less than 66% had a 2-year EFS of 21% compared with 79% for patients with ΔSUV_{max} greater than 66%. Other groups have reported optimal ΔSUV_{max} cutoffs varying from 72.9% to 91.8%.[51,58,67] In order to harmonize reporting criteria a group of experts initiated an international validation study to validate the quantitative methods. The results were presented at the Third International Workshop on Interim PET.[66] FDG-PET/CT scans were performed after 2 courses of chemoimmunotherapy in 120 patients. Three reviewers reported the

FDG-PET/CT scans according to Deauville 5PS and ΔSUV_{max} and found substantial interobserver agreement (k = 0.83) by a ΔSUV_{max} cutoff of 66% and moderate agreement (k = 0.66) according to Deauville 5PS differentiating PET negative (score 1–3) from PET positive (score 4–5).[68] Similar results were later published by Casasnovas and colleagues[69] who confirmed that ΔSUV_{max} reduction of 66% after 2 cycles and 70% after 4 cycles of chemoimmunotherapy were predictive of 2-year OS. Moreover, quantitative analysis was more predictive of outcome compared with visual interpretation. Pregno and colleagues[45] subsequently applied the same ΔSUV_{max} cutoff of 66% in a subset of 46 patients with DLBCL but they were not able differentiate between PET positive and PET negative using a quantitative approach.

Nevertheless, the ΔSUV_{max} of 66% is being used as a cutoff to evaluate interim results in the PETAL study. Patients with a ΔSUV_{max} less than 66% are randomized to receive either standard R-CHOP or an escalated acute lymphoblastic leukemia (ALL) regimen after 2 courses of R-CHOP.

To use ΔSUV_{max} for the prediction of outcome and in clinical trials requires a strict standardization of PET methods including cross-calibration of cameras, data analysis procedures, and quality control of imaging equipment. The European Association of Nuclear Medicine published a guideline on the minimal standard for the acquisition of FDG-PET in order to make quantitative applications feasible for clinical use.[70]

Apart from the different reporting criteria listed earlier it is important to question FDG-PET findings that do not correspond with the clinical situation and that are contradictory, with a good response in some areas and increased uptake in others. In these situations it is especially important that PET scans are assessed and discussed in a multidisciplinary setting with the participating imaging specialists and treating clinicians. A recent work studied a total of 241 interim and PET reports.[71] These written PET reports were blinded for personal data and given to 3 expert hematologists who had to interpret the reports as positive, negative, or indeterminate. Each PET/CT report was centrally labeled positive or negative if all 3 interpreters independently agreed. All others were considered indeterminate. In more than half the cases the reports were categorized as indeterminate. This study clearly underlines the important point that PET images need to be interpreted in the context of a clinical situation.

FDG-PET FOR POSTTREATMENT EVALUATION

Response evaluation after the completion of therapy is to date the most important role of

FDG-PET/CT scans in patients with lymphoma. Accurate information regarding tumor status after treatment is critical because DLBCL is a curable lymphoma. FDG-PET is clearly superior to CT alone when distinguishing fibrosis from residual active lymphoma tissue by the end of therapy.[72] This ability is particularly important in patients with bulky disease at diagnosis because they often have residual fibrosis at the conclusion of front-line therapy. Zijlstra and colleagues[73] performed a systematic review on FDG-PET on the diagnostic performance of posttreatment evaluation of malignant lymphoma. In a total of 15 studies of 705 patients including both HL and aggressive NHL they found pooled sensitivity of 72% and specificity of 100% for the detection of residual disease in patients with NHL. Terasawa and colleagues[74] repeated a systematic review a year later with a focus on the methodology and excluded a few studies that Zijlstra and colleagues[73] included because of mixed diagnosis. As well as investigating the accuracy of FDG-PET compared with CT for residual lesions, they also assessed the prediction of relapse and found a sensitivity of 33% to 77% and specificity of 82% to 100% for aggressive NHL. As a consequence, FDG-PET was incorporated into the International Working Group criteria in 2007 to accurately assess persistent lymphoma tissue.[75] The FDG-PET criteria eliminated the earlier definition of complete remission unconfirmed (Cru) from a better FDG characterization of active lymphoma tissue. Brespoels and colleagues[76] compared the CT-based IWC criteria with the revised FDG-PET International Workshop Criteria (IWC) and correlated the response at end of therapy with time to next treatment (TNT) in 69 patients with NHL. TNT as defined by CT-based IWC criteria was not significantly different in patients with complete response (CR)/Cru compared with those with partial response (PR), whereas for FDG-PET IWC criteria, TNT was significantly shorter in patients with PR compared with those with CR.

The revised response criteria for malignant lymphoma have adopted no FDG uptake on completion of therapy as the sole criterion for CR in lymphoma. However, in the presence of a PR, response is still mainly evaluated according to tumor size.

According to IHP recommendation, FDG-PET should be performed after at least 3 weeks of completion of therapy and after 8 to 12 weeks after radiotherapy in order for inflammatory reactions to subside. Updated criteria for staging and response evaluation in lymphoma are soon to be published and PET/CT scans will continue to play a major role in end-of-therapy response evaluation.

FDG-PET FOR SURVEILLANCE

Present guidelines recommend following patients with DLBCL after the completion of therapy with intervals of 3 to 6 months performing clinical examination and blood tests. Many centers also use routine imaging for aggressive lymphomas. The rationale for using imaging in routine surveillance is to detect an early relapse before it becomes symptomatic. CT has been the recommended choice for surveillance scans, but little evidence supports this practice because most relapses are detected by symptoms despite routine surveillance scans.[77,78] Because FDG-PET/CT has been shown to be more sensitive than CT in the staging setting, it is likely that it is able to detect a subclinical relapse. Previous studies show that FDG-PET/CT is both sensitive and specific for the detection of relapsed DLBCL[79–81] but the false-positive rate is high, causing many unnecessary biopsies and repeated tests, and much anxiety for the patients. Furthermore, it is unknown whether an early diagnosis of relapse translates into better outcome. It is likely that early detection gives a false impression of longer PFS because of lead time bias. However, a recent study by El-Galaly and colleagues[82] consisting of 258 patients with NHL and HL (173 DLBCL) found that patients with DLBCL who experienced imaging-detected relapse had lower disease stage and a trend toward a reduced risk of death. Nevertheless, it is possible that the use of FDG-PET only should apply to patients belonging to a high-risk group in order to keep costs and radiation exposure down. This approach was supported by Cheah and colleagues[83] who suggested that surveillance FDG-PET should be applied to patients with IPI greater than 3 during the first 18 months of follow-up when the risk of relapse is the greatest. In order to clearly define the role for surveillance imaging, prospective studies are needed.

SUMMARY

FDG-PET plays a major role in the management of patients with DLBCL. Baseline FDG-PET/CT provides enhanced staging accuracy and facilitates the interpretation of FDG-PET/CT studies after completion of therapy in patients with DLBCL. Staging and end-of-therapy PET/CT should be routinely performed according to the most recent international guidelines for imaging in lymphoma. Interim FDG-PET/CT has a strong predictive value and can be useful in monitoring early treatment response for patients with DLBCL. At present, the results of the clinical trials are awaited. Until the results of international randomized response adapted trials are available, interim PET is not recommended for therapy management outside clinical trials.

It is expected that the accuracy of FDG-PET/CT will increase because of refined interpretation methods but also stricter and more standardized acquisition of FDG-PET scans across institutions, which might allow a better comparison of quantitative data of multicenter results in future. It is likely that FDG-PET/CT will play a role in the surveillance of selected high-risk patients obtaining complete remission on first-line therapy and who are subsequently candidates for high-dose therapy. Recent studies suggest that FDG-PET imaging data obviates bone marrow biopsy in patients with HL, and routine bone marrow biopsy is no longer part of the recommendation in the diagnostic work-up for this group of patients. Although the clinical situation is different for patients with DLBCL, it is possible that new advances in interpretation and refinement of FDG-PET scans in future may also allow the omission of bone marrow biopsy in patients with DLBCL. Non-FDG tracers are now available for PET imaging and others are under preclinical development. Most of these tracers are designed based on cancer biomarkers that are more or less specific for DLBCL. Some tracers are designed based on increased DNA synthesis and others on upregulated amino acids transporters, CD20 expression in B cells, and cellular apoptosis. As advances are made in research into the molecular biology of lymphoma it might be possible to identify biomarkers in DLBCL that contribute to progression, which warrants the development of new specific lymphoma-targeted imaging tracers. This development might allow the assessment of additional aspects related to the prognosis and management of patients with DLBCL.

REFERENCES

1. Jaffe ES, Harris NL, Stein H, et al, editors. World Health Organization classification of tumours. Pathology and genetics of tumours of haematopoietic and lymphoid tissues. Lyon (France): IARC Press; 2001.
2. Watanabe R, Tomita N, Takeuchi K, et al. SUVmax in FDG-PET at the biopsy site correlates with the proliferation potential of tumor cells in non-Hodgkin lymphoma. Leuk Lymphoma 2010;51(2):279–83. http://dx.doi.org/10.3109/10428190903440953.
3. Weiler-Sagie M, Bushelev O, Epelbaum R, et al. (18)F-FDG avidity in lymphoma readdressed: a study of 766 patients. J Nucl Med 2010;51(1):25–30. http://dx.doi.org/10.2967/jnumed.109.067892.
4. Elstrom R, Guan L, Baker G, et al. Utility of FDG-PET scanning in lymphoma by WHO classification. Blood 2003;101(10):3875–6. http://dx.doi.org/10.1182/blood-2002-09-2778.
5. Carbone PP, Kaplan HS, Musshoff K, et al. Report of the Committee on Hodgkin's Disease Staging Classification. Cancer Res 1971;31(11):1860–1.
6. A predictive model for aggressive non-Hodgkin's lymphoma. The International Non-Hodgkin's Lymphoma Prognostic Factors Project. N Engl J Med 1993;329(14):987–94. http://dx.doi.org/10.1056/NEJM199309303291402.
7. Lister TA, Crowther D, Sutcliffe SB, et al. Report of a committee convened to discuss the evaluation and staging of patients with Hodgkin's disease: Cotswolds meeting. J Clin Oncol 1989;7(11):1630–6.
8. Zhou Z, Sehn LH, Rademaker AW, et al. An enhanced International Prognostic Index (NCCN-IPI) for patients with diffuse large B-cell lymphoma treated in the rituximab era. Blood 2014;123(6):837–42. http://dx.doi.org/10.1182/blood-2013-09-524108.
9. Schaefer NG, Hany TF, Taverna C, et al. Non-Hodgkin lymphoma and Hodgkin disease: coregistered FDG PET and CT at staging and restaging–do we need contrast-enhanced CT? Radiology 2004;232(3):823–9. http://dx.doi.org/10.1148/radiol.2323030985.
10. Hutchings M, Loft A, Hansen M, et al. Position emission tomography with or without computed tomography in the primary staging of Hodgkin's lymphoma. Haematologica 2006;91(4):482–9.
11. Isasi CR, Lu P, Blaufox MD. A metaanalysis of 18F-2-deoxy-2-fluoro-D-glucose positron emission tomography in the staging and restaging of patients with lymphoma. Cancer 2005;104(5):1066–74. http://dx.doi.org/10.1002/cncr.21253.
12. Raanani P, Shasha Y, Perry C, et al. Is CT scan still necessary for staging in Hodgkin and non-Hodgkin lymphoma patients in the PET/CT era? Ann Oncol 2006;17(1):117–22. http://dx.doi.org/10.1093/annonc/mdj024.
13. Naumann R, Beuthien-Baumann B, Reiss A, et al. Substantial impact of FDG PET imaging on the therapy decision in patients with early-stage Hodgkin's lymphoma. Br J Cancer 2004;90(3):620–5. http://dx.doi.org/10.1038/sj.bjc.6601561.
14. El-Galaly TC, Hutchings M, Mylam KJ, et al. Impact of 18F-FDG PET/CT staging in newly diagnosed classical Hodgkin lymphoma: less cases with stage I disease and more with skeletal involvement. Leuk Lymphoma 2013. http://dx.doi.org/10.3109/10428194.2013.875169.
15. Partridge S, Timothy A, O'Doherty MJ, et al. 2-Fluorine-18-fluoro-2-deoxy-D glucose positron emission tomography in the pretreatment staging of Hodgkin's disease: influence on patient

management in a single institution. Ann Oncol 2000;11(10):1273–9.

16. Pelosi E, Pregno P, Penna D, et al. Role of whole-body [18F] fluorodeoxyglucose positron emission tomography/computed tomography (FDG-PET/CT) and conventional techniques in the staging of patients with Hodgkin and aggressive non Hodgkin lymphoma. Radiol Med 2008;113(4):578–90. http://dx.doi.org/10.1007/s11547-008-0264-7.

17. Abdulqadhr G, Molin D, Astrom G, et al. Whole-body diffusion-weighted imaging compared with FDG-PET/CT in staging of lymphoma patients. Acta Radiol 2011;52(2):173–80. http://dx.doi.org/10.1258/ar.2010.100246.

18. Barrington SF, Mikhaeel NG, Kostakoglu L, et al. The role of imaging in the staging and response assessment of lymphoma: consensus of the ICML Imaging Working Group. J Clin Oncol 2014 [Accepted for publication].

19. Pakos EE, Fotopoulos AD, Ioannidis JP. 18F-FDG PET for evaluation of bone marrow infiltration in staging of lymphoma: a meta-analysis. J Nucl Med 2005;46(6):958–63.

20. Adams HJ, Kwee TC, de Keizer B, et al. FDG PET/CT for the detection of bone marrow involvement in diffuse large B-cell lymphoma: systematic review and meta-analysis. Eur J Nucl Med Mol Imaging 2013. http://dx.doi.org/10.1007/s00259-013-2623-4.

21. Adams HJ, Kwee TC, Fijnheer R, et al. Bone marrow F-fluoro-2-deoxy-d-glucose positron emission tomography/computed tomography cannot replace bone marrow biopsy in diffuse large B-cell lymphoma. Am J Hematol 2014. http://dx.doi.org/10.1002/ajh.23730.

22. Khan AB, Barrington SF, Mikhaeel NG, et al. PET-CT staging of DLBCL accurately identifies and provides new insight into the clinical significance of bone marrow involvement. Blood 2013;122(1):61–7. http://dx.doi.org/10.1182/blood-2012-12-473389.

23. Sehn LH, Scott DW, Chhanabhai M, et al. Impact of concordant and discordant bone marrow involvement on outcome in diffuse large B-cell lymphoma treated with R-CHOP. J Clin Oncol 2011;29(11):1452–7. http://dx.doi.org/10.1200/JCO.2010.33.3419.

24. Freeman C, Berg JW, Cutler SJ. Occurrence and prognosis of extranodal lymphomas. Cancer 1972;29(1):252–60.

25. Chua SC, Rozalli FI, O'Connor SR. Imaging features of primary extranodal lymphomas. Clin Radiol 2009; 64(6):574–88. http://dx.doi.org/10.1016/j.crad.2008.11.001.

26. Zucca E, Conconi A, Cavalli F. Treatment of extra-nodal lymphomas. Best Pract Res Clin Haematol 2002;15(3):533–47.

27. Moog F, Bangerter M, Diederichs CG, et al. Extra-nodal malignant lymphoma: detection with FDG PET versus CT. Radiology 1998;206(2):475–81. http://dx.doi.org/10.1148/radiology.206.2.9457202.

28. Buchmann I, Moog F, Schirrmeister H, et al. Positron emission tomography for detection and staging of malignant lymphoma. Recent Results Cancer Res 2000;156:78–89.

29. Abrey LE, Batchelor TT, Ferreri AJ, et al. Report of an international workshop to standardize baseline evaluation and response criteria for primary CNS lymphoma. J Clin Oncol 2005;23(22):5034–43. http://dx.doi.org/10.1200/JCO.2005.13.524.

30. O'Neill BP, Dinapoli RP, Kurtin PJ, et al. Occult systemic non-Hodgkin's lymphoma (NHL) in patients initially diagnosed as primary central nervous system lymphoma (PCNSL): how much staging is enough? J Neurooncol 1995;25(1):67–71.

31. Ferreri AJ, Reni M, Zoldan MC, et al. Importance of complete staging in non-Hodgkin's lymphoma presenting as a cerebral mass lesion. Cancer 1996; 77(5):827–33.

32. Karantanis D, O'Neill BP, Subramaniam RM, et al. Contribution of F-18 FDG PET-CT in the detection of systemic spread of primary central nervous system lymphoma. Clin Nucl Med 2007;32(4):271–4. http://dx.doi.org/10.1097/01.rlu.0000257269.99345.1b.

33. Mohile NA, Deangelis LM, Abrey LE. The utility of body FDG PET in staging primary central nervous system lymphoma. Neuro Oncol 2008;10(2):223–8. http://dx.doi.org/10.1215/15228517-2007-061.

34. Nakayama M, Okizaki A, Ishitoya S, et al. Dual-time-point F-18 FDG PET/CT imaging for differentiating the lymph nodes between malignant lymphoma and benign lesions. Ann Nucl Med 2013;27(2):163–9. http://dx.doi.org/10.1007/s12149-012-0669-1.

35. Kubota K, Itoh M, Ozaki K, et al. Advantage of delayed whole-body FDG-PET imaging for tumour detection. Eur J Nucl Med 2001;28(6):696–703.

36. Lan XL, Zhang YX, Wu ZJ, et al. The value of dual time point (18)F-FDG PET imaging for the differentiation between malignant and benign lesions. Clin Radiol 2008;63(7):756–64. http://dx.doi.org/10.1016/j.crad.2008.01.003.

37. Haw R, Sawka CA, Franssen E, et al. Significance of a partial or slow response to front-line chemotherapy in the management of intermediate-grade or high-grade non-Hodgkin's lymphoma: a literature review. J Clin Oncol 1994;12(5):1074–84.

38. Mikhaeel NG, Timothy AR, O'Doherty MJ, et al. 18-FDG-PET as a prognostic indicator in the treatment of aggressive non-Hodgkin's lymphoma–comparison with CT. Leuk Lymphoma 2000;39(5-6):543–53. http://dx.doi.org/10.3109/10428190009113384.

39. Jerusalem G, Beguin Y, Fassotte MF, et al. Persistent tumor 18F-FDG uptake after a few cycles of polychemotherapy is predictive of treatment failure in non-Hodgkin's lymphoma. Haematologica 2000; 85(6):613–8.

40. Spaepen K, Stroobants S, Dupont P, et al. Early re-staging positron emission tomography with (18)F-fluorodeoxyglucose predicts outcome in patients with aggressive non-Hodgkin's lymphoma. Ann Oncol 2002;13(9):1356–63.

41. Mikhaeel NG, Hutchings M, Fields PA, et al. FDG-PET after two to three cycles of chemotherapy predicts progression-free and overall survival in high-grade non-Hodgkin lymphoma. Ann Oncol 2005;16(9):1514–23. http://dx.doi.org/10.1093/annonc/mdi272.

42. Haioun C, Itti E, Rahmouni A, et al. [18F]fluoro-2-deoxy-D-glucose positron emission tomography (FDG-PET) in aggressive lymphoma: an early prognostic tool for predicting patient outcome. Blood 2005;106(4):1376–81. http://dx.doi.org/10.1182/blood-2005-01-0272.

43. Kostakoglu L, Coleman M, Leonard JP, et al. PET predicts prognosis after 1 cycle of chemotherapy in aggressive lymphoma and Hodgkin's disease. J Nucl Med 2002;43(8):1018–27.

44. Kostakoglu L, Goldsmith SJ, Leonard JP, et al. FDG-PET after 1 cycle of therapy predicts outcome in diffuse large cell lymphoma and classic Hodgkin disease. Cancer 2006;107(11):2678–87. http://dx.doi.org/10.1002/cncr.22276.

45. Pregno P, Chiappella A, Bello M, et al. Interim 18-FDG-PET/CT failed to predict the outcome in diffuse large B-cell lymphoma patients treated at the diagnosis with rituximab-CHOP. Blood 2012; 119(9):2066–73. http://dx.doi.org/10.1182/blood-2011-06-359943.

46. Zhao J, Qiao W, Wang C, et al. Therapeutic evaluation and prognostic value of interim hybrid PET/CT with (18)F-FDG after three to four cycles of chemotherapy in non-Hodgkin's lymphoma. Hematology 2007;12(5):423–30. http://dx.doi.org/10.1080/10245330701393840.

47. Querellou S, Valette F, Bodet-Milin C, et al. FDG-PET/CT predicts outcome in patients with aggressive non-Hodgkin's lymphoma and Hodgkin's disease. Ann Hematol 2006;85(11):759–67. http://dx.doi.org/10.1007/s00277-006-0151-z.

48. Fruchart C, Reman O, Le Stang N, et al. Prognostic value of early 18 fluorodeoxyglucose positron emission tomography and gallium-67 scintigraphy in aggressive lymphoma: a prospective comparative study. Leuk Lymphoma 2006;47(12):2547–57. http://dx.doi.org/10.1080/10428190600942959.

49. Ng AP, Wirth A, Seymour JF, et al. Early therapeutic response assessment by (18)FDG-positron emission tomography during chemotherapy in patients with diffuse large B-cell lymphoma: isolated residual positivity involving bone is not usually a predictor of subsequent treatment failure. Leuk Lymphoma 2007;48(3):596–600. http://dx.doi.org/10.1080/10428190601099965.

50. Lin C, Itti E, Haioun C, et al. Early 18F-FDG PET for prediction of prognosis in patients with diffuse large B-cell lymphoma: SUV-based assessment versus visual analysis. J Nucl Med 2007;48(10):1626–32. http://dx.doi.org/10.2967/jnumed.107.042093.

51. Itti E, Lin C, Dupuis J, et al. Prognostic value of interim 18F-FDG PET in patients with diffuse large B-Cell lymphoma: SUV-based assessment at 4 cycles of chemotherapy. J Nucl Med 2009;50(4):527–33. http://dx.doi.org/10.2967/jnumed.108.057703.

52. Han HS, Escalon MP, Hsiao B, et al. High incidence of false-positive PET scans in patients with aggressive non-Hodgkin's lymphoma treated with rituximab-containing regimens. Ann Oncol 2009;20(2):309–18. http://dx.doi.org/10.1093/annonc/mdn629.

53. Zinzani PL, Gandolfi L, Broccoli A, et al. Midtreatment 18F-fluorodeoxyglucose positron-emission tomography in aggressive non-Hodgkin lymphoma. Cancer 2011;117(5):1010–8. http://dx.doi.org/10.1002/cncr.25579.

54. Yoo C, Lee DH, Kim JE, et al. Limited role of interim PET/CT in patients with diffuse large B-cell lymphoma treated with R-CHOP. Ann Hematol 2011; 90(7):797–802. http://dx.doi.org/10.1007/s00277-010-1135-6.

55. Yang DH, Min JJ, Song HC, et al. Prognostic significance of interim (1)(8)F-FDG PET/CT after three or four cycles of R-CHOP chemotherapy in the treatment of diffuse large B-cell lymphoma. Eur J Cancer 2011;47(9):1312–8. http://dx.doi.org/10.1016/j.ejca.2010.12.027.

56. Cashen AF, Dehdashti F, Luo J, et al. 18F-FDG PET/CT for early response assessment in diffuse large B-cell lymphoma: poor predictive value of international harmonization project interpretation. J Nucl Med 2011;52(3):386–92. http://dx.doi.org/10.2967/jnumed.110.082586.

57. Safar V, Dupuis J, Itti E, et al. Interim [18F]fluorodeoxyglucose positron emission tomography scan in diffuse large B-cell lymphoma treated with anthracycline-based chemotherapy plus rituximab. J Clin Oncol 2012;30(2):184–90. http://dx.doi.org/10.1200/jco.2011.38.2648.

58. Yang DH, Ahn JS, Byun BH, et al. Interim PET/CT-based prognostic model for the treatment of diffuse large B cell lymphoma in the post-rituximab era. Ann Hematol 2013;92(4):471–9. http://dx.doi.org/10.1007/s00277-012-1640-x.

59. Gonzalez-Barca E, Canales M, Cortes M, et al. Predictive value of interim (1)(8)F-FDG-PET/CT for event-free survival in patients with diffuse large B-cell lymphoma homogenously treated in a phase II trial with six cycles of R-CHOP-14 plus pegfilgrastim as first-line treatment. Nucl Med Commun 2013;34(10):946–52. http://dx.doi.org/10.1097/MNM.0b013e328363c695.

60. Moskowitz CH. Interim PET-CT in the management of diffuse large B-cell lymphoma. Hematology Am Soc Hematol Educ Program 2012;2012:397–401. http://dx.doi.org/10.1182/asheducation-2012.1.397.

61. Juweid ME, Stroobants S, Hoekstra OS, et al. Use of positron emission tomography for response assessment of lymphoma: consensus of the Imaging Subcommittee of International Harmonization Project in Lymphoma. J Clin Oncol 2007;25(5):571–8. http://dx.doi.org/10.1200/JCO.2006.08.2305.

62. Itti E, Juweid ME, Haioun C, et al. Improvement of early 18F-FDG PET interpretation in diffuse large B-cell lymphoma: importance of the reference background. J Nucl Med 2010;51(12):1857–62. http://dx.doi.org/10.2967/jnumed.110.080556.

63. Meignan M, Gallamini A, Meignan M, et al. Report on the First International Workshop on Interim-PET-Scan in Lymphoma. Leuk Lymphoma 2009;50(8):1257–60. http://dx.doi.org/10.1080/10428190903040048.

64. Biggi A, Gallamini A, Chauvie S, et al. International Validation Study for Interim PET in ABVD-Treated, Advanced-Stage Hodgkin Lymphoma: interpretation criteria and concordance rate among reviewers. J Nucl Med 2013. http://dx.doi.org/10.2967/jnumed.112.110890.

65. Barrington SF, Qian W, Somer EJ, et al. Concordance between four European centres of PET reporting criteria designed for use in multicentre trials in Hodgkin lymphoma. Eur J Nucl Med Mol Imaging 2010;37(10):1824–33. http://dx.doi.org/10.1007/s00259-010-1490-5.

66. Meignan M, Gallamini A, Itti E, et al. Report on the Third International Workshop on Interim Positron Emission Tomography in Lymphoma held in Menton, France, 26-27 September 2011 and Menton 2011 consensus. Leuk Lymphoma 2012;53(10):1876–81. http://dx.doi.org/10.3109/10428194.2012.677535.

67. Fuertes S, Setoain X, Lopez-Guillermo A, et al. Interim FDG PET/CT as a prognostic factor in diffuse large B-cell lymphoma. Eur J Nucl Med Mol Imaging 2013;40(4):496–504. http://dx.doi.org/10.1007/s00259-012-2320-8.

68. Itti E, Meignan M, Berriolo-Riedinger A, et al. An international confirmatory study of the prognostic value of early PET/CT in diffuse large B-cell lymphoma: comparison between Deauville criteria and ΔSUVmax. Eur J Nucl Med Mol Imaging 2013;40(9):1312–20. http://dx.doi.org/10.1007/s00259-013-2435-6.

69. Casasnovas RO, Meignan M, Berriolo-Riedinger A, et al. SUVmax reduction improves early prognosis value of interim positron emission tomography scans in diffuse large B-cell lymphoma. Blood. 2011;118(1):37–43. Epub 2011/04/27. http://dx.doi.org/10.1182/blood-2010-12-327767. PubMed PMID: 21518924.

70. Boellaard R, O'Doherty MJ, Weber WA, et al. FDG PET and PET/CT: EANM procedure guidelines for tumour PET imaging: version 1.0. Eur J Nucl Med Mol Imaging 2010;37(1):181–200. http://dx.doi.org/10.1007/s00259-009-1297-4.

71. Mylam KJ, El-Galaly TC, Hutchings M, et al. Prognostic impact of clinician-based interpretation of F-fluorodeoxyglucose positron emission tomography/computed tomography reports obtained in patients with newly diagnosed diffuse large B-cell lymphoma. Leuk Lymphoma 2013. http://dx.doi.org/10.3109/10428194.2013.850165.

72. Surbone A, Longo DL, DeVita VT Jr, et al. Residual abdominal masses in aggressive non-Hodgkin's lymphoma after combination chemotherapy: significance and management. J Clin Oncol 1988;6(12):1832–7.

73. Zijlstra JM, Lindauer-van der Werf G, Hoekstra OS, et al. 18F-fluoro-deoxyglucose positron emission tomography for post-treatment evaluation of malignant lymphoma: a systematic review. Haematologica 2006;91(4):522–9.

74. Terasawa T, Nihashi T, Hotta T, et al. 18F-FDG PET for posttherapy assessment of Hodgkin's disease and aggressive non-Hodgkin's lymphoma: a systematic review. J Nucl Med 2008;49(1):13–21. http://dx.doi.org/10.2967/jnumed.107.039867.

75. Cheson BD, Pfistner B, Juweid ME, et al. Revised response criteria for malignant lymphoma. J Clin Oncol 2007;25(5):579–86. http://dx.doi.org/10.1200/JCO.2006.09.2403.

76. Brepoels L, Stroobants S, De Wever W, et al. Aggressive and indolent non-Hodgkin's lymphoma: response assessment by integrated international workshop criteria. Leukemia & lymphoma 2007;48(8):1522–30. http://dx.doi.org/10.1080/10428190701474365. PubMed PMID: 17701583.

77. Guppy AE, Tebbutt NC, Norman A, et al. The role of surveillance CT scans in patients with diffuse large B-cell non-Hodgkin's lymphoma. Leuk Lymphoma 2003;44(1):123–5. http://dx.doi.org/10.1080/1042819021000040323.

78. Elis A, Blickstein D, Klein O, et al. Detection of relapse in non-Hodgkin's lymphoma: role of routine follow-up studies. Am J Hematol 2002;69(1):41–4.

79. Zinzani PL, Stefoni V, Tani M, et al. Role of [18F]fluorodeoxyglucose positron emission tomography scan in the follow-up of lymphoma. J Clin Oncol 2009;27(11):1781–7. http://dx.doi.org/10.1200/jco.2008.16.1513.

80. Petrausch U, Samaras P, Haile SR, et al. Risk-adapted FDG-PET/CT-based follow-up in patients with diffuse large B-cell lymphoma after first-line therapy. Ann Oncol 2010;21(8):1694–8. http://dx.doi.org/10.1093/annonc/mdq015.

81. El-Galaly T, Prakash V, Christiansen I, et al. Efficacy of routine surveillance with positron emission

tomography/computed tomography in aggressive non-Hodgkin lymphoma in complete remission: status in a single center. Leuk Lymphoma 2011;52(4):597–603. http://dx.doi.org/10.3109/10428194.2010.547642.

82. El-Galaly TC, Mylam KJ, Bogsted M, et al. Role of routine imaging in detecting recurrent lymphoma; a review of 258 patients with relapsed aggressive non-Hodgkin and Hodgkin lymphoma. Am J Hematol 2014. http://dx.doi.org/10.1002/ajh.23688.

83. Cheah CY, Hofman MS, Dickinson M, et al. Limited role for surveillance PET-CT scanning in patients with diffuse large B-cell lymphoma in complete metabolic remission following primary therapy. Br J Cancer 2013;109(2):312–7. http://dx.doi.org/10.1038/bjc.2013.338.

FDG in Urologic Malignancies

Poul Flemming Høilund-Carlsen, MD, DMSc[a,b,*], Mads Hvid Poulsen, MD, PhD[b,c],
Henrik Petersen, MD[a], Søren Hess, MD[a], Lars Lund, MD, DMSci[b,c]

KEYWORDS

• Renal cancer • Bladder cancer • Prostate cancer • Radionuclide imaging • FDG

KEY POINTS

- The major urologic cancers, kidney, bladder, and prostate cancer, account for more than one-eighth of all yearly new cancer cases worldwide, but positron emission tomography (PET) imaging is not used nearly as much as in other cancers.
- Imaging in kidney cancer is dominated by computed tomography (CT); 18F-fluoro-deoxy-glucose (FDG)-PET/CT may have a future role for management decisions and prognostication.
- PET imaging in primary bladder cancer is impeded by urinary excretion of FDG and procedures to circumvent were so far not very successful; however, FDG-PET/CT may have a promising role in staging/restaging, primarily by detecting otherwise undiscovered metastases.
- The role of PET imaging has been far more examined in prostate than in other urologic cancers, albeit without clarification of what may be the most useful application.
- PET imaging of urologic cancers with FDG is often readily rejected, referring to a high frequency of false-negative results; not seldom these findings may instead reflect unrecognized underlying disease dynamics, as for example slow growth and a good prognosis.

INTRODUCTION

In comparison with multiple other applications, positron emission tomography (PET) and PET/computed tomography (PET/CT) imaging with 18F-fluorodeoxy-glucose (FDG) has never gained a strong foothold in urologic malignancies.[1] There are several reasons for this, some correct, some not. This review provides an overview of the reported use of FDG-PET/CT in the 3 major urologic cancers (kidney, bladder, and prostate), giving the pros and cons. Furthermore, modes of improvement, new applications, and the potential role of clinical molecular urologic imaging in years to come are reviewed. In doing so, we describe to what degree FDG-PET/CT imaging has contributed to characterization of these diseases so far, with regard to providing clinically useful information about primary diagnosis and staging, response evaluation, prognosis, and long-term follow-up.

FREQUENCY OF UROLOGIC CANCERS

By 2012, prostate cancer was the fourth most common cancer worldwide, with approximately 1.1 million new cases contributing almost 8% of the total number of new cases diagnosed this

This review was not funded.
The authors have nothing to disclose.
[a] Department of Nuclear Medicine, Odense University Hospital, Sønder Boulevard 29, Odense DK-5000, Denmark; [b] Institute of Clinical Research, University of Southern Denmark, Winsløwparken 19, DK-5000, Odense, Denmark; [c] Department of Urology, Odense University Hospital, Sønder Boulevard 29, Odense DK-5000, Denmark
* Corresponding author. Institute of Clinical Research, University of Southern Denmark, Sønder Boulevard 29, Odense, DK-5000, Denmark.
E-mail address: pfhc@rsyd.dk

PET Clin 9 (2014) 457–468
http://dx.doi.org/10.1016/j.cpet.2014.07.003
1556-8598/14/$ – see front matter © 2014 Elsevier Inc. All rights reserved.

year. Bladder cancer was the ninth, with approximately 430,000 new cases, and kidney cancer the twelfth most common cancer with approximately 338,000 new cases, contributing 3.1% and 2.4%, respectively, of the total number of new cases diagnosed in 2012. Taken together, worldwide these 3 cancers accounted in 2012 for more than one-eighth of all new cancer cases.[2]

In 2012, in men, prostate cancer was the second, bladder cancer the sixth, and kidney cancer the ninth most common cancer worldwide contributing 15.0%, 4.4%, and 2.9%, respectively. In women, kidney cancer was the 14th and bladder cancer the 19th most common cancer worldwide contributing 1.9% and 1.5% of the total new cancer cases diagnosed in 2012.[2] The highest cancer rate for men and women together is found in Denmark, with 338 people per 100,000 being diagnosed in 2012. The United States was in sixth place with 318, whereas the United Kingdom was number 23 on the list with 279 per 100,000.[2] The incidence rate of prostate cancer per 100,000 men per year has steadily increased when measured in 5-year intervals, from 70 in 1988 to 1992, to 151 in 2008 to 2012, albeit with an intermediate sharp decrease from 2009 to 2010, probably due to a change in the diagnostic behavior in general practice, where the frequency of prostate-specific antigen (PSA) testing declined after recommendation from the Danish Society of Urology. Following that, there have been only minor fluctuations in the rate from 2010 to 2012. In contrast, there has been no development in the incidence of the 2 other cancers, which taken together has remained approximately 68 to 70 per 100,000 for men and 23 to 24 for women during the same 5-year intervals.[3] All 3 cancers occur rarely in those younger than 45, and are almost nonexistent in individuals younger than 30. Rates

in 2011 for incidence, prevalence, and 5-year survival in Denmark are given in **Table 1**. From this, it appears that approximately 1.7% of the Danish population (which is about 1/53 of the US population) or 95,683 persons lived with 1 of these 3 cancers.[4]

KIDNEY CANCER

The by far most common type of kidney cancer in adults is the renal cell carcinoma (RCC), which accounts for approximately 80% of all kidney cancers. It is not a single entity, but rather a series of tumors, derived from the various parts of the nephron. In fact, the World Health Organization classification recognizes more than 40 subtypes of renal neoplasms.

Other types are papillary, chromophobe, oncolytic, and collecting duct cancers. More than 1 cell type may be present in a kidney cancer and all types can occasionally transform into sarcomatoid appearance (ie, having cells similar to those of supportive tissues). A special type is the transitional cell cancer of the renal pelvis, which resembles bladder cancer because the renal pelvis, the ureters, and the bladder are lined with the same type of cells. In children, kidney malignancies are seldom and 95% are the Wilms tumor type originating from uncontrolled growth of immature cells, sometimes associated with genetic disorders and birth defects.

Radiological investigations are essential when staging renal masses, whether due to local tumor or metastatic disease. Until recently, the only efficient treatment of local disease was surgery. In the era of targeted treatment with, for instance, tyrosin-kinase inhibitors (TKIs) one has the possibility to treat metastatic disease with good results, which was not the case a few years ago. CT or

Table 1
Urologic cancers in Denmark 2011

| Cancer Type | Incidence | | Prevalence | | Survival |
	Number	Crude	Number	Per Thousand of Male/Female Population	5-Year (%)
Kidney, males	477	17.3	2770	1.00	54
Kidney, females	240	8.6	1674	0.60	71
Bladder,[1] males	1334	48.3	12,076	4.37	54
Bladder,[1] females	478	17.0	4397	1.56	63
Prostate	4257	154.2	26,617	9.62	82

End of 2011 data in Denmark, population 2,766,178 males and 2,813,026 females, that is, total 5,579,204.

Data from Engholm G, Ferlay J, Christensen N, et al. NORDCAN: cancer incidence, mortality, prevalence and survival in the Nordic countries, Version 6.0. 2013. Association of the Nordic Cancer Registries; Danish Cancer Society. Available at: http://www.ancr.nu. Accessed May 20, 2014.

magnetic resonance imaging (MRI) are used to characterize the renal mass[5] with a sensitivity of 100% and a specificity of 88% to 95%.[6,7] Imaging must be performed with intravenous contrast to demonstrate enhancement, a change of 20 Hounsfield units (HU) is a strong evidence of enhancement.[8] The CT scan allows diagnosis of RCC and provides information of function and morphology of the contralateral kidney, primary tumor extension, and extrarenal spread, venous involvement, enlargement of lymph nodes, and the relationship to the adrenal gland. Thus, the assessment of renal masses and primary staging of RCC are the domain of modern CT.

FDG-PET/CT may be helpful in the evaluation of "equivocal findings" by conventional imaging, including bone scan, and also in the differentiation between recurrence and post-therapy changes.[9] The detection rate of retroperitoneal lymph node metastases by CT scanning may be as high as 95%,[10] but even if a nodal size of 1 cm or greater is a criterion for disease, false-positive findings can range from 3% to 43% mainly due to reactive hyperplasia.[11]

Preoperative Use

The aim of any preoperative imaging in RCC is to differentiate benign from malignant lesions, to adequately assess tumor size and to identify lymph node metastases.[12] CT is considered the most appropriate imaging modality to differentiate benign from malignant lesions.[13] However, RCCs can appear as isodense, hyperdense, or hypodense lesions on native CT scans, but often have a contrast enhancement of approximately 115 ± 48 HU in the corticomedullary phase and of 62 ± 25 HU in the excretory phase.[5] Using a cutoff value of 84 HU in the former and of 44 HU in latter phase, the sensitivity and specificity for the differentiation

of RCC from other subtypes of renal tumors was 74% and 100%, and 84% and 91%, respectively.[5]

Few studies have used FDG-PET/CT for the detection of primary disease since the appearance of the first one comprising only 5 patients.[14] There have been a few since, but overall the PET sensitivity and specificity for the detection of primary RCC were 60% and 100% (CT: 92% and 100%) (**Fig. 1**).[9] It has previously been demonstrated that dual time point FDG-PET/CT technique is able to reveal differences of FDG uptake in benign versus malignant lesions to increase the specificity of diagnosis for lesions occurring in a variety of anatomic sites[15] and this can be of use in difficult and rare cases like Xanthogranulomatous pyelonephritis.[16] In a recent retrospective study of 19 patients (with 25 known solid malignant renal masses), who underwent FDG-PET/CT qualitative blinded visual analysis of PET revealed that of the 25 solid malignant renal masses (18 RCC, 3 lymphoma, 4 metastases), 22 were detectable, and, in addition, all correctly spatially localized. Fifteen of 18 with RCC were detectable, and so were all renal lymphomas and metastases. The investigators concluded that the FDG-PET had a sensitivity of 88% for detection of solid malignant renal lesions in patients with known renal malignancy, and that PET revealed differences in metabolic activity based on histopathological type, which may be useful for purposes of individualized medicine.[17]

Metastatic Disease

The detection of metastases appears to be crucial, as it has been shown that even patients with metastatic disease might benefit from radical nephrectomy followed by systemic immunotherapy or TKI treatment in cases of a good performance status. A new study involving 60 patients

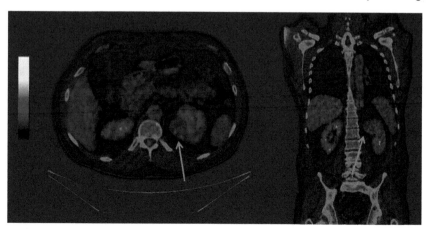

Fig. 1. FDG-PET/CT in a patient with a renal mass with very little FDG avidity (*arrow*). Biopsy confirmed that the mass was a renal cell carcinoma.

tried to assess the influence of FDG-PET/CT on the treatment decision in renal cell carcinoma and the prognostic value of the FDG accumulation assessments.[18] All patients underwent FDG-PET/CT, including 2-phase CT-angiography of the kidneys. The level of the FDG accumulation within the tumor was compared with the histologic grading, and the development of the disease was assessed 12 months after FDG-PET/CT. The overall mortality reached 46.7%, the highest FDG accumulation showed tumor of grade 4 (mean maximum standardized uptake value [SUVmax] = 10.7, range = 5–23), and the highest mortality was found for tumors exceeding an SUVmax value of 10 (mortality 62.5%). New information was brought by FDG-PET/CT in 85% of cases. The conclusion was that FDG-PET/CT has a potential to estimate survival judged from the measured SUVmax.

Depiction of occult metastatic disease has an emerging role in decision-making regarding surgery.[18] Since the start of TKI treatment, it has been important to assess the effect of the different drugs. A new study with 35 patients evaluated for RCC response to TKI treatment (sunitinib 19 cases, sorafenib 16 cases) by tumor size and FDG uptake using FDG-PET/CT before and after 1 month.[19] The study showed that PET can predict not only the duration of response to TKIs, but also survival duration, and that early assessment by FDG-PET/CT provides useful information for determining strategies for individual management of patients with advanced RCC.[19]

FDG-PET/CT also has potency as an "imaging biomarker," which can be helpful in clinical decision-making. Thus, a study from 2010 of 26 patients with advanced RCC was the first to demonstrate that a high SUVmax signaled a poor prognosis ($P = .005$, hazard ratio 1.326, 95% confidence interval 1.089–1.614) and that the survival of patients with an SUVmax of 8.8 or higher was significantly shorter than that of patients with an SUVmax less than 8.8 ($P = .0012$).[20]

The investigators of a recent meta-analysis of the sensitivity and specificity of FDG-PET and FDG-PET/CT searched for relevant studies published since 2001 and found 14.[21] The pooled sensitivity and specificity of FDG-PET were 62% and 88%, respectively, for the detection of renal lesions. The pooled rates for detection of extrarenal lesions were 79% and 90%, respectively, on a per-patient basis, and 84% and 91% on a per-lesion basis. The use of a hybrid FDG-PET/CT to detect extrarenal lesions (reported in only 2 studies) increased the pooled sensitivity and specificity to 91% and 88%, respectively, albeit with good consistency. The investigators concluded that for RCC, the adjunct of FDG-PET/CT is more helpful for detecting extrarenal metastasis than renal lesions.[21]

In summary, CT, and so far not PET, is the method of choice for the detection and staging of primary RCC. FDG-PET/CT may have an emerging role for the choice between surgery or targeted treatment before the start of TKI treatment and during follow-up. FDG-PET/CT has the potential to estimate patient survival.

BLADDER CANCER

Bladder cancer is the most common malignancy in the urinary tract and represents 7% of all malignancies in men and 2% in women[2,22] and 30% of cases present with muscle-invasive disease at time of diagnosis and a subsequently poorer prognosis.[23] More than 90% of bladder carcinomas are transitional cell (urothelial) carcinomas, whereas 5% are squamous cell carcinomas and less than 2% are adenocarcinomas.

Diagnosis/Staging

If muscle-invasive bladder cancer (MIBC) is suspected from bimanual palpation and cystoscopy, appropriate imaging should be performed before trans-urethral resection of the bladder wall. The European Association of Urology (EAU) guidelines[24] recommend multidetector-row CT (MDCT) of the chest, abdomen, and pelvis, including CT-urography in confirmed muscle-invasive bladder cancer. If MDCT is not available, a conventional excretory urography and a chest radiograph can be used. For patients with locoregional disease suitable for radical treatment, local staging can be performed using MRI and contrast-enhanced MDCT. The National Comprehensive Cancer Network recommends MDCT or MRI with nonspecified chest imaging (radiograph and CT) for staging of MIBC, and contrast-enhanced CT and MRI for staging of locoregional disease.[25]

The role of FDG-PET in detection and local staging of MIBC is somewhat compromised by the often intense excretion of FDG in the urine. Unlike glucose, FDG is not reabsorbed in the kidneys, and, therefore, only avid tumors may be visible (**Fig. 2**). In a recent meta-analysis of the use of FDG-PET/CT in staging and restaging of bladder cancer, Lu and colleagues[26] found in 6 studies comprising 236 patients a pooled sensitivity of 82% and a pooled specificity of 89%. Two of the studies[27,28] used delayed pelvic imaging after administration of diuretics and oral hydration to examine the value of FDG-PET for primary detection of MIBC. Anjos and colleagues[28] found a sensitivity and specificity of both 100% for detection of bladder wall lesions, whereas Harkirat and

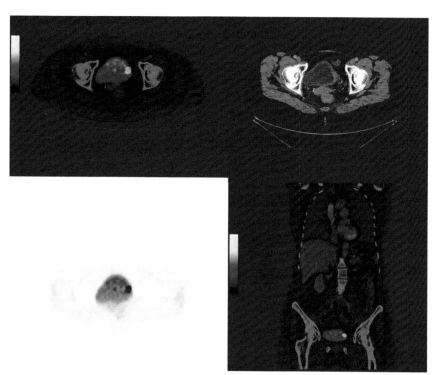

Fig. 2. FDG-PET/CT in a patient with muscle-invasive bladder cancer. Unlike glucose, FDG is not reabsorbed in the kidneys and, therefore, with time FDG is cleared from these. Simultaneously, the accumulation in the bladder increases, so that only very avid tumors may become readily visible; note the focus to the left in the bladder wall.

colleagues[27] reported values of 86.7% and 100%, respectively. This gives us a pooled sensitivity/specificity of 90%/100%. Furthermore, the analysis concluded that using FDG-PET/CT instead of FDG-PET increases the diagnostic value.

In a study by Goodfellow and colleagues,[29] 233 patients with MIBC or high-risk non-MIBC underwent preoperative FDG-PET and CT scan of the chest, abdomen, and pelvis to asses pelvic nodal involvement and distant metastases. FDG-PET was able to detect distant metastasis outside the pelvis with a sensitivity of 54% compared with 41% with CT. Specificities were 97% and 98% respectively. FDG-PET detected 13 lesions that were not visualized by CT. Six of them were metastatic bladder cancers; 1 was a primary colonic cancer, 1 colonic adenoma, 1 a basal cell tumor of the parotid gland, and 4 were inflammatory lesions. They found that the combination of FDG-PET and CT increased the sensitivity to 69%, with only a small reduction in the specificity to 95%.

Finally, Kibel and colleagues[30] studied 43 patients due for radical cystoprostatectomy. All had a negative bone and CT scan and all underwent a whole-body FDG-PET/CT. PET-positive lesions were confirmed by percutaneous biopsy or surgical exploration and negative findings by complete lymphadenectomy. Median follow-up

was 14.9 months. One patient did not undergo lymphadenectomy and was excluded. FDG-PET/CT showed occult metastatic disease in 7 of the 42 remaining patients, and, thus, the positive and negative predictive values were 78% (7/9) and 91% (30/33), whereas sensitivity and specificity were 70% and 94%, respectively. The investigators found that PET findings were strongly correlated with survival.

In summary, neither the EAU nor the National Comprehensive Cancer Network guidelines do currently consider PET in their current staging algorithms.[26,31] Further studies are seriously needed to establish the future role of FDG-PET/CT for staging and restaging of bladder cancer. The application of FDG-PET/CT for primary detection and locoregional staging of bladder cancer is challenging because of the urinary excretion of FDG. Several interventions, such as delayed imaging with diuretics and oral hydration, have been tried to overcome this obstacle,[24,27,28] so far without reaching a consensus, let alone a proposal for a standard procedure for FDG-PET/CT imaging of bladder cancer. However, several studies have shown a role for FDG-PET in staging and restaging of metastatic disease. In the study by Kibel and colleagues,[30] unrecognized metastatic disease was detected by PET in 7 (17%) of 42 patients, and the PET findings were strongly correlated with survival. In their meta-analysis, Lu and colleagues[26] concluded that FDG-PET or FDG-PET/CT have a good diagnostic accuracy with regard to staging and restaging, but the number of suitable studies was too small to allow assessment of the capability of FDG-PET or FDG-PET/CT for diagnosing primary bladder wall cancer. The literature seems to reflect a common consensus that staging and restaging of MIBC should be performed by FDG-PET/CT rather than by FDG-PET.

PROSTATE CANCER

The role of PET imaging has been examined far more extensively in this than in other urologic cancers. It is well-known that the ability of FDG-PET/CT to detect cancer is based on an elevated glucose metabolism in the malignant compared with nonmalignant tissues originally described as the Warburg effect.[32] The hypermetabolism is facilitated by an increased expression of glucose transporters (GLUTs) in the cell membrane and enhanced by intracellular hexokinase activity.[33] In prostate cancer, the GLUT expression is higher in poorly differentiated and androgen-resistant cells than in the well-differentiated and hormone-sensitive cancer cells, and the GLUT expression is downregulated when the cells are deprived of androgen (**Fig. 3**).[34] This expression is significantly higher in prostatic cancer than in benign prostatic hyperplasia tissue and is correlated with the Gleason score.[35] Together, these findings may explain the observation of higher FDG uptake in castration-resistant than in castration-sensitive tumors, and the decreased glucose metabolism observed in castration-sensitive tumors after androgen deprivation. Many previous studies have demonstrated that in most cases the FDG avidity of prostate cancers is insufficient to produce hotspots, by which we can readily detect the cancer.[36–38] The list of literature is long and reaches back to the time of standalone PET. But with the introduction of hybrid PET/CT imaging at the millennium and the gradual takeover of this technique we will in the following concentrate on results from studies applying FDG-PET/CT for prostate cancer.

Primary Diagnosis

In 2008, Jadvar and colleagues[39] examined the glucose metabolism of the normal prostate gland. In 145 male patients, who had undergone FDG-PET/CT imaging for indications unrelated to prostate pathology and none of whom had calcifications in the prostate gland or an elevated PSA, they found in the prostate gland a mean SUVmean of 1.3 ± 0.4 (range 0.1–2.7) and a mean SUVmax of 1.6 ± 0.4 (range 1.1–3.7). There was no histologic confirmation that the patients did not harbor a prostate cancer. Following this, 3 clinical trials studied the value of FDG-PET/CT for primary staging. In 2010, Minamimoto and colleagues[40] did so in 50 patients who were scanned before prostate biopsy for suspicion of prostate cancer because of an elevated PSA. Their median age was 68.2 years and their median PSA was 15.9 ng/mL. The investigators reported a sensitivity of 51.9% and a specificity of 75.7% and concluded that FDG-PET/CT was appropriate for detection of peripheral zone cancer in patients with a greater than intermediate risk. The year after, Shiiba and colleagues[41] reported from a prospective study comparing ^{11}C-methionine and FDG in 20 men with suspicion of cancer because of elevated PSA. The median age was 72.4 years and the median PSA was 181.3 ng/mL. The sensitivity and specificity of FDG-PET/CT with standard 60-minute acquisition was 35.8% and 92.3%, respectively, and the investigators concluded that in patients with a high Gleason score the 2 tracers performed equally well, whereas for Gleason scores less than 8, FDG-PET/CT was inferior. In 2012, Minamimoto and colleagues[42] reported again, but this time from a 4-year (2006–2009) multicenter screening program in asymptomatic subjects applying "FDG-PET" (ie, FDG-PET in 39% and FDG-PET/CT in 61% of studies). A total of 155,456 persons were included, and positive findings were noted in 16,955. Of these, 1912 were diagnosed with cancers, and 165 men with prostate cancer. The overall sensitivity of "FDG-PET" for the detection of any cancer was 78% (1491/1912), but as low as 37% for prostate cancer. There was no description of the characteristics of these patients with prostate cancer, but the detection rate was higher with PET/CT than with PET only.[42] In summary, although these studies were different in setup and patient groups, their results point in the same direction that FDG-PET/CT detects some prostate cancers, especially the more aggressive ones, whereas it misses most of the cancers, and, therefore, is not appropriate for the primary diagnosing of prostate cancer. The results of these 3 articles are summarized in **Table 2**.

Incidental Focal Uptake

From time to time, patients are referred to our and other clinics because of an incidental focal uptake in the prostate gland seen by FDG-PET/CT performed for reasons not related to the prostate gland. Three retrospective clinical trials have shed light on this specific issue. Han and

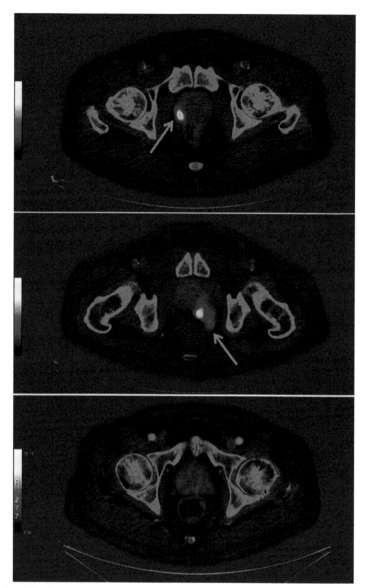

Fig. 3. Variable FDG avidity in prostate cancer. The top image shows localized, focal FDG uptake in the right prostate lobe in a patient scanned for multiple myeloma. Biopsy confirmed the unknown prostate cancer. The middle image from another patient demonstrates mixed focal/diffuse uptake in the left prostate lobe (*arrow*) possibly affecting the seminal vesicles. The bottom image is from a patient with known prostate cancer, who is under active surveillance and was scanned on suspicion of infection. There was no FDG uptake anywhere in the prostate gland.

colleagues[43] reported in 2010 an evaluation of 5119 FDG-PET/CT scans. Cases of known prostate cancer were excluded, after which 63 cases remained in which the patients had an incidental focal uptake in the prostate gland (ie, an incidence equal to 1.2% of all FDG-PET/CT scans performed). Eight patients were lost to follow-up. Of the remaining 55 patients, 52 were found to have a benign prostate gland and 3 (5.4%) had prostate cancer. The patients had been evaluated by various examinations, including additional PET/CT, MR, transrectal ultrasound, and biopsies. The investigators concluded that in case of an incidental focal uptake in the prostate gland, further evaluation would be prudent. Hwang and colleagues[44] conducted in 2012 a reevaluation of 12,037 FDG-PET/CT scans. After patients with known prostate cancer or a recent prostatic procedure had been excluded, 184 (or 1.5% of the whole material) had hypermetabolism in the prostate gland. Sixty-four were lost to follow-up, and in the remaining 120 patients, 23 were diagnosed

Table 2
Detection of prostate cancer with FDG-PET/CT

Author, Year	No. of Patients	Objective	Modality	PSA (Mean), ng/mL	Sensitivity (%)	Specificity (%)
Minamimoto et al,[40] 2011	50	Detection	FDG-PET/CT	12.0	51.9	75.7
Shiiba et al,[41] 2012	20	Detection	FDG and ^{11}C-methionine PET/CT	181.3	35.8	92.3
Minamimoto et al,[42] 2013	155,456	Screening	FDG-PET and FDG-PET/CT	N/A	37.0	N/A

Abbreviations: CT, computed tomography; FDG, 18F-fluoro-deoxy-glucose; N/A, not applicable; PET, positron emission tomography; PSA, prostate-specific antigen.
Data from Refs.[40–42]

with prostate cancer on transrectal ultrasound-guided biopsy. Of these, 91.3% had a Gleason score of 7 or higher. The investigators concluded that patients with hypermetabolism in the prostate should not be ignored but instead evaluated with rectal exploration and PSA. Bhosale and colleagues[45] reevaluated in 2013 the scans from 1440 patients who had undergone FDG-PET/CT imaging due to a known cancer other than prostate. Sixty-five patients (4.5%) had a hotspot within the prostate gland. Of these, 12 patients were lost to follow-up, whereas 53 patients could be evaluated further. Thirty-nine were biopsied, and of them 15 were diagnosed with prostate cancer. Thus, 28.3% of the patients with hotspots who were accessible to follow-up had actually cancer. The investigators concluded that patients with a hotspot in their prostate gland have a high risk of occult prostate cancer and a urology consult should be obtained. The results of these 3 studies on incidental focal uptake appear in **Table 3**.

In summary, although different in patient populations, the studies do align with respect to

relevant detection rates of occult prostate cancer. As a consequence, patients with hotspots in the prostate gland by FDG-PET/CT imaging should be further evaluated. Whether a PSA and rectal examination are sufficient have yet to be proven. Recently, a case series was published by Bartoletti ands colleagues,[46] who reported on 6 patients who had hotspots with FDG-PET/CT despite a normal PSA. All 6 harbored prostate cancer as confirmed by biopsy.

Staging

Few studies have directly addressed this subject. Three articles should be mentioned. In 2010, Tiwari and colleagues[47] examined 16 patients with FDG-PET/CT and bone scintigraphy and found 197 bone lesions by conventional bone scintigraphy and 97 (49% of 197) by FDG-PET/CT imaging. Most lesions (ie, 95%) seen by FDG-PET/CT had a matching lesion on bone scintigraphy. Unfortunately, the study did not present reference data for validation of the potentially metastatic

Table 3
Incidental focal uptake by FDG-PET/CT imaging and detection of prostate cancer

Author, Year	No. of Patients	Patient Population	Patients with Hotspots in Prostate (Fraction)	Patients with Hotspots and Follow-up Prostate	Patients with Cancer in Follow Patients (Fraction)
Han et al,[43] 2010	5119	Cancer evaluation or health check-up	64 (1.3%)	52	3 (5.4%)
Hwang et al,[44] 2013	12,037	Cancer screening or known nonprostate cancer	184 (1.5%)	120	23 (19.2%)
Bhosale et al,[45] 2013	1440	Known nonprostate cancer	65 (4.5%)	53	15 (28.3%)

Abbreviations: CT, computed tomography; FDG, 18F-fluoro-deoxy-glucose; PET, positron emission tomography.
Data from Refs.[43–45]

deposits, and, nonetheless, the investigators stated that FDG-PET/CT imaging "compliments" bone scintigraphy.[47] The year after Yu and colleagues[48] published a small pilot series of 8 patients comparing FDG and ^{11}C-acetate PET/CT and reported that ^{11}C-acetate PET/CT found more metastases in most of the patients than did FDG-PET/CT. In 2013, Damle and colleagues[49] compared FDG-PET/CT, ^{18}F-sodium fluoride PET/CT and bone scintigraphy for detection of bone metastases in prostate, lung, and breast cancer. In 49 patients with prostate cancer, they found with FDG-PET/CT a sensitivity, specificity, and accuracy of 71.9%, 100%, and 81.6%, respectively. This placed FDG-PET/CT somewhat in-between the 2 other modalities, with sodium fluoride at the top. However, the precise circumstances were not fully described, the study was small, the confidence intervals were overlapping, and, thus, no clear conclusions could be drawn.

In summary, with regard to FDG-PET/CT for staging of prostate cancer, there are currently no studies addressing the N-stage. The sparse data on M-staging apparently point to FDG-PET/CT as being inferior to other modalities, including conventional bone scintigraphy and ^{18}F-sodium fluoride PET/CT, but the data are sparse and the true interrelationship, in particular with regard to bone metastases, may be completely different from what is traditionally anticipated. An example is the study from India in which comparison of conventional whole-body bone scans with FDG-PET/CT imaging of bone metastases apparently leans in favor of the bone scan,[47] but where a succeeding comment by the same group pinpointed the complicated individual circumstances of the study and its material, without which one cannot interpret the results and is easily led astray.[50] Thus, in untreated patients, FDG-PET/CT was actually superior to the bone scan, whereas in hormone-treated cases, where the FDG uptake tend to normalize rapidly, it appeared to be inferior, although in fact FDG most likely demonstrates

the true condition, as it depicts the very early bone *marrow* metastases long before they become visible as bone *matrix* metastases by means of a bone scan tracer.[51] The latter is prone to happen months or years later, and only when the bone matrix becomes affected, but at a time when active cancer cells may have disappeared a long time earlier due to chemotherapy or radiotherapy. So, what seems a simple discrepancy and an apparent superiority may at times be an expression of the exact opposite.

Restaging

At present, 3 studies have surfaced regarding FDG-PET/CT for restaging of prostate cancer (**Table 4**). They all compared FDG with another PET tracer. García and colleagues[52] included 38 patients and found a focal uptake in 34% with FDG-PET/CT and in 68% with ^{11}C-choline PET/CT, leading to the conclusion that FDG-PET/CT was inferior. Richter and colleagues[53] examined 73 patients with the same tracers and reported similar data (ie, a sensitivity with FDG of 31% compared with one of 60% with ^{11}C-choline). More recently, Jadvar and coworkers[54] used FDG and ^{18}F-sodium fluoride PET/CT in 37 patients and found sensitivities as low as 8.1% and 16.2%, respectively. In all studies, the investigators concluded that clinical yield of FDG-PET/CT for restaging prostate cancer was limited. However, before rejecting FDG-PET/CT for this purpose, a study from the National Oncologic PET Registry in the United States deserves mentioning.[55] Scans were performed for staging, restaging, or detection of suspected recurrence in patients with pathologically proven cancers. A total of 40,863 FDG-PET and FDG-PET/CT scans were included, of which 5309 were performed in men with prostate cancer (ie, in 2042 for initial staging, in 1477 for restaging, and in 1790 for detection of suspected recurrence). These scans resulted in a change of the intended management of the cancer

Table 4
Restaging by FDG PET/CT in patients with prostate cancer

Author, Year	No. of Patients	Reference Method	PSA (Mean), ng/mL	Sensitivity (%)
Garcia et al,[52] 2009	38	Biopsy, PSA, MR	4.7	34
Richter et al,[53] 2010	73	Biopsy, PSA	2.7	31
Jadvar et al,[54] 2012	37	Imaging and biochemistry	3.2 (median)	8.1

Abbreviations: CT, computed tomography; FDG, 18F-fluoro-deoxy-glucose; MT, magnetic resonance; PET, positron emission tomography; PSA, prostate-specific antigen.
Data from Refs.[52–54]

in 35.1% of cases; in 25.3% in a change from nontreatment to treatment and in 9.7% from treatment to nontreatment. The change in management within the subgroups of staging, restaging, or detection of suspected recurrence was 32.0%, 34.0%, and 39.4%, respectively. The change in management for all cancers was 38%, which was significantly higher than for prostate cancer management.[55] Similar trends have been reported from the first 6056 PET/CT scans performed from 2006 to 2009 at our institution, where we recorded a constantly increasing use that caused a change in management in 36% of cases. At that time, only 274 scans had been performed for urologic diseases and of these, 182 (66%) were for staging of mainly prostate cancer.[56]

In summary, the sensitivity of FDG-PET/CT for staging and restaging seems suboptimal, and other tracers may be preferable if available. The rather high impact of FDG-PET/CT on management of prostate cancer in the National Oncologic PET Registry is, however, noteworthy, regardless of the lack of clinical data. Results of the latter 3 studies are compared in **Table 3**.

Prognostic Value

One study pursued the question whether FDG-PET/CT is beneficial for predicting outcome in prostate cancer. This study was published in 2013 by Jadvar and colleagues,[57] who included 87 patients with castration-resistant metastatic prostate cancer and followed them for a median of 22.2 months, during which 61 patients died. By means of univariate and multivariable Cox regression analyses of continuous PET parameters adjusted for standard clinical parameters (age, serum PSA level, alkaline phosphatase, use of pain medication, prior chemotherapy, and Gleason score at initial diagnosis), they examined the impact of SUVmax, sum of SUVmax, and average SUVmax on overall survival and found that the sum of SUVmax of all metabolically active lesions (after subtraction of a patient-specific background-liver average SUV) contributed independent prognostic information on overall survival in men with castration-resistant metastatic prostate cancer, and that this information might be useful in assessing the comparative effectiveness of various conventional and emerging treatment strategies.

SUMMARY

FDG-PET/CT is not yet the primary choice for detection of urologic cancers, primarily because of a presumed low sensitivity, which may or may not be a product of a true metabolic underlying metabolic state of tissues and abnormalities studied. In all 3 major types of cancer, there is a need to examine systematically the huge potential of molecular imaging in the shape of PET/CT with FDG or other potentially more-specific tracers. In kidney cancer, FDG-PET/CT may have an emerging role for the choice between surgery and targeted treatment before the start of TKI treatment and during follow-up. In bladder cancer, FDG-PET/CT appears to be useful for staging and restaging, whereas the clinical value of its present use for this purpose in prostate cancer is more doubtful, although accidentally detected increased uptake in the prostate gland should probably be evaluated further to rule out cancer. In all 3 cancers, FDG-PET/CT may have the potential to estimate patient survival. The choice of imaging procedure and of PET tracer probably should be tailored to each individual patient and with a definitive clinical question in mind. A better appreciation of the underlying theoretic concepts would enhance understanding of the possibilities of molecular imaging and serve as a basis for a more efficient use of this powerful technology in urologic cancers.

REFERENCES

1. Hess S, Blomberg BA, Zhu HJ, et al. The pivotal role of FDG-PET/CT in modern medicine. Acad Radiol 2014;21:232–49.
2. Ferlay J, Soerjomataram I, Ervik M, et al. GLOBO-CAN 2012 v1.0, cancer incidence and mortality worldwide: IARC cancer base no. 11. Lyon (France): International Agency for Research on Cancer; 2013 [Internet]. Available at: http://globocan.iarc.fr. Accessed May 20, 2014.
3. Cancer registry 2012: Numbers and analysis. Copenhagen (Denmark): Danish Health and Medicines Authority; 2013.
4. Engholm G, Ferlay J, Christensen N, et al. NORD-CAN: cancer incidence, mortality, prevalence and survival in the Nordic countries, version 6.0. Association of the Nordic Cancer Registries; Danish Cancer Society; 2013. Available at: http://www.ancr.nu. Accessed May 20, 2014.
5. Kim JK, Kim TK, Ahn HJ, et al. Differentiation of subtypes of renal cell carcinoma on helical CT scans. AJR Am J Roentgenol 2002;178:1499–506.
6. Schreyer HH, Uggowitzer MM, Ruppert-Kohlmayr A. Helical CT of the urinary organs. Eur Radiol 2002;12:575–91.
7. Kopka L, Fischer U, Zoeller G, et al. Dual-phase helical CT of the kidney: value of the corticomedullary and nephrographic phase for evaluation of renal lesions and preoperative staging of renal cell carcinoma. AJR Am J Roentgenol 1997;169:1573–8.

8. Israel GM, Bosniak MA. Pitfalls in renal mass evaluation and how to avoid them. Radiographics 2008;28:1325–38.

9. Schöder H, Larson SM. Positron emission tomography for prostate, bladder, and renal cancer. Semin Nucl Med 2004;34:274–92.

10. Hilton S. Imaging of renal cell carcinoma. Semin Oncol 2000;27:150–9.

11. Zagoria RJ, Bechtold RE, Dyer RB. Staging of renal adenocarcinoma: role of various imaging procedures. Am J Roentgenol 1995;164:363–70.

12. Heidenreich A, Ravery V. Preoperative imaging in renal cell cancer. World J Urol 2004;22:307–15.

13. Isreal GM, Bosniak MA. Renal imaging for diagnosis and staging of renal cell carcinoma. Urol Clin North Am 2003;30:499–514.

14. Wahl RL, Harney J, Hutchins G, et al. Imaging of renal cancer using positron emission tomography with 2-deoxy-2-(18F)-fluoro-D-glucose: pilot animal and human studies. J Urol 1991;146:1470–4.

15. Cheng G, Torigian DA, Alavi A. FDG PET/CT and MRI findings in a patient with focal xanthogranulomatous pyelonephritis mimicking cystic renal malignancy. Clin Nephrol 2013;76:484–6.

16. Huang H, Pourdehnad M, Lambright ES, et al. Dual time point 18F-FDG PET imaging for differentiating malignant from inflammatory processes. J Nucl Med 2001;42:1412–7.

17. Nakhoda Z, Torigian DA, Saboury B, et al. Assessment of the diagnostic performance of (18)F-FDG-PET/CT for detection and characterization of solid renal malignancies. Hell J Nucl Med 2013;16:19–24.

18. Ferda J, Ferdova E, Hora M, et al. FDG-PET/CT in potentially advanced renal cell carcinoma: a role in treatment decisions and prognosis estimation. Anticancer Res 2013;33:2665–72.

19. Ueno D, Yao M, Tateishi U, et al. Early assessment by FDG-PET/CT of patients with advanced renal cell carcinoma treated with tyrosine kinase inhibitors is predictive of disease course. BMC Cancer 2012;162:2–8.

20. Namura K, Minamimoto R, Yao M, et al. Impact of maximum standardized uptake value (SUVmax) evaluated by 18-Fluoro-2-deoxy-D-glucose positron emission tomography/computed tomography (18F-FDG-PET/CT) on survival for patients with advanced renal cell carcinoma: a preliminary report. BMC Cancer 2010;10:667–75.

21. Wang HY, Ding HJ, Chen JH, et al. Meta-analysis of the diagnostic performance of [18F]FDG-PET and PET/CT in renal cell carcinoma. Cancer Imaging 2012;12:464–74.

22. Jemal A, Bray F, Center MM, et al. Global cancer statistics. CA Cancer J Clin 2011;61:69–90.

23. Kaufman DS, Shipley WU, Feldman AS. Bladder cancer. Lancet 2009;374:239–49.

24. Stenzl A, Cowan NC, De Santis M, et al. The updated EAU guidelines on muscle-invasive and metastatic bladder cancer. Eur Urol 2009;55:815–25.

25. Lawrentschuk N, Lee ST, Scott AM. Current role of PET, CT, MR for invasive bladder cancer. Curr Urol Rep 2013;14:84–9.

26. Lu YY, Chen JH, Liang JA, et al. Clinical value of FDG PET or PET/CT in urinary bladder cancer: a systemic review and meta-analysis. Eur J Radiol 2012;81:2411–6.

27. Harkirat S, Anand S, Jacob M. Forced diuresis and dual-phase F-fluorodeoxyglucose-PET/CT scan for restaging of urinary bladder cancers. Indian J Radiol Imaging 2010;20:13–9.

28. Anjos DA, Etchebehere EC, Ramos CD, et al. 18F-FDG PET/CT delayed images after diuretic for restaging invasive bladder cancer. J Nucl Med 2007;48:764–70.

29. Goodfellow H, Viney Z, Hughes P, et al. Role of fluorodeoxyglucose positron emission tomography (FDG PET)-computed tomography (CT) in the staging of bladder cancer. BJU Int 2013. [Epub ahead of print].

30. Kibel AS, Dehdashti F, Katz MD, et al. Prospective study of [18F]fluorodeoxyglucose positron emission tomography/computed tomography for staging of muscle-invasive bladder carcinoma. J Clin Oncol 2009;27:4314–20.

31. Lee ST, Lawrentschuk N, Scott AM. PET in prostate and bladder tumors. Semin Nucl Med 2012;42:231–46.

32. Warburg O, Wind F, Negelein E. Über den Stoffwechsel von Tumoren im Körper. Klin Wochenschr 1926;5:829–32.

33. Kroemer G, Pouyssegur J. Tumor cell metabolism: cancer's Achilles's heel. Cancer cell 2008;13:472–82.

34. Jadvar H. Imaging of prostate cancer with 18F fluorodeoxyglucose PET/CT: utility and limitations. Eur J Nucl Med Mol Imaging 2013;40:5–10.

35. Oyama N, Akino H, Suzuki Y, et al. The increased accumulation of [18F] fluorodeoxyglucose in untreated prostate cancer patients. Jpn J Clin Oncol 1999;29:623–9.

36. Schöder H, Herrmann K, Gönen M, et al. 2-[18F]fluoro-2-deoxyglucose positron emission tomography for the detection of disease in patients with prostate-specific antigen relapse after radical prostatectomy. Clin Cancer Res 2005;1(11):4761–9.

37. Watanabe H, Kanematsu M, Kondo H, et al. Preoperative detection of prostate cancer: a comparison with 11C-choline PET, 18F-fluorodeoxyglucose PET and MR imaging. J Magn Reson Imaging 2010;31:1151–6.

38. Larson SM, Morris M, Gunther I, et al. Tumor localization of 16beta-18F-fluoro-5alpha-dihydrotestosterone versus 18F-FDG in patients with progressive,

metastatic prostate cancer. J Nucl Med 2004;45: 366–73.

39. Jadvar H, Ye W, Groshen S, et al. [F-18]-fluoro-deoxyglucose PET-CT of the normal prostate gland. Ann Nucl Med 2008;22:787–93.

40. Minamimoto R, Uemura H, Sano F, et al. The potential of FDG-PET/CT for detecting prostate cancer in patients with an elevated serum PSA level. Ann Nucl Med 2011;25:21–7.

41. Shiiba M, Ishihara K, Kimura G, et al. Evaluation of primary prostate cancer using 11C-methionine-PET/CT and 18F-FDG-PET/CT. Ann Nucl Med 2012;26:138–45.

42. Minamimoto R, Senda M, Jinnouchi S, et al. The current status of an FDG-PET cancer screening program in Japan, based on a 4-year (2006-2009) nationwide survey. Ann Nucl Med 2013;27:46–57.

43. Han EJ, HO J, Choi WH, et al. Significance of incidental focal uptake in prostate on 18-fluoro-2-deoxyglucose positron emission tomography CT images. Br J Radiol 2010;83:915–20.

44. Hwang I, Chong A, Jung SI, et al. Is further evaluation needed for incidental focal uptake in the prostate in 18-fluoro-2-deoxyglucose positron emission tomography-computed tomography images? Ann Nucl Med 2013;27:140–5.

45. Bhosale P, Balachandran A, Vikram R, et al. What is the clinical significance of FDG unexpected uptake in the prostate in patients undergoing PET/CT for other malignancies? Int J Mol Imaging 2013;2013: 476786.

46. Bartoletti R, Meliani E, Bongini A, et al. Fluorodeoxyglucose positron emission tomography may aid the diagnosis of aggressive primary prostate cancer: a case series study. Oncol Lett 2014;7:381–6.

47. Tiwari BP, Jangra S, Nair N, et al. Complimentary role of FDG-PET imaging and skeletal scintigraphy in the evaluation of patients of prostate carcinoma. Indian J Cancer 2010;47:385–90.

48. Yu EY, Muzi M, Hackenbracht JA, et al. C11-acetate and F-18 FDG PET for men with prostate cancer bone metastases: relative findings and response to therapy. Clin Nucl Med 2011;36:192–8.

49. Damle NA, Bal C, Bandopadhyaya GP, et al. The role of 18F-fluoride PET-CT in the detection of bone metastases in patients with breast, lung and prostate carcinoma: a comparison with FDG PET/CT and 99mTc-MDP bone scan. Jpn J Radiol 2013;31: 262–9.

50. Basu S, Tiwari BP. Complimentary role of FDG-PET imaging and skeletal scintigraphy in the evaluation of patients of prostate carcinoma. Indian J Cancer 2011;48:513–4.

51. Suva LJ, Washam C, Nicholas RW, et al. Bone metastasis: mechanisms and therapeutic opportunities. Nat Rev Endocrinol 2011;7:208–18.

52. García JR, Soler M, Blanch MA, et al. PET/CT with (11)C-choline and (18)F-FDG in patients with elevated PSA after radical treatment of a prostate cancer. Rev Esp Med Nucl 2009;28:95–100.

53. Richter JA, Rodríguez M, Rioja J, et al. Dual tracer 11C-choline and FDG-PET in the diagnosis of biochemical prostate cancer relapse after radical treatment. Mol Imaging Biol 2010;12:210–7.

54. Jadvar H, Desai B, Ji L, et al. Prospective evaluation of 18F-NaF and 18F-FDG PET/CT in detection of occult metastatic disease in biochemical recurrence of prostate cancer. Clin Nucl Med 2012;37: 637–43.

55. Hillner BE, Siegel BA, Shields AF, et al. Relationship between cancer type and impact of PET and PET/CT on intended management: findings of the national oncologic PET registry. J Nucl Med 2008; 49:1928–35.

56. Høilund-Carlsen PF, Gerke O, Vilstrup MH, et al. PET/CT without capacity limitations: a Danish experience from a European perspective. Eur Radiol 2011;21:1277–85.

57. Jadvar H, Desai B, Ji L, et al. Baseline 18F-FDG PET/CT parameters as imaging biomarkers of overall survival in castrate-resistant metastatic prostate cancer. J Nucl Med 2013;54:1195–201.

[^{18}F]Fluorodeoxyglucose PET for Interventional Oncology in Liver Malignancy

CrossMark

Morsal Samim, MD[a], Ghassan E. El-Haddad, MD, PhD[b], Izaak Quintes Molenaar, MD, PhD[a], Warner Prevoo, MD[c], Maurice A.A.J. van den Bosch, MD, PhD[d], Abass Alavi, MD, PhD, DSc[e], Marnix G.E.H. Lam, MD, PhD[d],*

KEYWORDS

- FDG-PET • Liver • Interventional oncology • Imaging • Staging • Radiofrequency ablation
- Radioembolization • Chemoembolization

KEY POINTS

- FDG-PET(/CT) seems to be superior to conventional imaging for the detection of extrahepatic lesions during the work-up of patients for liver resection and ablative therapy.
- The size of the lesion and chemotherapy before liver resection influence the sensitivity of the test.
- FDG-PET(/CT) can be used for surveillance after RFA for detection of incomplete ablation or early recurrence.
- FDG-PET(/CT) is an useful diagnostic modality in the workup of patients before Yttrium-90 radioembolization.
- FDG-PET(/CT) in the follow-up of patients after Yttrium-90 radioembolization seems to be a predictor of tumor response and the survival of patients.
- Directly following Yttrium-90 radioembolization, Yttrium-90-PET/CT imaging can be used to quantify the distribution of the microspheres.

INTRODUCTION

In recent years, many new treatment modalities have been established in liver-directed oncologic intervention. Examples are radiofrequency ablation (RFA), radioembolization, transarterial chemoembolization (TACE), and high-intensity focused ultrasonography (HIFU). The development of minimally invasive image-guided procedures in tandem with improvements in existing methods has resulted in improved prognosis of oncology patients.[1–3] These advances provide medical consultants with more treatment options but also require individualized treatment strategies. Therefore, careful selection of patients before the intervention remains of paramount importance in determining the optimal treatment strategy.

Besides patient selection and treatment planning, there is an increasing demand for monitoring

Funding Sources: None.
Conflict of Interest: None.
[a] Department of Surgery, University Medical Center Utrecht, Heidelberglaan 100, Utrecht 3584 CX, The Netherlands; [b] Department of Interventional Radiology, Moffitt Cancer Center, 12902 Magnolia Drive, Tampa, FL 33612, USA; [c] Department of Interventional Radiology, Antoni van Leeuwenhoek Hospital, Plesmanlaan 121, Amsterdam 1066 CX, The Netherlands; [d] Department of Radiology and Nuclear Medicine, University Medical Center Utrecht, Heidelberglaan 100, Utrecht 3584 CX, The Netherlands; [e] Division of Nuclear Medicine, University of Pennsylvania Perelman School of Medicine, 3535 Market Street, Philadelphia, PA 19104, USA
* Corresponding author.
E-mail address: m.lam@umcutrecht.nl

PET Clin 9 (2014) 469–495
http://dx.doi.org/10.1016/j.cpet.2014.07.004

the effectiveness of minimally invasive image-guided procedures. Early evaluation of the effectiveness of the treatment is important, as patients might benefit from interventions or alternative treatment regimens in cases of recurrent or residual disease.

Computed tomography (CT) and magnetic resonance (MR) imaging, although widely used, are of limited sensitivity, specificity, and accuracy with regard to the detection of residual or recurrent disease.[4] The main limitation is the morphologic character of these diagnostic modalities.[4] Other limitations, particularly in ablative treatment, include the nonmalignant procedure-related causes of enhancement in the treatment zone (peritumoral reaction to the thermal injury and local flow disturbances).[5,6]

Over the past decade, PET using [^{18}F]fluoro-2-deoxy-D-glucose (FDG) has been established as a major component in the management of patients with cancer in general.[7] A recent report from the National Oncologic PET Registry (NOPR) elaborated on how FDG-PET has affected the care decision. Reported FDG-PET–based change of management in various forms of cancer ranged from 30% to 40%.[7]

FDG-PET is a functional imaging tool that provides metabolic information. It may be effective for (1) staging and selection of patients by detection of intrahepatic and extrahepatic disease; (2) detection of residual disease in ablative therapy; (3) detection of recurrent disease; (4) stratification of patients before the procedure; and (5) response assessment following the procedure.[8] FDG is a glucose analogue, which uses the same metabolic pathways as glucose. It enters the cell via glucose transporters; it is phosphorylated by hexokinase and converted to FDG-6-phosphate. As such it is trapped in the cell, preferentially in those cells with high glucose uptake and low glucose-6-phosphatase enzymatic activity, such as tumor cells. Hence, metabolic alterations in tissues can accurately be depicted by FDG-PET. It is known that metabolic changes usually precede anatomic changes, so FDG-PET may detect a lesion before it becomes anatomically apparent. This ability constitutes a strong argument for using FDG-PET/CT in the management of oncology patients.

Many studies have investigated the accuracy of FDG-PET or FDG-PET/CT for these purposes. However, most studies have a small sample size based on a retrospective cohort. This article aims to provide an overview of the role of FDG-PET or FDG-PET/CT in patients with liver malignancies treated by means of surgical resection, ablative therapy, chemoembolization, radioembolization, and brachytherapy, all of which are liver-directed oncologic interventions.

METHODS

A comprehensive literature search was performed from inception to December 2013 for articles assessing the diagnostic accuracy of FDG-PET or FDG-PET/CT in diagnosis, staging, and follow-up of patients with liver malignancies. The literature search was performed in PubMed, Embase, and the Cochrane library, and included synonyms for liver resection; ablation therapy; radioembolization; chemoembolization; external-beam radiotherapy (EBRT); HIFU; and FDG-PET. From the studies identified by the initial literature search, all titles and abstracts were screened to select studies reporting on FDG-PET/CT imaging in liver-directed interventional oncology treatments. Subsequently, full-text articles of the selected studies were screened to assess eligibility. All cross-references were screened for potential relevant studies not identified by the initial literature search. Inclusion and exclusion criteria included studies on FDG-PET, any primary cancer or metastatic disease of the liver, preoperative baseline imaging for comparison, and original data. Exclusion criteria included animal studies, reviews, studies with fewer than 5 patients, and case reports. The search flowchart is shown in **Fig. 1**.

Given the extent of the literature available for liver resection, and to provide an up-to-date overview of the data on this topic, the authors have selected the relevant studies published in the last 10 years. For the remaining topics, the full set of available literature was used.

RESULTS
Liver Resections

Liver surgery is considered the gold standard for curative treatment of liver malignancies, with 5-year survival rates between 24% and 58% for colorectal carcinoma (CRC) liver metastases,[9–12] and up to 70% in carefully selected patients with hepatocellular carcinoma (HCC).[13] Complete surgical resection of liver malignancies is confirmed by pathologic examination of the specimen margins during the operation or immediately after surgery. Nevertheless, local tumor recurrence or intrahepatic tumor recurrence appears in up to 35% of patients, which jeopardizes the disease-free survival (DFS) of these patients significantly.[14,15] Intrahepatic tumor recurrence can be the result of micrometastases in the periphery of the target lesion that are not visible on preoperative imaging. Moreover, tumor lesions not detectable on preoperative imaging have been found intraoperatively by means of ultrasonographic imaging.[16–18] In addition to preoperative imaging,

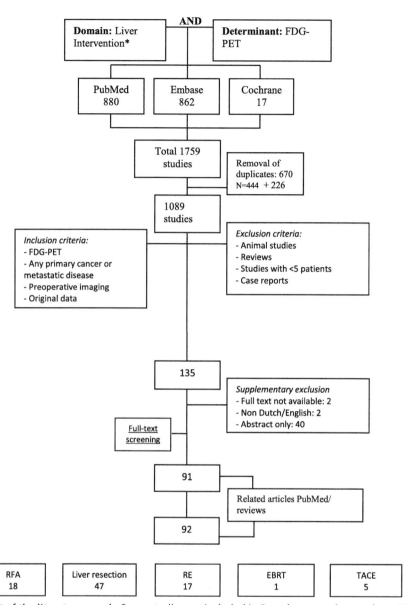

Fig. 1. Flowchart of the literature search. Some studies are included in 2 study groups (eg, study on RFA and liver resection combined). [a] The search was performed separately for each intervention: liver resection, radiofrequency ablation (RFA), radioembolization (RE), chemoembolization (TACE), external-beam radiotherapy (EBRT), and high-intensity focused ultrasonography.

contrast-enhanced intraoperative ultrasonography has been shown to yield significant new information, and changes the operative plan in up to 50% of patients.[17,18] The latter emphasizes the need for more accurate preoperative imaging.

To achieve adequate decision making in surgery, it is important to assess the precise extent of the disease. Both intrahepatic and extrahepatic disease influences the decision-making process. In the past, extrahepatic disease was considered a contraindication for liver resection.[19,20] However, the limits of resectable disease are shifting. Several

centers have reported results of simultaneous liver resection and the resection of extrahepatic disease,[21–23] with a 5-year survival of 29% reported by Elias and colleagues.[24] There was also a significant ($P = .021$) difference in the prognosis of patients who had an R0 resection compared with an R1-R2 resection (all sites of extrahepatic disease).[24] Hence, not only the localization of the extrahepatic disease but also the completeness of resection is important. Therefore it is recommended that patients with disease not amenable to a complete resection should not be offered combined metastasectomy of intrahepatic and extrahepatic disease.[25] In general, there is no gold-standard treatment algorithm available for liver malignancy, and different centers each have their own distinct treatment policy. However, the recommended treatment algorithm for liver resection indicates that patients with intrahepatic and extrahepatic disease should initially be treated with systematic chemotherapy, and that patients with progressive disease are not candidates for surgery and should be treated with systemic chemotherapy and palliative support.[25] When stable or responsive disease is achieved, patients should be evaluated for surgery. Those in whom R0 resection is not possible are not candidates for surgery and should continue with chemotherapy.[25] Patients with simultaneous intrahepatic and extrahepatic CRC metastases should be selected for surgery, aiming to achieve R0 resection in all sites.[25]

Preoperative imaging is important not only for presurgical planning to determine resectability but also for the detection of extrahepatic disease. In the following sections this article focuses on the value of FDG-PET in relation to: (1) preoperative staging of patients and change of management based on intrahepatic versus extrahepatic disease; (2) the follow-up of patients; (3) cost-effectiveness of FDG-PET; and (4) tumor cell type.

Preoperative staging

In the past, many studies have focused on the additional value of FDG-PET in the selection of patients for liver resection.[26–31] As already mentioned, selection of patients for surgery depends on the number and localization of the intrahepatic lesions in addition to the presence of extrahepatic disease.[25,32]

Intrahepatic disease The published results on FDG-PET(/CT) regarding presurgical hepatic staging show large variability in the sensitivity and specificity of the detection of intrahepatic lesions (Table 1). For the detection of intrahepatic lesions, FDG-PET(/CT) has a sensitivity and specificity ranging from 45% to 98% and 25% to 71%, respectively. Comparison with conventional imaging modalities resulted in a sensitivity and specificity for CT, MR imaging, and ultrasonography of 71% to 100% and 50% to 94%, 67% to 100% and 57% to 100%, and 63% and 50%, respectively (see Table 1). Only few studies reported a significant difference between FDG-PET(/CT) and conventional imaging.[26,42,43] In the studies from Seo and colleagues[42] and Servois and colleagues,[43] FDG-PET(/CT) was respectively compared with gadoxetate disodium–enhanced MR imaging and plain MR imaging. Both studies were in favor of

MR imaging with regard to the detection of intrahepatic disease. Ramos and colleagues[26] compared FDG-PET/CT with conventional imaging (CT or MR imaging), and also reported a significant ($P<.001$) difference in favor of conventional imaging. Although these 3 studies reported data in favor of conventional imaging, other studies did not report any difference between both imaging strategies,[33,34,37,44] or even superior results for FDG-PET when compared with conventional imaging.[27] One of the largest prospective studies consisted of a cohort of 131 patients who were selected for liver surgery.[44] CT was compared with FDG-PET and compared with findings during laparotomy and follow-up data. A total of 128 patients had liver lesions identified at laparotomy. CT detected 127 true-positive lesions and FDG-PET 126 true positives. There were 3 false-positive lesions and 1 false-negative lesion detected by CT, and no false-positive and 2 false-negative lesions using FDG-PET. Both CT and FDG-PET missed lesions (25%) between 10 and 20 mm.[44]

The sensitivity of FDG-PET for the detection of intrahepatic disease is influenced by tumor size less than 1 cm, tumor cell type, and neoadjuvant chemotherapy.[27,28,33,37,42] When looking at predictive factors of the utility of FDG-PET/CT for the selection of patients for hepatic resection, neoadjuvant chemotherapy affected the results in a negative way.[26,37,45,46] A history of insufficient surgery (number of lymphatic nodes in histopathologic analysis <12, infiltration of radial margin) seemed to increase the probability that the change of management as suggested by FDG-PET was appropriate.[26] The former was also confirmed by a recent meta-analysis on the preoperative imaging of CRC liver metastases after neoadjuvant chemotherapy.[28] In patients with liver metastases who received neoadjuvant chemotherapy, the diagnostic accuracy of FDG-PET and FDG-PET/CT was strongly affected by chemotherapy (sensitivity decreased from 81.3% to 54.5%, and 71% to 51.7% for FDG-PET and FDG-PET/CT, respectively).[28] In the neoadjuvant setting, MR imaging seemed to be most accurate in the selection of patients for liver resection based on intrahepatic lesion detection. The pooled sensitivity reported in the literature was 85.7% for MR imaging and 69.9% for CT.[28] A reported explanation for the decreased diagnostic performance of FDG-PET in this setting is the induced necrosis, which may give initially solid metastases a more cystic appearance. MR imaging and CT might still visualize these lesions during the arterial phase in the form of rim enhancement. On FDG-PET, however, there is no FDG uptake in areas with necrosis, and therefore lesions may be missed.[28]

Table 1
Liver resection studies: role of FDG-PET in the detection of intrahepatic disease

Authors,[Ref.] Year	N[a] 1 = Patients 2 = Lesions	Comparison	% Change of Management with FDG-PET	Accuracy (%)	Sensitivity (%)	Specificity (%)
Bohm et al,[27] 2004	2 = 174	FDG-PET; CT; MRI; US	18[b]	FDG-PET 80[c]; CT 70[c]; MRI 54[c]; US 63[c]	FDG-PET 82; CT 71; MRI 83; US 63	FDG-PET 25; CT 50; MRI 57; US 50
Ramos et al,[26] 2011	2 = 225	FDG-PET/CT CT/MRI	8 useful[b]; 9 harmful[d]	—	FDG-PET/CT 55; CT/MRI 82.9; P<.001	—
Kong et al,[33] 2008	1 = 65	FDG-PET/CT; CT; Mn-DPDP MRI	17[b]	—	FDG-PET/CT 94; MRI 99	FDG-PET/CT 100; MRI 100
Truant et al,[34] 2005	2 = 119	FDG-PET; CT	9 useful[b]; 6 harmful[b]	Intrahepatic: FDG-PET 79; CT 77; Overall: FDG-PET 88; CT 86	Intrahepatic: FDG-PET 79; CT 79; Overall: FDG-PET 78; CT 76	Intrahepatic: FDG-PET 80; CT 25; Overall: FDG-PET 97; CT 94
Grassetto et al,[35] 2010	1 = 43	FDG-PET/CT; US; CT	28[d]	—	—	—
Sorensen et al,[36] 2007	1 = 54	FDG-PET; CT	19[d]	—	—	—
Selzner et al,[37] 2004	1 = 76	FDG-PET/CT	21[b]	—	FDG-PET/ CT 91 CT 95	FDG-PET/ CT 90 CT 70
Kochhar et al,[38] 2010[e]	1 = 157	FDG-PET/CT MRI/CT	33.8[d]; P<.0001[f]	FDG-PET/CT 87.3; MRI/ CT NR	FDG-PET/CT 87.1; MRI/ CT NR	FDG-PET/CT 88; MRI/ CT NR
Briggs et al,[39] 2011	1 = 102 (94 liver)	FDG-PET/CT; MRI/CT	30 useful[b]; 10 harmful[b]	—	—	—
McLeish et al,[40] 2012	1 = 54	FDG-PET; CT	66.7[d]	—	—	—
Georgakopoulos et al,[41] 2013	1 = 35 (19 resection)	FDG-PET/CT; CEUS	36.8[b]	—	—	—
Seo et al,[42] 2011	1 = 68	FDG-PET/CT; EOB-MRI	—	FDG-PET/CT 81; EOB-MRI 94; P<.001	FDG-PET/CT 93; EOB-MRI 100; P = .375	FDG-PET/CT 71; EOB-MRI 71; P = .375
Servois et al,[43] 2010	2 = 28	FDG-PET; MRI	—	FDG-PET 43[c]; MRI 64[c]	FDG-PET 45; MRI 67; P = .01	FDG-PET 100[c]; MRI⁻
Wiering et al,[44] 2007	1 = 131	FDG-PET; CT	—	FDG-PET 98[c]; CT 98[c]	FDG-PET 98[c]; CT 100[c]	FDG-PET 100[c]; CT⁻

In all studies, histology, clinical, and imaging follow-up data were used as reference test. P value is given if it was reported.

Abbreviations: CEUS, contrast-enhanced ultrasonography; CT, contrast-enhanced computed tomography unless otherwise specified; EOB, gadoxetate disodium–enhanced; FDG, [¹⁸F]fluoro-2-deoxy-D-glucose; Mn-DPDP MRI, magnetic resonance imaging with liver-specific contrast medium; MRI, magnetic resonance imaging; NR, not reported; US, ultrasonography.

[a] Analysis performed based on number of patients or number of lesions.
[b] Based on extrahepatic disease detection.
[c] Calculated using the available data.
[d] Not specified.
[e] Data analysis for intrahepatic and extrahepatic disease.
[f] Significant correlation between pre-PET/CT conventional imaging and PET/CT results on the clinical impact on patient management.

Data from Refs.[26,27,33–40,42–44]

Extrahepatic disease FDG-PET does seem to be superior to CT and MR imaging in the detection of extrahepatic disease during staging of patients before liver resection (**Fig. 2**).[26,27,29,30,33,34,37,44,47,48] In terms of detection of the location of the extrahepatic disease, FDG-PET seems most useful in the detection of small malignant mesenteric and peritoneal nodules,[26,33] uncommon sites such as bone and spleen,[26] and mediastinal and vertebral lesions.[34] The reported sensitivity and specificity for the detection of extrahepatic disease shows a wide range of 60% to 100% and 14% to 98% for FDG-PET(/CT), and 17% to 100% and 25% to 100% for CT, respectively (**Table 2**).

The only randomized controlled trial was conducted by Ruers and colleagues[29] in a cohort of 150 patients with CRC liver metastases who were randomly assigned to CT only or CT plus FDG-PET. The primary outcome of this study was the number of futile laparotomies (defined as any laparotomy that did not result in complete tumor treatment) that revealed benign disease, or did not result in DFS longer than 6 months.[29] There were fewer futile laparotomies in the FDG-PET plus CT group (28% vs 45%). The relative risk reduction of futile laparotomy was 38% (95% confidence interval 4%–60%; $P = .042$). Follow-up of the patients showed that FDG-PET correctly predicted benign disease in 2 patients and unresectable extrahepatic disease in 3 patients.[29] Overall, in 7 patients FDG-PET was able to detect additional extrahepatic disease that was missed on the CT scan (pulmonary metastasis, mediastinal metastases, and abdominal lymph nodes). The 3-year survival showed no significant difference between survival of patients in both groups, so although fewer laparotomies were performed in the experimental group than in the conventional group, this was not at the expense of a decrease in survival.[29]

Change of management
Change of management is a frequently reported end point in studies on FDG-PET(/CT) in patients scheduled for liver resection, ranging from 8% to 67%. Throughout the literature, change of management is defined as change in the treatment algorithm based on additional information obtained by FDG-PET(/CT), for example, first-line systemic chemotherapy instead of curative liver resection after irresectable extrahepatic disease has been detected on FDG-PET. In essence, change of management is considered as all cases whereby the treatment of choice selected from the therapy algorithm is reconsidered, sometimes resulting in

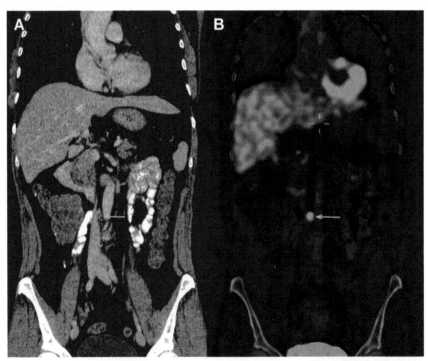

Fig. 2. Workup imaging by means of FDG-PET/CT and contrast-enhanced CT (CECT) in a patient with colorectal carcinoma liver metastases. The CECT showed 2 solitary liver metastases. However, FDG-PET/CT showed one para-aortal lymph node (*arrow*) that was not seen on the CECT scan (*B*). Retrospectively, the lymph node could be detected on the CECT and measured 0.9 cm (*arrow in A*). The patient underwent liver resection plus resection of the lymph node. Histopathologic examination of the resected lymph node showed metastatic disease.

Table 2
Liver resection studies: role of FDG-PET in the detection of extrahepatic disease

Authors,[Ref.] Year	N[a] 1 = Patients 2 = Lesions	Comparison	Accuracy (%)	Sensitivity (%)	Specificity (%)	Site
Bohm et al,[27] 2004	2 = 174	FDG-PET CT MRI US	FDG-PET 63[b] CT 48[b] MRI 43[b] US 28[b]	FDG-PET 63 CT 47 MRI 40 US 29	FDG-PET 60 CT 50 MRI 50 US 25	Intra-abdominal cavity and extra-abdominal organs
Ramos et al,[26] 2011	2 = 225	FDG-PET/CT CT or MRI	NR	FDG-PET/CT 67 CT 17 $P = .257$	FDG-PET/CT 96 CT 99 $P = .251$	Locoregional recurrence of primary
Truant et al,[34] 2005	2 = 119	FDG-PET CT	Intra-abdominal: FDG-PET 93 CT 82 Extra-abdominal: FDG-PET 97 CT 100	Intra-abdominal: FDG-PET 63 CT 25 Extra-abdominal: FDG-PET 100 CT 100	Intra-abdominal: FDG-PET 98 CT 91 Extra-abdominal: FDG-PET 97 CT 100	Intra-abdominal cavity and extra-abdominal organs
Selzner et al,[37] 2004	1 = 76	FDG-PET/CT CT	NR	1. FDG-PET/CT 93 CT 53 $P = .03$ 2. FDG-PET/CT 89 CT 64 $P = .02$	NR	1. Locoregional recurrence of primary 2. Extrahepatic disease
Wiering et al,[44] 2007	1 = 131	FDG-PET CT	FDG-PET 41[b] CT 50[b]	FDG-PET 60[b] CT 100[b]	FDG-PET 14[b] CT 25[b]	Extrahepatic intra-abdominal

Histology, clinical, and imaging follow-up data were used as reference test. *P* value is given if it was reported.
[a] Analysis performed based on number of patients or number of lesions.
[b] Calculated using the available data.
Data from Refs.[26,27,34,37,44]

palliative treatment instead of curative treatment. The reported change of management is mostly the result of the detection of extrahepatic disease (see **Table 1**).[26,27,33,34,37,39,41] In a recent prospective study in a combined cohort of RFA and liver resection in patients with CRC liver metastases, the results of FDG-PET/CT altered the management in 36.8% of patients by the detection of extrahepatic disease.[41] McLeish and colleagues,[40] who performed a retrospective study of 54 patients considered for liver resection of CRC liver metastases, reported a high rate of change of management (66.7%). However, the investigators did not report whether the change of management was based on the detection of intrahepatic or extrahepatic disease.[40] Of note, FDG-PET proved very useful in equivocal CT cases. In patients with equivocal hepatic lesions on CT images, FDG-PET was able to definitely assess lesions in 92% of patients, hence aiding in the management decision.[40]

However, not all changes in the management of patients were desirable. Some studies also emphasized the downside of patient selection using FDG-PET.[26,34,39] In a prospective study in 97 patients, new findings in FDG-PET/CT resulted in a change of therapeutic strategy in 17 patients (17%); however, the additional information was correct in only 8 cases.[26] Other studies also reported false-negative and false-positive results of FDG-PET, ranging from 6% to 10%.[34,39] Possible explanations are false-negative results owing to the small size of lesions, tumor cell type, neoadjuvant chemotherapy, and false-positive results in the case of benign lesions, such as inflammation.

Role of FDG-PET in the follow-up

Using conventional imaging techniques it may be difficult to differentiate between malignant and benign lesions, particularly distinguishing scar tissue from tumor recurrence in previously resected patients (**Fig. 3**). Many studies have reported on the role of FDG-PET in the preoperative setting, such as already mentioned. However, limited data are available on the role of FDG-PET in the follow-up of patients. Selzner and colleagues[37] investigated the value of FDG-PET/CT for the detection of recurrent disease after hepatic resection of CRC liver metastases. Although CT and PET/CT provided comparable results for the detection of intrahepatic metastases (sensitivity of 95% and 91%, respectively), PET/CT was superior in establishing the diagnosis of intrahepatic recurrences in patients with prior hepatectomy (specificity 50% vs 100%, $P = .04$). Furthermore, CT and PET/CT detected local recurrences at the primary colorectal resection site with a sensitivity of 53% and 93%, respectively ($P = .03$).[37]

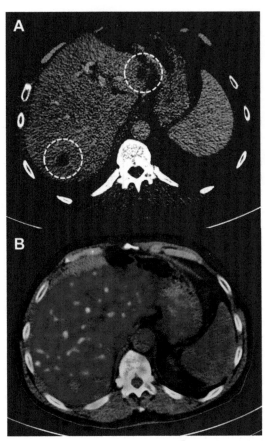

Fig. 3. Follow-up imaging (1 year) in a patient with colorectal carcinoma liver metastases who was treated with liver resection (segment II and V, see *dotted circles*) and RFA for a lesion in segment VII. CECT shows the lesion in segment II and postablative lesion in segment VII (*A*). FDG-PET/CT did not show increased FDG uptake in these lesions (*B*).

Several studies reported on the survival of patients staged by means of FDG-PET compared with conventional imaging before liver resection for CRC liver metastases.[30,49,50] Finkelstein and colleagues[49] included 100 patients staged by FDG-PET before liver resection. The results indicated that early recurrences after liver resection for CRC liver metastases are much more likely to be found in the liver, and later recurrences are much more likely to be found in extrahepatic sites. The investigators collected all available case series on survival after liver resection in patients who were staged by conventional imaging methods. In contrast to FDG-PET, none of the 18 large case series reported a time-specific or site-specific pattern of recurrence.[49] A possible explanation could be that FDG-PET has a higher sensitivity for the detection of extrahepatic disease. The same group also reported a 5-year overall survival of 58% (95% confidence interval 46%–72%) in patients staged with FDG-PET, compared with only 30% 5-year survival in patients staged without FDG-PET.[50] Preoperative screening with FDG-PET was associated with a preferable postoperative 5-year survival and resulted in longer progression-free survival in terms of extrahepatic disease.[50]

Role of FDG-PET(/CT) in hepatocellular carcinoma

The sensitivity of FDG-PET in hepatocellular carcinoma (HCC) differs from the sensitivity in CRC liver metastases. In early HCC without portal vein invasion, curative resection can be achieved. However, HCC often presents late with a poor prognosis. Therefore, diagnostic confirmation and assessment of the extent of disease are important for management.[51] In studies that investigated the diagnostic accuracy of FDG-PET in staging HCC, the reported sensitivity was only 70% to 80%.[27,52] Some studies reported a decrease in sensitivity of FDG-PET when used for staging of well-differentiated HCC.[27,53,54] Other studies, however, did not find any association between FDG activity and differentiation level of the lesion.[52] Possible explanation for the reduced sensitivity may be the similarity in glucose uptake of well-differentiated HCC cells and normal hepatocytes. Differences in FDG uptake of the lesions in comparison with the healthy liver parenchyma were only apparent with moderately or poorly differentiated HCC lesions.[27] A recent study by Kitamura and colleagues[54] investigated the usefulness of preoperative FDG-PET as a tool for predicting recurrence patterns following liver resection in 63 patients with HCC. In this study, the tumor-to-nontumor ratio was an independent predictive factor of the recurrence pattern (1.6 ± 0.8 vs 1.3 ± 2.7 in the group with recurrence after 1 year and in the group with recurrence within 1 year, respectively).[54]

Cost-effectiveness

The cost-effectiveness of FDG-PET was compared with that of conventional imaging techniques by Wiering and colleagues.[31] A randomized multicenter study was conducted in 145 patients with CRC liver metastases (75 patients in the conventional arm and 70 patients in the FDG-PET arm). Overall, after comparing the diagnostic strategies, the average total costs were lower in the PET group. Three years after randomization, the mean costs (range) for the conventional workup and FDG-PET group were 92,836 (7516–290,308) and 81,776 (68,087–341,012) euros, respectively. Excluding the costs of chemotherapy, the mean costs in the conventional workup and FDG-PET groups were 15,874 (5974–34,143) and 18,664 (1984–87,930) euros,

respectively. Hence this study demonstrated that the addition of FDG-PET to the conventional workup of patients results in a better selection of patients and avoidance of futile laparotomies, thus reducing costs.[31] Zubeldia and colleagues[55] analyzed the costs of adding FDG-PET to CT preoperatively in patients with potentially resectable CRC liver metastases. CT with and without FDG-PET was compared among patients with CRC liver metastases in staging for surgical resection of liver metastases. Patients who were found positive for extrahepatic disease by either or both modalities were assumed to be surgically resectable. If one of the modalities detected extrahepatic disease, patients were assigned to palliative therapy.[55] Patients assigned to be surgical candidates were exposed to 3 possible outcomes: uncomplicated surgery, complicated surgery, or death. The primary outcome of the study was expected costs for adding FDG-PET in the preoperative diagnostic workup of patients with CRC liver metastases. The average expected surgical costs per patient when FDG-PET was used to determine the presence of extrahepatic disease was US$16,278, compared with $21,547 for conventional management. Thus, a net saving of $5269 was realized when FDG-PET was integrated in the diagnostic workup of patients.[55] These substantial net savings are the result of cost avoidance by excluding patients with extrahepatic disease, and thus avoiding unnecessary surgical expense. Lejeune and colleagues[56] conducted a similar study in patients with CRC liver metastases, and reported an expected incremental cost saving of approximately $3213 per patient for the same level of expected effectiveness as CT alone when compared with CT plus FDG-PET.

Summary

The data on the added value of FDG-PET(/CT) show wide heterogeneity. There are discrepancies in the reported results on the added value of FDG-PET(/CT) for staging patients and the detection of intrahepatic lesions. FDG-PET(/CT) does seem to be superior to conventional imaging for the detection of extrahepatic disease. The size of the lesions and chemotherapy before liver resection influence the sensitivity of the test. In terms of change of management, the results vary widely. Although FDG-PET(/CT) does seem to contribute to a useful change of management, several studies warn of false-positive and false-negative results that might lead to wrong decisions. The role of FDG-PET(/CT) in the follow-up of patients after liver resection has not been investigated broadly. However, the available data are promising, and report good sensitivity for the detection of recurrent disease and excellent survival in patients who have been staged by means of FDG-PET(/CT) imaging.

A more selective application of FDG-PET/CT seems preferable when using this modality for the selection of patients for surgery. Some investigators suggested that FDG-PET is more useful in specific settings: for example, patients with specific risk factors for tumor recurrence,[34,57] patients with recent suboptimal surgery of the primary tumor,[26] or patients in whom abdominal extrahepatic disease is suspected.[34,37]

Thermal Ablation Therapy

Local tumor destruction by RFA has emerged as a safe and effective treatment modality for patients with liver tumors that are irresectable.[58] RFA is considered a safe technique with the ability to accomplish local disease control, as shown in large cohort studies and meta-analyses.[58-61] Furthermore, RFA is frequently performed in combination with concomitant liver resection at laparotomy.[62] The identification of patients eligible for local ablative therapy is based on pretreatment imaging.[63] Intrahepatic tumor staging is mainly based on contrast dynamics in contrast-enhanced CT (CECT) or intraoperative ultrasonography. Despite improvements and developments in diagnostic imaging, surgeons can still detect intrahepatic tumor lesions not detected on preoperative imaging, resulting in change of the extent of the surgical approach in up to 55% of patients.[63] Furthermore, local tumor recurrence is a major limitation of RFA, with lesion recurrence rates of up to 60%.[58] The aforementioned problems emphasize the need for more accurate preinterventional and postinterventional imaging.

One major limitation in imaging following RFA is the evaluation of the completeness of the resultant thermal lesions.[58,63] It remains difficult to determine whether the target tumor lesion has been completely ablated when monitored immediately after the RFA procedure.[58] In addition, during follow-up of patients it is difficult to accurately distinguish on CT imaging between residual tumor and necrosis.[64] This aspect, however, is very important, as patients with remnant tumor cells might be candidates for repeated RFA treatment and improvement of their progression-free survival. FDG-PET/CT is a sensitive tool for the diagnosis of metastatic liver tumors based on increased metabolic rate measured in the tumor lesions.[8] **Table 2** provides an overview of studies on the role of PET imaging for RFA treatment.

Preinterventional staging

Patients eligible for RFA should carefully be selected, as guidelines recommend the following selection criteria: (1) lesions should not exceed 3 cm at their longest diameter; (2) no evidence of vascular invasion or extrahepatic spread; (3) no tumor located less than 1 cm from the main biliary tract; (4) no dilation of intrahepatic bile duct; (5) no bilioenteric anastomosis; and (6) no untreatable coagulopathy.[65] Accurate imaging is very important in recognizing patients with contraindications, as mentioned earlier.

Several studies have investigated the role of FDG-PET/CT for the selection and staging of patients who are considered for RFA treatment of liver lesions (**Table 3**).[41,66,67] The studies reported a change of management of 25% to 82% of cases when pretreatment FDG-PET was added to the diagnostic workup of patients. With 238 patients, Sahin and colleagues[67] conducted the largest study to investigate the role of FDG-PET(/CT) for the staging of patients before RFA. The routine follow-up after laparoscopic RFA included triphasic liver CT scan at 1 week, followed by the postoperative CT scans according to their protocol. PET/CT scans in the follow-up were ordered at the discretion of the oncologist or surgeon. Candidates for RFA were patients with unresectable disease with fewer than 8 lesions and less than 20% of total volume involved. The patients had either no or minimal extrahepatic disease. The results demonstrated that in comparison with CT, FDG-PET provided additional information in almost 25% of the patients and that this information changed the management in most patients (82%).[67] The only study that mentioned the diagnostic accuracy of FDG-PET in comparison with CT reported sensitivity, specificity and accuracy of respectively 54%, 100%, and 57% for FDG-PET, 96%, 100%, and 97% for FDG-PET/CT, and 98%, 0%, and 93% for CT in the detection of intrahepatic lesions.[66] For the detection of extrahepatic lesions the sensitivity, specificity, and accuracy were respectively 57%, 98%, and 93% for FDG-PET, 86%, 100%, and 98% for FDG-PET/CT, and 85%, 96%, and 95% for CT.[66] Thus, for detection of intrahepatic lesions CT imaging was superior to FDG-PET and FDG-PET/CT. However, for detection of extrahepatic disease, FDG-PET/CT was more accurate than FDG-PET alone or CT imaging alone.

Detection of residual tumor/incomplete ablation

A major problem in RFA is the occurrence of local tumor recurrence because of incomplete ablation. In general, an ablation procedure is considered to be complete when the ablated area (either through a single ablation or with multiple overlapping ablations) encompasses the target tumor by including

Table 3
Radiofrequency ablation studies for role of FDG-PET in preinterventional staging

Authors,[Ref.] Year	N[a] 1 = Patients 2 = Lesions	Comparison	% Change of Management with FDG-PET	Sensitivity (%)	Specificity (%)	Accuracy (%)	Time Interval RFA and Follow-Up PET	Time to Detection of LTP (mo)
Kuehl et al,[66] 2008	1 = 58	FDG-PET/CT CT	PET 57 (45 wrong) PET/CT 26 (2 wrong) CT 22 (5 wrong)	PET 54 PET/CT 96 CT 98	PET 100 PET/CT 100 CT 0	PET 57 PET/CT 97 CT 93	NR	PET/CT = 4.1 CECT = 5.85
Sahin et al,[67] 2012	1 = 238 (134 PET and 104 PET/CT)	FDG-PET/CT FDG-PET CT	PET/CT 82	—	—	—	Baseline Follow-up[b,c]	NR
Georgakopoulos et al,[41] 2013	1 = 35 (16 RFA)	FDG-PET/CT CT	FDG-PET/CT 25 (RFA only)	—	—	—	Baseline	NR

Histology, clinical, and imaging follow-up data were used as reference test.
Abbreviations: LTP, local tumor progression; RFA, radiofrequency ablation.
[a] Analysis performed based on number of patients or number of lesions.
[b] Interval between RFA and follow-up PET was not further specified.
[c] Interventional therapy: radiofrequency ablation; percutaneous ethanol injection therapy; transcatheter arterial chemoembolization.
Data from Refs.[41,66,67]

at least a 0.5- to 1.0-cm ablative margin, as determined by a lack of contrast enhancement on post-RFA CT.[65] Follow-up imaging after RFA is mainly focused on detection of complete ablation and local tumor recurrence. However, the appearance of incomplete ablation on follow-up imaging is still a matter of discussion. In general, follow-up is conducted using CECT or MR imaging.[65] The enhancing rim that may be observed around the periphery of the ablation zone is a uniform process in an area with smooth inner margins.[65] This transient finding represents a benign physiologic response of the liver parenchyma to the thermal injury. It is important to distinguish benign periablational enhancement from irregular peripheral enhancement caused by residual tumor. A general shortcoming of CECT is the difficulty to differentiate the posttreatment effect in the ablation margin (benign periablational enhancement) from local tumor recurrence in the periphery of the ablation zone.

Many studies have investigated the value of FDG-PET/CT in the detection of incomplete tumor ablation following RFA (**Table 4**).[5,47,68–72] The interval between RFA and posttreatment FDG-PET varies widely between the different studies, from directly after RFA (within 10–15 minutes)[72] to less than 8 weeks following RFA.[70] Several studies demonstrated that tissue regeneration and inflammation in the periphery of the ablation zone could be seen as early as 2 days after the RFA procedure.[68,69] This observation suggested that FDG-PET/CT should be performed early or at least within 2 days following the RFA procedure. However, the data on which these results are based came from small sample sizes, which might bias the results. Other studies that investigated FDG-PET/CT following RFA in a series of time intervals did not find any relation between time interval of RFA to FDG-PET/CT and true or false results. Kim and colleagues[71] investigated the correlation between the time interval of FDG-PET scan and the RFA procedure and true or false imaging results. The interval between RFA and imaging was 8.8 ± 8.3 days for true results and 10.4 ± 9.8 days for false results. There was no significant difference in the interval between the 2 groups ($P = .689$).[71]

Chen and colleagues[70] and Langenhoff and colleagues[47] studied the largest cohorts on this matter to date, comprising 28 and 23 patients, respectively. Both studies reported the superiority of FDG-PET over CT or MR imaging for the detection of incomplete ablation shortly after RFA treatment. Langenhoff and colleagues[47] recommended the combination of FDG-PET with diagnostic CT for more precise anatomic localization. In daily practice, FDG-PET can determine the need for further imaging and may guide diagnostic CT reading. This combined information offers the opportunity to retreat residual tumors at an early stage. When interpreting the results, however, one should be aware of false-positive FDG-PET results in the case of inflammatory processes, especially following RFA.[47] It is recommended to postpone the PET scan in cases where there is evidence of active focal inflammation.[47] Another limitation of FDG-PET is the limited spatial resolution, which may lead to false-negative reports in cases of lesions smaller than 1 cm.[47]

Khandani and colleagues[68] also investigated the diagnostic accuracy of FDG-PET for the assessment of complete ablation following RFA, and concluded that early (2–41 hours after RFA) FDG-PET has the potential to evaluate the efficacy of RFA by defining total photopenia as macroscopic tumor-free margin and focal FDG uptake as macroscopic residual tumor.[68] Veit and colleagues[69] confirmed these results.

Another interesting end point investigated was the ablation adequacy measured by intraprocedural dissipation of FDG uptake induced by thermal ablation.[72] The hypothesis was that tissue vaporization, which occurs during ablation therapy, could conceivably release FDG into veins and lymphatic and surrounding tissue, and could decrease absolute FDG activity in an ablated tumor. The aim of the study was to determine whether tumor FDG activity was dissipated by RFA during PET/CT-guided ablation.[72] Ultimately the goal was to find out whether it could be possible to detect incomplete ablation before completion of the procedure. Twelve patients were included (10 liver metastasis, 1 perihepatic lesion, and 1 lung lesion), of whom 6 underwent percutaneous RFA treatment and 6 only biopsy for suspected liver metastasis (control patients).[72] FDG-PET/CT was performed 10 to 15 minutes following the ablation. Preprocedural FDG-PET/CT was also performed. The mean interval between both scans was 83.4 minutes.[72] The standardized uptake value (SUV) ratio (tumor maximum SUV to liver average SUV) was analyzed to interpret the FDG-PET/CT results. The target tumor maximum SUV (Target SUV_{max}) based on the region of interest was also calculated. The mean increase in the Target SUV_{max} for the experimental group was 32.5% (range 8.2%–46.7%) compared with 24.6% (range 3.7%–42.4%) in the control group. The mean increase in SUV ratio for the experimental group was 47.9% (range 18.8%–69.6%) compared with 37.6% (9.4%–65%) in the control group.[72] These results demonstrated that ablation-induced tissue heating and

Table 4
Radiofrequency ablation studies for role of FDG-PET in detection of residual disease

Authors,[Ref.] Year	N[a] 1 = Patients 2 = Lesions	Comparison	Sensitivity (%)	Specificity (%)	Accuracy (%)	Time Interval RFA and Follow-Up PET	Time to Detection of LTP (mo)
Khandani et al,[68] 2007	2 = 8	FDG-PET CT	PET 67[b,c]	PET 80[b]	PET 75[b]	Baseline 2–41 h 3–16 mo	NR
Veit et al,[69] 2006	2 = 16	FDG-PET/CT FDG-PET CT	PET 65 PET/CT 65 CT 44	—	PET 68 PET/CT 68 CT 47	Baseline 2 d	NR
Langenhoff et al,[47] 2002	1 = 22	FDG-PET CT	FDG-PET 80[b]	—	—	<3 wk	FDG-PET 3.8 CT 8.5
Chen et al,[70] 2013	2 = 33	FDG-PET or FDG-PET/CT CT MRI	FDG-PET 94 MRI 67 CT 67 P<.05	FDG-PET 81 MRI 88 CT 63 P>.05	FDG-PET 88 MRI 75 CT 64 P<.05	<8 wk	NR
Kim et al,[71] 2012	2 = 45	FDG-PET/CT CT	FDG-PET/CT 87.5	FDG-PET/CT 71.4	FDG-PET/CT 80	<1 mo	NR

Histology, clinical, and imaging follow-up data were used as reference test.
[a] Analysis performed based on number of patients or number of lesions.
[b] Calculated using the available data.
[c] Interventional therapy: radiofrequency ablation; percutaneous ethanol injection therapy; transcatheter arterial chemoembolization.
Data from Refs.[47,68–71]

vaporization does not result in measurable dissipation of FDG activity from the ablation zone. The lack of thermal effects on FDG activity (injected before the RFA procedure) within the target tumors during PET/CT-guided RFA indicated that changes in FDG activity cannot be used to monitor ablation coverage or completeness of the therapy.[72]

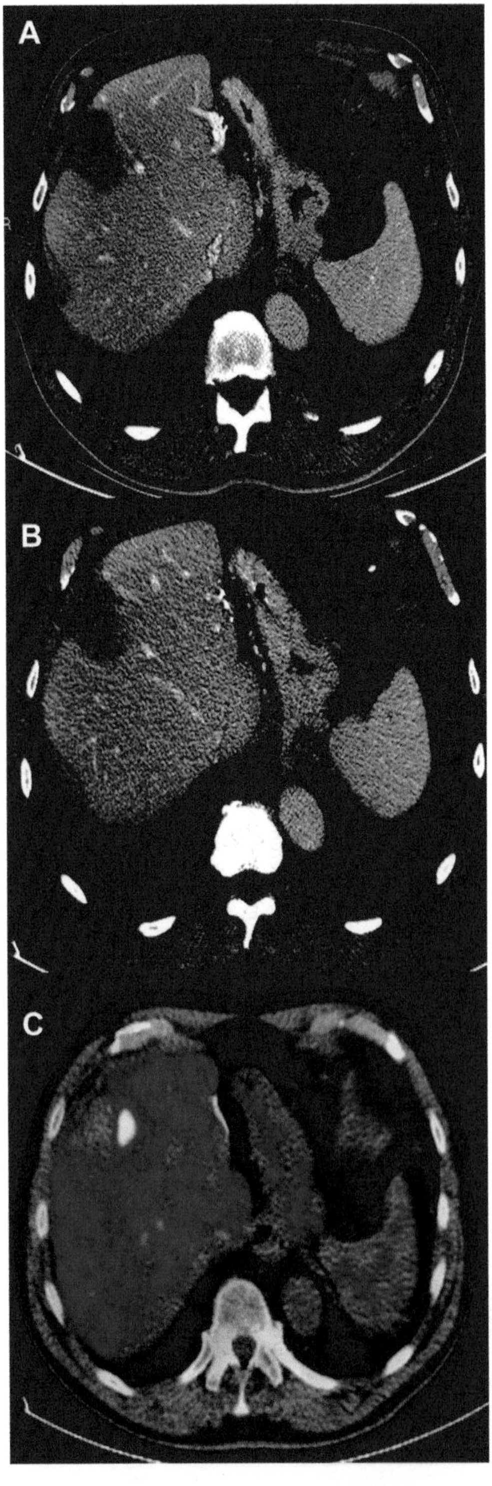

Early detection of tumor recurrence

Incomplete tumor ablation may result in local tumor progression. Incomplete ablation is defined as the presence of residual unablated tumor, which is seen as peripheral irregular enhancement on imaging.[65] Local tumor progression is defined as appearance at follow-up of foci of untreated disease in tumors that were previously considered to be completely ablated.[65,73] Not only incomplete ablation, but also micrometastases that are not detectable on preintervention imaging, may result in local tumor recurrence. In general, the term local tumor recurrence includes both local tumor progression as a result of incomplete ablation and outgrowth of the micrometastases. Detecting these local tumor recurrences as early as possible influences the prognosis because retreatment is only possible in limited disease (**Fig. 4**). Studies that have investigated the value of PET imaging for early detection of tumor recurrence reported superior results obtained by FDG-PET when compared with conventional imaging methods.[5,47,70,74–79]

Kuehl and colleagues[79] compared the results of FDG-PET/CT, FDG-PET alone, and contrast-enhanced MR imaging with the standard of reference (histology, clinical data, and CECT) to investigate the accuracy of detecting local tumor recurrence after CT-guided RFA of CRC liver metastases. The results showed a significant advantage of FDG-PET/CT over single FDG-PET; however, no difference between FDG-PET/CT and contrast-enhanced MR imaging was detected.[79] Combined morphologic and functional imaging was recommended for treatment planning of repeated percutaneous intervention for patients with recurrent tumors, because the combination of CT and FDG-PET information enables exact localization of the tumor recurrence in relation to the existing ablation zone.[79] The same research group studied the accuracy of FDG-PET/CT for the staging and follow-up of patients treated with RFA for

Fig. 4. Follow-up imaging after 6 months (*A*) and 9 months (*B, C*) in a patient with colorectal carcinoma liver metastases who was treated with RFA. FDG-PET/CT and CECT at 9 months' follow-up were performed on the same day. CECT images (portal-venous phase) did not detect any residual disease or recurrent intrahepatic disease at 6 months or 9 months (*A, B*). The first post-RFA FDG-PET/CT scan at 9 months' follow-up showed increased FDG uptake at the medial side of the RFA lesion (maximum standardized uptake value 5.1), suggesting recurrent disease.

primary (HCC) liver malignancy or CRC liver metastases.[80] In patients with a PET-positive lesion on preinterventional imaging, FDG-PET/CT was performed during follow-up. Patients with PET-negative lesions were followed by means of CECT only. In addition, the investigators assessed predictive factors of local tumor progression, including lesion size, metastatic disease, localization, and PET positivity.[80] However, no significant difference in the mean time to detection of local tumor progression after RFA was found between FDG-PET/CT and CECT.

When focused on the correlation between FDG uptake and the histologic findings after RFA, FDG-PET was able to detect recurrence earlier than CT.[77] The mean time to recurrence was not reported. In 2 patients, recurrence was detected between 4 and 6 months following RFA by means of FDG-PET, while having a negative CT scan. Moreover, 6 patients were positive on FDG-PET performed between 7 and 9 months, whereas CT showed only 4 of 6 to be positive for recurrence.[77]

In studies where patients with HCC were included, a significant difference was observed in the SUV of well-differentiated and moderately differentiated HCC. As expected, SUV was higher in moderately differentiated and poorly differentiated HCC.[74,77] Furthermore, the correlation between the SUV and recurrent disease was investigated. A significant correlation was found between the SUV of the HCC lesion before RFA and the interval between RFA and the time of recurrence detected by FDG-PET. A significant difference was noted in the SUV between patients who showed recurrence during 4 to 6 and 7 to 9 months (5.29 ± 0.50 vs 3.44 ± 1.02, $P = .027$), 4 to 6 and 10 to 18 months (5.29 ± 0.50 vs 1.69 ± 0.45, $P = .013$), and 7 to 9 and 10 to 18 months (3.44 ± 1.02 vs 1.69 ± 0.45, $P = .007$).[77]

Data on mean time to local tumor recurrence was reported in 3 studies.[47,75,78] FDG-PET detected local tumor recurrence after a mean follow-up time of 3.8 to 6.8 months, with the time to detection by CT being 8.5 to 9.8 months.[47,78] Although the time to recurrence is longer for CT than for FDG-PET, it is not clear whether these results are significant. The diagnostic accuracy of FDG-PET(/CT) varied between 71% and 95%.[5,74,79] The sensitivity and specificity of FDG-PET(/CT) varied between 61% and 100% and 83% and 100%, respectively (Table 5). The diagnostic accuracy of the conventional imaging modalities varied from 64% to 91% (MR imaging or contrast-enhanced ultrasonography), and the sensitivity and specificity varied between 25% and 100% and 75% and 100%, respectively (see Table 5).

FDG-PET reading

In most studies, the assessment of residual disease or local recurrence was based on FDG focal uptake around the ablation zone. FDG uptake in the area surrounding the ablation zone may also occur as result of postablative inflammation. However, this can be distinguished from residual tumor, because FDG uptake resulting from postablative inflammation shows a homogeneous tracer distribution surrounding the area that turned necrotic after ablative therapy.[75,81]

A photopenic area in the ablated zone with no adjacent focal irregular nodular uptake was defined as successful ablation in most studies.[70,71] Nevertheless, the FDG-uptake pattern should be evaluated accurately to relate the FDG activity to clinical conclusions. Inflammatory/physiologic postablative reaction may lead to false-positive results. Conversely, there is a risk of false-negative results as increased glucose metabolism, owing to tissue regeneration, may superimpose on small areas of residual tumor, resulting in images on which small residual tumor deposits overlap with rim-shaped FDG uptake.[71]

Role of FDG-PET(/CT) in HCC

FDG-PET/CT is generally more accurate than conventional imaging modalities in detecting local tumor recurrence following RFA. However, it has some limitations in HCC, owing to a low diagnostic sensitivity for the detection of intrahepatic lesions. The reason for this low detection rate is found in the difference of HCC tumor differentiation. FDG uptake in well-differentiated HCC lesions is similar to that in normal liver parenchyma, which makes the detection of tumor cells difficult. The diagnostic accuracy is higher for the detection of intrahepatic tumor recurrence because recurrent HCC has a higher degree of malignancy.[74,77] In a study with 24 patients, detection of intrahepatic and extrahepatic disease during follow-up was more accurate by means of FDG-PET in comparison with CT. During the follow-up period, FDG-PET detected intrahepatic and extrahepatic recurrence in 14 patients, 8 of which within the first 9 months following RFA. CT was able to detect the recurrence in only 8 patients, half of these within the first 9 months following RFA.[77] The advantage of FDG-PET lies mainly in the fact that it is a whole-body imaging method that enables more accurate detection of extrahepatic disease.

Cost-effectiveness analyses

The results of a cost-effectiveness analysis of FDG-PET in comparison with the more conventional imaging modalities were recently reported by Chen and colleagues.[70] Twenty-eight patients

Table 5
Radiofrequency ablation studies for role of FDG-PET in detection of recurrent disease

Authors, Ref. Year	N[a] 1 = Patients 2 = Lesions	Comparison	Sensitivity (%)	Specificity (%)	Accuracy (%)	Time Interval RFA and Follow-Up PET	Time to Detection of LTP (mo)
Kuehl et al,[79] 2008	2 = 25	FDG-PET/CT PET MRI	PET 61 PET/CT 84 MRI 73	PET 98 PET/CT 100 MRI 100	PET 79 PET/CT 92 MRI 91	Baseline 1 mo 3 mo	NR
Donckier et al,[5] 2003	1 = 17	FDG-PET CT	PET 100[b,c] CT 25[b]	PET 100[b] CT 100[b]	PET 71[b]	Baseline 7 d 1 mo 3 mo	NR
Sahin et al,[67] 2012	1 = 238	FDG-PET/CT FDG-PET CT	LTR: PET/CT 92 CT 83 EHD: PET/CT 97 CT 71	LTR: PET/CT 100 CT 100 EHD: PET/CT 100 CT 75	—	Baseline Follow-up[d]	NR
Langenhoff et al,[47] 2002	1 = 23	FDG-PET CT	LTR: FDG-PET 100[b] CT 100[b] EHD: FDG-PET 100[b] CT 89[b]	—	—	<3 wk	FDG-PET 3.8 CT 8.5
Anderson et al,[76] 2003	1 = 13	FDG-PET CT	FDG-PET 100 CT 43 MRI 50	FDG-PET 100	—	9 ± 5 mo	NR
Wang et al,[74] 2013	1 = 36	FDG-PET/CT CEUS	FDG-PET/CT 96.7 CEUS 56.7	FDG-PET/CT 83.3 CEUS 100	FDG-PET/CT 94.4 CEUS 63.9	2–3 mo	NR

Histology, clinical, and imaging follow-up data were used as reference test.
Abbreviations: EHD, extrahepatic disease; LTR, local tumor recurrence.
[a] Analysis performed based on number of patients or number of lesions.
[b] Calculated using the available data.
[c] Interventional therapy: radiofrequency ablation; percutaneous ethanol injection therapy; transcatheter arterial chemoembolization.
[d] Interval between RFA and follow-up PET was not further specified.
Data from Refs.[5,47,67,74,76,79]

were included in the study and analyses were performed for 33 lesions. Whenever a postintervention scan (FDG-PET, CT, or MR imaging) resulted in misdiagnosis, the imaging modality was repeated until the correct diagnosis (recurrent disease) was achieved. The total number of scans per case was used to calculate the average scan number for each imaging modality. An average scan number needed for PET, MR imaging, and CT to achieve a final accurate diagnosis of respectively 1.12, 1.32, and 1.25 with a corresponding reimbursement cost of $1455.20, $1845.80, and $933.80 was reported.[70] Hence, FDG-PET was found to be more cost-effective than MR imaging, but not in comparison with CT. However, the investigators emphasized that a cost-effectiveness analysis should not only focus on the initial imaging procedure (which was the case in this study) but should also include potential reintervention, further follow-up imaging, additional therapy, patient survival, and change of management.[70] Considering that FDG-PET is more accurate in the detection of incomplete ablation and early detection of intrahepatic tumor recurrence in comparison with conventional imaging methods, the cost-effectiveness analysis would probably be in favor of FDG-PET. When the results of FDG-PET imaging lead to reintervention and additional procedures, the costs will increase in comparison with those for patients who have had CT alone. However, with improved survival of patients resulting from the additional therapy, the final health costs will eventually be lower.

Summary

At present, there is no indication for the standard use of FDG-PET(/CT) during staging and follow-up of patients treated with RFA. It is mainly used to exclude the presence of extrahepatic disease or to evaluate equivocal or negative findings on MR imaging or CT. Therefore, as in liver surgery, the role of FDG-PET(/CT) before the RFA procedure is mainly determined by the detection of extrahepatic disease and prevention of unnecessary surgery. Concerning the role of FDG-PET/CT during follow-up, available data suggest that FDG-PET/CT imaging could be used as the primary method for surveillance after RFA. Additional conventional imaging techniques may be used to more precisely localize the findings identified by FDG-PET.

FDG-PET being a whole-body imaging technique confers another advantage in that extrahepatic disease may be detected, which is very important in the staging of patients before intervention. In HCC patients and patients treated with chemotherapy, FDG-PET for the workup of patients is not totally reliable, owing to the biological behavior of the tumor lesions in relation to their FDG uptake.

In the follow-up setting, sensitivity of FDG-PET/CT is higher that of the conventional diagnostic modalities for early detection of local tumor recurrence and is related to the size of the lesion, with decreasing sensitivity in lesions smaller than 1 cm.[69,82] Detection of complete ablation can also be achieved by FDG-PET/CT, although the time between ablation and the FDG-PET scan may be problematic because in surgical ablation, patients are usually not fit enough to perform an FDG-PET scan directly (same day) after the procedure. In the percutaneous approach it is more feasible to perform FDG-PET directly after the procedure. However, FDG-PET/CT for the detection of complete ablation may be performed up to 3 to 4 weeks following the RFA treatment.[47]

Radioembolization

Hepatic radioembolization with yttrium-90 (^{90}Y) is a form of brachytherapy whereby radioactive resin or glass microspheres are injected into the hepatic arterial vessels to target malignant lesions. Over the past 2 decades more than 18,000 patients in more than 150 centers worldwide have been treated with ^{90}Y radioembolization, either in a salvage setting or in combination with chemotherapy.[83,84]

Before radioembolization, each patient receives preprocedural screening by means of hepatic angiography and technetium-99m-labeled albumin macroaggregates (^{99m}Tc-MAA) injection, followed by planar imaging and single-photon emission CT (SPECT). The preprocedural angiography permits visualization of the anatomy of the vessels and provides an opportunity to coil-embolize arteries to extrahepatic tissue if necessary. ^{99m}Tc-MAA SPECT/CT allows for visualization and quantification of extrahepatic uptake/shunting to the lungs, stomach, duodenum, and pancreas.[83]

Because of the potential risk for major toxicity to the liver, lungs, and the gastrointestinal tract, in addition to costs, proper patient selection is of utmost importance.[85] In the case of radioembolization, accurate staging procedures are mandatory to rule out extrahepatic disease progression.[84] Furthermore, a careful risk assessment has to be performed concerning the maintenance of sufficient liver function, because exposure of liver parenchyma to radiation cannot be avoided.[84,85] When patients are considered eligible for radioembolization, diagnostic modalities are needed to gather distinct information about the individual hepatic arterial anatomy, and to define perfusion territories from the chosen location of administration.[83,85]

Preinterventional staging

Kennedy and colleagues[86] reported the results of a consensus panel from the Radioembolization Brachytherapy Oncology Consortium. In this report, recommendations were given for a diagnostic algorithm of the workup. However, a clear sequence of the procedures and the definite prerequisites for decision making and planning of radioembolization was not provided.

Denecke and colleagues[87] aimed to set up a standardized, sequential diagnostic approach for the staging of patients eligible for radioembolization by using radiologic and nuclear medicine imaging procedures. In 22 patients with histologically proven irresectable liver metastasis from colorectal cancer, CT, MR imaging, FDG-PET/CT, and angiography with perfusion scintigraphy were sequentially performed. The impact of each test on treatment management was recorded. The chosen sequence of imaging modalities was effective by depiction of contraindications or indication of alternative locally ablative treatment options in approximately one-third of evaluated patients. The results showed that CT alone was not sufficient enough in the workup of patients, because PET and MR imaging (the second step of patient evaluation) showed additional cases with progressive extrahepatic disease, not depicted by CT alone.[87] Rosenbaum and colleagues[88] compared CT with FDG-PET for the workup of 42 patients, and found a 17% change of management attributable to the direct results of FDG-PET/CT (7 of 42 patients; in 6 patients additional extrahepatic disease was detected, and in 1 patient intrahepatic disease in an additional segment).

Becker and colleagues[89] investigated the value of C-arm CT imaging compared with FDG-PET/CT and CT alone to display liver metastases during the workup and staging of patients for radioembolization. Although the study showed that C-arm CT was useful for determining the eligibility and feasibility of radioembolization, it was not as sensitive as FDG-PET/CT and CT alone for the detection of liver tumors.[89] According to the available data, whole-body FDG-PET(/CT) has been proved to be useful for comprehensive assessment of intrahepatic and extrahepatic tumor manifestation during the staging of patients for radioembolization.

Posttreatment imaging

Following ^{90}Y radioembolization, bremsstrahlung SPECT images are made to assess the distribution of the microspheres. Although bremsstrahlung imaging is rapid and convenient, it has some major limitations. Low counts, energy distribution, and scatter restrict the spatial resolution. Quantitative analysis on bremsstrahlung SPECT is challenging.[90,91] D'Arienzo and colleagues[92] conducted a study to demonstrate the feasibility of ^{90}Y PET imaging for the assessment of radiation absorbed dose after radioembolization with ^{90}Y microspheres, and showed the potential of high spatial resolution of ^{90}Y PET.

Two studies compared ^{90}Y PET/CT imaging with bremsstrahlung SPECT in patients after ^{90}Y radioembolization to assess the particle uptake and evaluate the efficacy of the procedure.[90,91] Padia and colleagues[91] studied 13 patients, including 7 patients with portal vein thrombus (PVT). Patients underwent ^{90}Y PET/CT 4 hours after the procedure. The results were in line with the study performed by D'Arienzo and colleagues.[91,92] PET provided images with less scatter and at least equivalent spatial resolution compared with bremsstrahlung SPECT, and was superior in terms of quantitative analysis.[91] Quantitative analysis showed significantly less uptake in nontumor areas in comparison with bremsstrahlung images.[91] This result confirmed other findings on the value of postimplantation PET/CT for distribution analysis of ^{90}Y microspheres.[90,93] Another advantage of PET/CT over SPECT was that, in contrast with PET/CT, the SPECT images showed uptake of the microspheres in the liver but could not elucidate their precise location within the liver.[91] In the patients with PVT, PET/CT was able to demonstrate that the activity in the portal vein correlated to the tumor thrombus on baseline imaging. On follow-up imaging, there was resolution of enhancement of PVT.[91]

Response assessment and prognostication

The usefulness of FDG-PET/CT was confirmed by the results of studies that investigated the prognostic value of FDG-PET/CT for the survival of patients with liver malignancies.[94,95] These studies showed that the median survival from the first ^{90}Y radioembolization in patients with low metabolic tumor burden measured by FDG-PET/CT was significantly higher than that of patients with high metabolic tumor burden.[94,95] However, the reported influence on changes in SUV on survival was variable (**Fig. 5**).[94,96] Fendler and colleagues[94] reported no influence of the change in SUV peak or SUV_{max} pretreatment and posttreatment on the survival of patients with CRC liver metastases treated with ^{90}Y radioembolization. Haug and colleagues[96] reported that changes in SUV_{max} as assessed by FDG-PET/CT before and 3 months after ^{90}Y radioembolization was the only independent

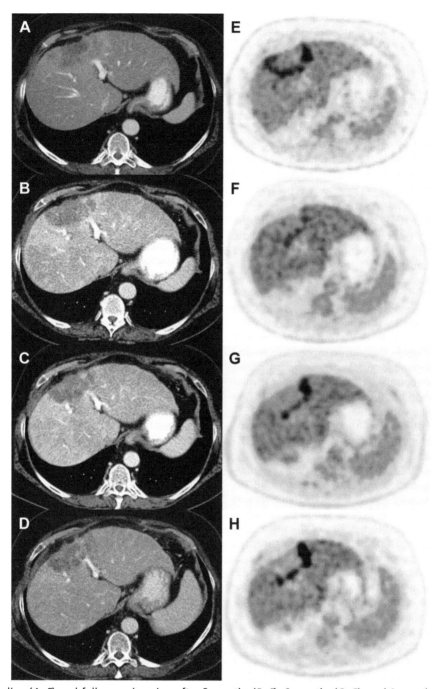

Fig. 5. Baseline (*A, E*) and follow-up imaging after 3 months (*B, F*), 6 months (*C, G*), and 9 months (*D, H*) in a patient with cholangiocarcinoma who was treated with hepatic radioembolization. CECT images (portal-venous phase) show stable disease according to RECIST (Response Evaluation Criteria In Solid Tumors) while FDG-PET images show partial metabolic response at 3 months followed by gradual progression.

predictor of survival in patients with hepatic metastases of breast cancer. The study by Zerizer and colleagues,[97] which included 25 patients who underwent FDG-PET/CT before and during follow-up after ^{90}Y radioembolization, showed that the response according to the European Organization for Research and Treatment of Cancer (EORTC) PET criteria correlated with the response of the tumor markers ($P<.0001$ for lactate dehydrogenase, $P = .01$ for carcinoembryonic antigen, and $P = .02$ for cancer antigen 19-9), in addition to the progression-free survival of patients. This finding contrasts with the responses on contrast-enhanced CT studies that used both RECIST (Response Evaluation Criteria In Solid Tumors) and tumor density criteria, which were not significantly correlated with the responses of tumor markers or survival.[97] These findings were further confirmed by Zalom and colleagues,[98] who found that FDG-PET/CT during follow-up proved to be a predictor of long-term survival. Although the sample size was relatively small (31 patients), no new extrahepatic lesions at 3 months portended a favorable prognosis, indicating that posttreatment FDG-PET/CT is a significant tool in determining survival.[98]

Imaging studies play an essential role in the assessment of response to ^{90}Y radioembolization. Several studies have investigated the response to ^{90}Y radioembolization.[99–102] Tochetto and colleagues[102] evaluated the correlation between the change in attenuation on CT and the tumor metabolic activity assessed by FDG-PET/CT in CRC liver metastases. In 11 patients, 74 lesions were evaluated semiquantitatively using SUV analysis. The lesions were categorized according to the EORTC definitions for metabolic response[103]: responders with complete or partial response (a minimum reduction of 25% in tumor FDG SUV), and nonresponders with stable (an increase of <25% or decrease of <25% in tumor FDG SUV) or progressive (an increase of >25% in tumor FDG SUV) disease. In responder lesions, SUV_{max}, measured on the preintervention and postintervention images, decreased by a mean of 48.7% (8.73 ± 3.0 to 4.26 ± 1.2, $P<.001$). There was no significant decrease in SUV_{max} in nonresponder lesions.[102] In contrast to the size of the lesion, the percentage change in attenuation levels detected by CT had a high correlation with the metabolic activity assessed by FDG-PET. Hence, the change in attenuation may reflect changes in tumor composition not detected by changes in tumor size. Necrosis within the tumor mass was one of the key explanations for these findings.[102]

Another study tried to compare the existing guidelines for tumor response evaluation (RECIST and World Health Organization [WHO]) with other imaging criteria such as lesion necrosis and FDG uptake on FDG-PET.[101] The results of the FDG-PET scan were compared with clinical and biochemical follow-up data. The response on FDG-PET scanning was also assessed quantitatively using the SUV to compare the number of lesions, and the distribution and activity of the tumors.[101] The combined criteria resulted in a higher response rate when compared with WHO and RECIST alone (50% vs 19% and 24%, respectively). Necrosis and PET positivity seemed

important in the evaluation of response to radioembolization therapy.[101]

Summary

FDG-PET/CT is a useful diagnostic modality in the workup of patients before ^{90}Y radioembolization. According to recommendations made by Denecke and colleagues, FDG-PET/CT should be performed following the baseline CECT. The major added value of FDG-PET/CT in the workup concerns the selection of patients. In most cases, CT is sufficient to detect intrahepatic lesions; however, FDG-PET/CT is proven to be superior in the detection of extrahepatic disease. In addition, FDG-PET/CT during follow-up of patients seems to be a predictor of tumor response and the survival of patients. [90]Y PET/CT imaging can also be used directly following treatment to quantify the distribution of the microspheres.

Transarterial Chemoembolization

Most of the blood supply to a malignant liver lesion is derived from the hepatic artery rather than the portal vein. This characteristic has led to the development of techniques designed to eliminate the tumor blood supply by particle embolization or to directly infuse cytotoxic chemotherapy into the branch of the hepatic artery that feeds the tumor. The role of FDG-PET imaging has been investigated in a few studies. Zhao and colleagues[104] assessed the accuracy of early post-therapeutic FDG-PET/CT after TACE combined with RFA for HCC, with a 90.9% positive detection rate of residual disease after treatment with TACE combined with RFA. These results were similar to those of Kim and colleagues.[71] However, the latter group investigated the efficacy of FDG-PET/CT in a mixed group of patients who received TACE, RFA, or percutaneous ethanol injection for the treatment of HCC. In this study, 26 of 40 lesions were treated with TACE; however, the diagnostic accuracy of FDG-PET(/CT) was measured for all interventional procedures (TACE, RFA, and percutaneous ethanol injection). Posttreatment FDG-PET/CT using visual analysis resulted in a sensitivity, specificity, and accuracy of 87.5%, 71.4%, and 80.0%. The interobserver reliability was high, with an interclass correlation coefficient value of 0.907 ($P<.001$).[71]

Cascales Campos and colleagues[105] investigated the use of FGD-PET/CT before and after TACE to predict the percentage of tumor necrosis (the time interval between TACE and FDG-PET scan was not reported). The study consisted of a small sample size (6 cirrhotic patients selected for liver transplantation), and reported good performance of FDG-PET for the detection of necrosis following therapy.[105] Among patients with SUV post-TACE of less than 3, the percentage of necrosis was greater than 80%.[105] The results of an older study by Vitola and colleagues[106] in only 4 patients (34 lesions) were in agreement with the results reported by Cascales Campos and colleagues.[105] Seventy-four percent of the lesions showed decreased FDG uptake (mean SUV of 8 $\pm$ 2 vs 3 $\pm$ 1, $P<.00001$), as was expected following a successful TACE procedure. The results were in agreement with a decrease of the tumor marker level of 271 $\pm$ 103 ng/mL before treatment compared with 45 $\pm$ 17 ng/mL following TACE.[106] Kim and colleagues[71] noted that chemoembolization materials cause an overestimation of FDG activity when using CT information for PET-attenuation correction. Non–attenuation-corrected PET images should be considered to avoid a misdiagnosis in patients treated with TACE.[71]

External-Beam Radiation Therapy

EBRT can achieve local control of liver tumors when sufficient radiation-absorbed doses are applied. The radiation-absorbed dose that may be applied is limited by the potential risk of radiation-induced liver disease. Until recently, EBRT was not used to treat liver tumors because of the low tolerance of the liver parenchyma to radiation. However, recent advances in technology allow more precise delivery of radiation to the tumor while minimizing radiation doses to the surrounding liver parenchyma. Kim and colleagues[107] investigated the role of FDG-PET in assessing the significance of the ratio between SUV of tumor and normal functional liver tissue in predicting the response of HCC patients treated with EBRT. In this study, 51 patients with HCC were treated with EBRT, all having undergone FDG-PET imaging before the procedure. Following EBRT, the objective response rate 1 month after completion of the therapy was 63%.[107] Objective radiologic response was measured 1 month after completion of EBRT by means of CT imaging according to the RECIST criteria. A significant difference in objective response rates between the high-SUV ratio group and the low-SUV ratio group (46% vs 17%, $P = .015$) was found.[107] However, no differences were observed in either tumor marker level or median survival.[107]

DISCUSSION

The purpose of this review is to provide an overview of the studies that have investigated the diagnostic accuracy of FDG-PET(/CT) for: (1) staging and selection of patients by detection of intrahepatic and extrahepatic disease; (2) detection of residual disease in ablative therapy; (3) detection of recurrent disease during follow-up; (4) stratification of patients before the procedure; and (5) response assessment following the procedure. The role of FDG-PET(/CT) has been investigated in the most frequently used oncologic interventions in the current era, namely liver resection, RFA, radioembolization, chemoembolization, and EBRT.

Reviewing the available literature on the role of FDG-PET(/CT) in liver resection, it is clear that there is a large variability among the available data. FDG-PET(/CT) seems most effective when used for the workup of patients before liver resection, and the diagnostic accuracy seems superior to that of conventional imaging methods for the detection of extrahepatic disease. Just as in liver resection, in RFA FDG-PET(/CT) has an important role in the detection of extrahepatic disease during the staging and workup of patients. The available literature also suggests that FDG-PET(/CT) can be used for early detection of residual or recurrent intrahepatic disease during follow-up of patients after RFA. With regard to radioembolization, FDG-PET(/CT) seems to be a useful diagnostic modality in the workup of patients before treatment, again especially for the detection of extrahepatic disease. The small number of studies that investigated the role of FDG-PET(/CT) in chemoembolization concluded that this modality is useful for posttreatment response assessment. The role of FDG-PET(/CT) in patients selected for chemoembolization and EBRT needs to be further studied before any conclusions can be drawn about its diagnostic accuracy. The available data on the role of FDG-PET(/CT) in HIFU are too insufficient to be of relevance. The usefulness of FDG-PET(/CT) imaging has not yet been investigated in HIFU, and future studies should attempt to better define the role of this imaging modality.

The primary strength of FDG-PET/CT is the combination of a whole-body imaging modality with high sensitivity. In the management of liver-directed treatments, this may especially be useful to detect extrahepatic lesions during the workup. Many studies showed a considerable change of management based on FDG-PET/CT findings, although the differences in results were sometimes large. This variability may be logical when considering the heterogeneity of the patient cohorts included in the various studies, in addition to the differences in patients selected for particular treatments.

For example, Ruers and colleagues[29] randomized a cohort of patients with CRC liver metastases in group A (only conventional imaging was performed for workup) and group B (with FDG-PET added to the diagnostic workup). Inclusion criteria for this study included patients with fewer than 4 resectable CRC liver metastases, without evidence of extrahepatic metastatic disease (with the exception of a maximum of 2 resectable lung metastases).[29] In this study, the addition of FDG-PET to the workup for surgical resection was found to be superior to conventional imaging alone. Other studies that investigated the role of FDG-PET(/CT) in radioembolization or chemoembolization included patients with less favorable disease extension.[71,87,88] In a study by Denecke and colleagues,[87] patients were referred for radioembolization of CRC liver metastases in a salvage setting after third-line chemotherapy, which indicates the extent of the disease and the clear difference from the cohort studied by Ruers and colleagues.[29] It may be expected that patients who are selected for liver resection have a lower a priori chance of having extrahepatic disease in comparison with patients selected for radioembolization, and this is likely to influence the value of FDG-PET/CT imaging in these settings.

Overall, this article provides an extensive overview of the available data on the role of FDG-PET(/CT) in the interventional oncology of liver malignancy. Although the results are not always consistent, the available data suggest that FDG-PET(/CT) can be useful in a selected group of patients for the detection of extrahepatic disease during workup of patients to prevent unnecessary surgery or ablative therapy and, hence, prevention of unnecessary costs; and for early detection of recurrent intrahepatic disease and, more importantly, extrahepatic disease, to aid in evaluating the indications for reintervention or additional systemic therapy.

REFERENCES

1. Fusai G, Davidson BR. Strategies to increase the resectability of liver metastases from colorectal cancer. Dig Surg 2003;20(6):481–96.
2. Adam R, Delvart V, Pascal G, et al. Rescue surgery for unresectable colorectal liver metastases downstaged by chemotherapy: a model to predict long-term survival. Ann Surg 2004;240(4):644–57 [discussion: 657–8].
3. Vauthey JN, Zorzi D, Pawlik TM. Making unresectable hepatic colorectal metastases resectable–does it work? Semin Oncol 2005;32(6 Suppl 9):S118–22. http://dx.doi.org/10.1053/j.seminoncol.2005.04.030.
4. Frankel TL, Do RK, Jarnagin WR. Preoperative imaging for hepatic resection of colorectal cancer metastasis. J Gastrointest Oncol 2012;3(1):11–8.
5. Donckier V, Van Laethem JL, Goldman S, et al. [F-18] fluorodeoxyglucose positron emission tomography as a tool for early recognition of incomplete tumor destruction after radiofrequency ablation for liver metastases. J Surg Oncol 2003; 84(4):215–23. http://dx.doi.org/10.1002/jso.10314.
6. Antoch G, Vogt FM, Veit P, et al. Assessment of liver tissue after radiofrequency ablation: findings with different imaging procedures. J Nucl Med 2005; 46(3):520–5.
7. Hillner BE, Siegel BA, Liu D, et al. Impact of positron emission tomography/computed tomography and positron emission tomography (PET) alone on expected management of patients with cancer: initial results from the National Oncologic PET Registry. J Clin Oncol 2008;26(13):2155–61. http://dx.doi.org/10.1200/JCO.2007.14.5631.
8. Alavi A, Kung JW, Zhuang H. Implications of PET based molecular imaging on the current and future practice of medicine. Semin Nucl Med 2004;34(1): 56–69.
9. Fernandez FG, Drebin JA, Linehan DC, et al. Five-year survival after resection of hepatic metastases from colorectal cancer in patients screened by positron emission tomography with F-18 fluorodeoxyglucose (FDG-PET). Ann Surg 2004;240(3): 438–47 [discussion: 447–50].
10. Nordlinger B, Guiguet M, Vaillant JC, et al. Surgical resection of colorectal carcinoma metastases to the liver. A prognostic scoring system to improve case selection, based on 1568 patients. Association Francaise de Chirurgie. Cancer 1996;77(7): 1254–62.
11. Abdalla EK, Vauthey JN, Ellis LM, et al. Recurrence and outcomes following hepatic resection, radiofrequency ablation, and combined resection/ablation for colorectal liver metastases. Ann Surg 2004;239(6):818–25 [discussion: 825–7].
12. Morris EJ, Forman D, Thomas JD, et al. Surgical management and outcomes of colorectal cancer liver metastases. Br J Surg 2010;97(7):1110–8. http://dx.doi.org/10.1002/bjs.7032.
13. Shi M, Guo RP, Lin XJ, et al. Partial hepatectomy with wide versus narrow resection margin for solitary hepatocellular carcinoma: a prospective randomized trial. Ann Surg 2007;245(1):36–43. http://dx.doi.org/10.1097/01.sla.0000231758.07868.71.
14. Ruers T, Bleichrodt RP. Treatment of liver metastases, an update on the possibilities and results. Eur J Cancer 2002;38(7):1023–33.
15. Gomez D, Sangha VK, Morris-Stiff G, et al. Outcomes of intensive surveillance after resection of hepatic colorectal metastases. Br J Surg 2010;97(10): 1552–60. http://dx.doi.org/10.1002/bjs.7136.
16. Schulz A, Dormagen JB, Drolsum A, et al. Impact of contrast-enhanced intraoperative ultrasound on operation strategy in case of colorectal liver metastasis. Acta Radiol 2012;53(10):1081–7. http://dx.doi.org/10.1258/ar.2012.120049.

17. Leen E, Ceccotti P, Moug SJ, et al. Potential value of contrast-enhanced intraoperative ultrasonography during partial hepatectomy for metastases: an essential investigation before resection? Ann Surg 2006;243(2):236–40. http://dx.doi.org/10.1097/01.sla.0000197708.77063.07.

18. Fioole B, de Haas RJ, Wicherts DA, et al. Additional value of contrast enhanced intraoperative ultrasound for colorectal liver metastases. Eur J Radiol 2008; 67(1):169–76. http://dx.doi.org/10.1016/j.ejrad.2007.03.017.

19. Fong Y, Cohen AM, Fortner JG, et al. Liver resection for colorectal metastases. J Clin Oncol 1997; 15(3):938–46.

20. Scheele J, Stangl R, Altendorf-Hofmann A, et al. Indicators of prognosis after hepatic resection for colorectal secondaries. Surgery 1991;110(1):13–29.

21. Shah SA, Haddad R, Al-Sukhni W, et al. Surgical resection of hepatic and pulmonary metastases from colorectal carcinoma. J Am Coll Surg 2006;202(3): 468–75. http://dx.doi.org/10.1016/j.jamcollsurg.2005.11.008.

22. Glehen O, Kwiatkowski F, Sugarbaker PH, et al. Cytoreductive surgery combined with perioperative intraperitoneal chemotherapy for the management of peritoneal carcinomatosis from colorectal cancer: a multi-institutional study. J Clin Oncol 2004;22(16):3284–92. http://dx.doi.org/10.1200/JCO.2004.10.012.

23. da Silva RG, Sugarbaker PH. Analysis of prognostic factors in seventy patients having a complete cytoreduction plus perioperative intraperitoneal chemotherapy for carcinomatosis from colorectal cancer. J Am Coll Surg 2006;203(6):878–86. http://dx.doi.org/10.1016/j.jamcollsurg.2006.08.024.

24. Elias D, Ouellet JF, Bellon N, et al. Extrahepatic disease does not contraindicate hepatectomy for colorectal liver metastases. Br J Surg 2003;90(5): 567–74. http://dx.doi.org/10.1002/bjs.4071.

25. Pawlik TM, Schulick RD, Choti MA. Expanding criteria for resectability of colorectal liver metastases. Oncologist 2008;13(1):51–64. http://dx.doi.org/10.1634/theoncologist.2007-0142.

26. Ramos E, Valls C, Martinez L, et al. Preoperative staging of patients with liver metastases of colorectal carcinoma. Does PET/CT really add something to multidetector CT? Ann Surg Oncol 2011;18(9):2654–61. http://dx.doi.org/10.1245/s10434-011-1670-y.

27. Bohm B, Voth M, Geoghegan J, et al. Impact of positron emission tomography on strategy in liver resection for primary and secondary liver tumors. J Cancer Res Clin Oncol 2004;130(5):266–72.

28. van Kessel CS, Buckens CF, van den Bosch MA, et al. Preoperative imaging of colorectal liver metastases after neoadjuvant chemotherapy: a meta-analysis. Ann Surg Oncol 2012;19(9):2805–13. http://dx.doi.org/10.1245/s10434-012-2300-z.

29. Ruers TJ, Wiering B, van der Sijp JR, et al. Improved selection of patients for hepatic surgery of colorectal liver metastases with (18)F-FDG PET: a randomized study. J Nucl Med 2009;50(7):1036–41. http://dx.doi.org/10.2967/jnumed.109.063040.

30. Strasberg SM, Dehdashti F. Role of FDG-PET staging in selecting the optimum patient for hepatic resection of metastatic colorectal cancer. J Surg Oncol 2010;102(8):955–9. http://dx.doi.org/10.1002/jso.21729.

31. Wiering B, Adang EM, van der Sijp JR, et al. Added value of positron emission tomography imaging in the surgical treatment of colorectal liver metastases. Nucl Med Commun 2010;31(11):938–44. http://dx.doi.org/10.1097/MNM.0b013e32833fa9ba.

32. Adams RB, Aloia TA, Loyer E, et al. Selection for hepatic resection of colorectal liver metastases: expert consensus statement. HPB (Oxford) 2013; 15(2):91–103.

33. Kong G, Jackson C, Koh DM, et al. The use of ^{18}F-FDG PET/CT in colorectal liver metastases–comparison with CT and liver MRI. Eur J Nucl Med Mol Imaging 2008;35(7):1323–9. http://dx.doi.org/10.1007/s00259-008-0743-z.

34. Truant S, Huglo D, Hebbar M, et al. Prospective evaluation of the impact of [18]fluoro-2-deoxy-D-glucose positron emission tomography of resectable colorectal liver metastases. Br J Surg 2005; 92(3):362–9.

35. Grassetto G, Fornasiero A, Bonciarelli G, et al. Additional value of FDG-PET/CT in management of "solitary" liver metastases: preliminary results of a prospective multicenter study. Mol Imaging Biol 2010;12(2):139–44.

36. Sorensen M, Mortensen FV, Hoyer M, et al, Liver Tumour Board at Aarhus University Hospital. FDG-PET improves management of patients with colorectal liver metastases allocated for local treatment: a consecutive prospective study. Scand J Surg 2007;96(3):209–13.

37. Selzner M, Hany TF, Wildbrett P, et al. Does the novel PET/CT imaging modality impact on the treatment of patients with metastatic colorectal cancer of the liver? Ann Surg 2004;240(6):1027–34 [discussion: 1035–6].

38. Kochhar R, Liong S, Manoharan P. The role of FDG PET/CT in patients with colorectal cancer metastases. Cancer Biomark 2010;7(4–5):235–48.

39. Briggs RH, Chowdhury FU, Lodge JP, et al. Clinical impact of FDG PET-CT in patients with potentially operable metastatic colorectal cancer. Clin Radiol 2011;66(12):1167–74. http://dx.doi.org/10.1016/j.crad.2011.07.046.

40. McLeish AR, Lee ST, Byrne AJ, et al. Impact of ^{18}F-FDG-PET in decision making for liver metastectomy of colorectal cancer. ANZ J Surg 2012; 82(1–2):30–5.

41. Georgakopoulos A, Pianou N, Kelekis N, et al. Impact of ^{18}F-FDG PET/CT on therapeutic decisions in patients with colorectal cancer and liver metastases. Clin Imaging 2013;37(3):536–41.

42. Seo HJ, Kim MJ, Lee JD, et al. Gadoxetate disodium-enhanced magnetic resonance imaging versus contrast-enhanced ^{18}F-fluorodeoxyglucose positron emission tomography/computed tomography for the detection of colorectal liver metastases. Invest Radiol 2011;46(9):548–55. http://dx.doi.org/10.1097/RLI.0b013e31821a2163.

43. Servois V, Mariani P, Malhaire C, et al. Preoperative staging of liver metastases from uveal melanoma by magnetic resonance imaging (MRI) and fluorodeoxyglucose-positron emission tomography (FDG-PET). Eur J Surg Oncol 2010;36(2):189–94.

44. Wiering B, Ruers TJ, Krabbe PF, et al. Comparison of multiphase CT, FDG-PET and intra-operative ultrasound in patients with colorectal liver metastases selected for surgery. Ann Surg Oncol 2007; 14(2):818–26. http://dx.doi.org/10.1245/s10434-006-9259-6.

45. Adie S, Yip C, Chu F, et al. Resection of liver metastases from colorectal cancer: does preoperative chemotherapy affect the accuracy of PET in preoperative planning? ANZ J Surg 2009;79(5):358–61.

46. Akhurst T, Kates TJ, Mazumdar M, et al. Recent chemotherapy reduces the sensitivity of [^{18}F]fluorodeoxyglucose positron emission tomography in the detection of colorectal metastases. J Clin Oncol 2005;23(34):8713–6. http://dx.doi.org/10.1200/JCO.2005.04.4222.

47. Langenhoff BS, Oyen WJ, Jager GJ, et al. Efficacy of fluorine-18-deoxyglucose positron emission tomography in detecting tumor recurrence after local ablative therapy for liver metastases: a prospective study. J Clin Oncol 2002;20(22):4453–8.

48. Rappeport ED, Loft A, Berthelsen AK, et al. Contrast-enhanced FDG-PET/CT vs. SPIO-enhanced MRI vs. FDG-PET vs. CT in patients with liver metastases from colorectal cancer: a prospective study with intraoperative confirmation. Acta Radiol 2007;48(4):369–78. http://dx.doi.org/10.1080/02841850701294560.

49. Finkelstein SE, Fernandez FG, Dehdashti F, et al. Unique site- and time-specific patterns of recurrence following resection of colorectal carcinoma hepatic metastases in patients staged by FDG-PET. J Hepatobiliary Pancreat Surg 2008;15(5):483–7.

50. Fernandez FG, Drebin JA, Linehan DC. Five-year survival after resection of hepatic metastases from colorectal cancer in patients screened by positron emission tomography with F-18 fluorodeoxyglucose (FDG-PET): Commentary. Dis Colon Rectum 2005;48(1):181.

51. Bruix J, Sherman M, American Association for the Study of Liver Diseases. Management of hepatocellular carcinoma: an update. Hepatology 2011;53(3):1020–2. http://dx.doi.org/10.1002/hep.24199.

52. Wolfort RM, Papillion PW, Turnage RH, et al. Role of FDG-PET in the evaluation and staging of hepatocellular carcinoma with comparison of tumor size, AFP level, and histologic grade. Int Surg 2010; 95(1):67–75.

53. Ijichi H, Shirabe K, Taketomi A, et al. Clinical usefulness of ^{18}F-fluorodeoxyglucose positron emission tomography/computed tomography for patients with primary liver cancer with special reference to rare histological types, hepatocellular carcinoma with sarcomatous change and combined hepatocellular and cholangiocarcinoma. Hepatol Res 2013;43(5):481–7.

54. Kitamura K, Hatano E, Higashi T, et al. Preoperative FDG-PET predicts recurrence patterns in hepatocellular carcinoma. Ann Surg Oncol 2012;19(1):156–62.

55. Zubeldia JM, Bednarczyk EM, Baker JG, et al. The economic impact of [18]FDG positron emission tomography in the surgical management of colorectal cancer with hepatic metastases. Cancer Biother Radiopharm 2005;20(4):450–6.

56. Lejeune C, Bismuth MJ, Conroy T, et al. Use of a decision analysis model to assess the cost-effectiveness of ^{18}F-FDG PET in the management of metachronous liver metastases of colorectal cancer. J Nucl Med 2005;46(12):2020–8.

57. Schussler-Fiorenza CM, Mahvi DM, Niederhuber J, et al. Clinical risk score correlates with yield of PET scan in patients with colorectal hepatic metastases. J Gastrointest Surg 2004;8(2):150–8.

58. Wong SL, Mangu PB, Choti MA, et al. American Society of Clinical Oncology 2009 clinical evidence review on radiofrequency ablation of hepatic metastases from colorectal cancer. J Clin Oncol 2010;28(3):493–508. http://dx.doi.org/10.1200/JCO.2009.23.4450.

59. Gillams AR, Lees WR. Five-year survival in 309 patients with colorectal liver metastases treated with radiofrequency ablation. Eur Radiol 2009;19(5):1206–13. http://dx.doi.org/10.1007/s00330-008-1258-5.

60. Van Tilborg AA, Meijerink MR, Sietses C, et al. Long-term results of radiofrequency ablation for unresectable colorectal liver metastases: a potentially curative intervention. Br J Radiol 2011; 84(1002):556–65. http://dx.doi.org/10.1259/bjr/78268814.

61. Hompes D, Prevoo W, Ruers T. Radiofrequency ablation as a treatment tool for liver metastases of colorectal origin. Cancer Imaging 2011;11:23–30. http://dx.doi.org/10.1102/1470-7330.2011.0004.

62. Gleisner AL, Choti MA, Assumpcao L, et al. Colorectal liver metastases: recurrence and survival

following hepatic resection, radiofrequency ablation, and combined resection-radiofrequency ablation. Arch Surg 2008;143(12):1204–12. http://dx.
doi.org/10.1001/archsurg.143.12.1204.

63. Wallace JR, Christians KK, Quiroz FA, et al. Ablation of liver metastasis: is preoperative imaging sufficiently accurate? J Gastrointest Surg 2001;5(1):
98–107.

64. Limanond P, Zimmerman P, Raman SS, et al. Interpretation of CT and MRI after radiofrequency ablation of hepatic malignancies. AJR Am J Roentgenol
2003;181(6):1635–40. http://dx.doi.org/10.2214/ajr.
181.6.1811635.

65. Crocetti L, de Baere T, Lencioni R. Quality improvement guidelines for radiofrequency ablation of liver
tumours. Cardiovasc Intervent Radiol 2010;33(1):
11–7. http://dx.doi.org/10.1007/s00270-009-9736-y.

66. Kuehl H, Rosenbaum-Krumme S, Veit-Haibach P,
et al. Impact of whole-body imaging on treatment
decision to radio-frequency ablation in patients
with malignant liver tumors: comparison of [18F]flu-
orodeoxyglucose-PET/computed tomography, PET
and computed tomography. Nucl Med Commun
2008;29(7):599–606. http://dx.doi.org/10.1097/
MNM.0b013e3282f8144d.

67. Sahin DA, Agcaoglu O, Chretien C, et al. The utility of
PET/CT in the management of patients with colorectal
liver metastases undergoing laparoscopic radiofrequency thermal ablation. Ann Surg Oncol 2012;
19(3):850–5. http://dx.doi.org/10.1245/s10434-011-
2059-7.

68. Khandani AH, Calvo BF, O'Neil BH, et al. A pilot study
of early 18F-FDG PET to evaluate the effectiveness of
radiofrequency ablation of liver metastases. AJR Am
J Roentgenol 2007;189(5):1199–202. http://dx.doi.
org/10.2214/AJR.07.2126.

69. Veit P, Antoch G, Stergar H, et al. Detection of residual tumor after radiofrequency ablation of liver
metastasis with dual-modality PET/CT: Initial results. Eur Radiol 2006;16(1):80–7.

70. Chen W, Zhuang H, Cheng G, et al. Comparison of
FDG-PET, MRI and CT for post radiofrequency
ablation evaluation of hepatic tumors. Ann Nucl
Med 2013;27(1):58–64. http://dx.doi.org/10.1007/
s12149-012-0656-6.

71. Kim SH, Won KS, Choi BW, et al. Usefulness of F-
18 FDG PET/CT in the evaluation of early treatment
response after interventional therapy for hepatocellular carcinoma. Nucl Med Mol Imaging 2012;
46(2):102–10.

72. Sainani NI, Shyn PB, Tatli S, et al. PET/CT-guided
radiofrequency and cryoablation: is tumor
fluorine-18 fluorodeoxyglucose activity dissipated
by thermal ablation? J Vasc Interv Radiol 2011;
22(3):354–60.

73. Goldberg SN, Grassi CJ, Cardella JF, et al. Image-
guided tumor ablation: standardization of

terminology and reporting criteria. J Vasc Interv
Radiol 2009;20(7 Suppl):S377–90. http://dx.doi.
org/10.1016/j.jvir.2009.04.011.

74. Wang XY, Chen D, Zhang XS, et al. Value of
18F-FDG-PET/CT in the detection of recurrent hepatocellular carcinoma after hepatectomy or radiofrequency ablation: a comparative study
with contrast-enhanced ultrasound. J Dig Dis
2013;14(8):433–8.

75. Travaini LL, Trifiro G, Ravasi L, et al. Role of [18F]
FDG-PET/CT after radiofrequency ablation of liver
metastases: preliminary results. Eur J Nucl Med
Mol Imaging 2008;35(7):1316–22.

76. Anderson GS, Brinkmann F, Soulen MC, et al. FDG
positron emission tomography in the surveillance of
hepatic tumors treated with radiofrequency ablation. Clin Nucl Med 2003;28(3):192–7.

77. Paudyal B, Oriuchi N, Paudyal P, et al. Early diagnosis of recurrent hepatocellular carcinoma with
18F-FDG PET after radiofrequency ablation therapy.
Oncol Rep 2007;18(6):1469–73.

78. Blokhuis TJ, van der Schaaf MC, van den Tol MP,
et al. Results of radio frequency ablation of primary
and secondary liver tumors: long-term follow-up
with computed tomography and positron emission
tomography-18F-deoxyfluoroglucose scanning.
Scand J Gastroenterol Suppl 2004;(241):93–7.

79. Kuehl H, Antoch G, Stergar H, et al. Comparison of
FDG-PET, PET/CT and MRI for follow-up of colorectal liver metastases treated with radiofrequency
ablation: Initial results. Eur J Radiol 2008;67(2):
362–71. http://dx.doi.org/10.1016/j.ejrad.2007.11.
017.

80. Kuehl H, Stattaus J, Hertel S, et al. Mid-term
outcome of positron emission tomography/
computed tomography-assisted radiofrequency
ablation in primary and secondary liver tumours–
a single-centre experience. Clin Oncol (R Coll Radiol) 2008;20(3):234–40. http://dx.doi.org/10.1016/
j.clon.2007.11.011.

81. Antoch G, Kaiser GM, Mueller AB, et al. Intraoperative radiation therapy in liver tissue in a pig model:
monitoring with dual-modality PET/CT. Radiology
2004;230(3):753–60.

82. Fong Y, Saldinger PF, Akhurst T, et al. Utility of
18F-FDG positron emission tomography scanning
on selection of patients for resection of hepatic
colorectal metastases. Am J Surg 1999;178(4):
282–7.

83. Nicolay NH, Berry DP, Sharma RA. Liver metastases from colorectal cancer: radioembolization with
systemic therapy. Nat Rev Clin Oncol 2009;6(12):
687–97. http://dx.doi.org/10.1038/nrclinonc.2009.
165.

84. Coldwell D, Sangro B, Wasan H, et al. General selection criteria of patients for radioembolization of
liver tumors: an international working group report.

Am J Clin Oncol 2011;34(3):337–41. http://dx.doi.org/10.1097/COC.0b013e3181ec61bb.

85. Salem R, Thurston KG. Radioembolization with yttrium-90 microspheres: a state-of-the-art brachytherapy treatment for primary and secondary liver malignancies: Part 3: comprehensive literature review and future direction. J Vasc Interv Radiol 2006;17(10):1571–93. http://dx.doi.org/10.1097/01.RVI.0000236744.34720.73.

86. Kennedy A, Nag S, Salem R, et al. Recommendations for radioembolization of hepatic malignancies using yttrium-90 microsphere brachytherapy: a consensus panel report from the radioembolization brachytherapy oncology consortium. Int J Radiat Oncol Biol Phys 2007;68(1):13–23. http://dx.doi.org/10.1016/j.ijrobp.2006.11.060.

87. Denecke T, Ruhl R, Hildebrandt B, et al. Planning transarterial radioembolization of colorectal liver metastases with yttrium 90 microspheres: evaluation of a sequential diagnostic approach using radiologic and nuclear medicine imaging techniques. Eur Radiol 2008;18(5):892–902.

88. Rosenbaum CE, van den Bosch MA, Veldhuis WB, et al. Added value of FDG-PET imaging in the diagnostic workup for yttrium-90 radioembolisation in patients with colorectal cancer liver metastases. Eur Radiol 2013;23(4):931–7. http://dx.doi.org/10.1007/s00330-012-2693-x.

89. Becker C, Waggershauser T, Tiling R, et al. C-arm computed tomography compared with positron emission tomography/computed tomography for treatment planning before radioembolization. Cardiovasc Intervent Radiol 2011;34(3):550–6.

90. Elschot M, Vermolen BJ, Lam MG, et al. Quantitative comparison of PET and bremsstrahlung SPECT for imaging the in vivo yttrium-90 microsphere distribution after liver radioembolization. PLoS One 2013;8(2):e55742. http://dx.doi.org/10.1371/journal.pone.0055742.

91. Padia SA, Alessio A, Kwan SW, et al. Comparison of positron emission tomography and bremsstrahlung imaging to detect particle distribution in patients undergoing yttrium-90 radioembolization for large hepatocellular carcinomas or associated portal vein thrombosis. J Vasc Interv Radiol 2013;24(8):1147–53.

92. D'Arienzo M, Chiaramida P, Chiacchiararelli L, et al. 90Y PET-based dosimetry after selective internal radiotherapy treatments. Nucl Med Commun 2012;33(6):633–40. http://dx.doi.org/10.1097/MNM.0b013e3283524220.

93. Gates VL, Esmail AA, Marshall K, et al. Internal pair production of 90Y permits hepatic localization of microspheres using routine PET: proof of concept. J Nucl Med 2011;52(1):72–6. http://dx.doi.org/10.2967/jnumed.110.080986.

94. Fendler WP, Philippe Tiega DB, Ilhan H, et al. Validation of several SUV-based parameters derived from 18F-FDG PET for prediction of survival after SIRT of hepatic metastases from colorectal cancer. J Nucl Med 2013;54(8):1202–8. http://dx.doi.org/10.2967/jnumed.112.116426.

95. Piduru SM, Schuster DM, Barron BJ, et al. Prognostic value of 18F-fluorodeoxyglucose positron emission tomography-computed tomography in predicting survival in patients with unresectable metastatic melanoma to the liver undergoing yttrium-90 radioembolization. J Vasc Interv Radiol 2012;23(7):943–8.

96. Haug AR, Tiega Donfack BP, Trumm C, et al. 18F-FDG PET/CT predicts survival after radioembolization of hepatic metastases from breast cancer. J Nucl Med 2012;53(3):371–7. http://dx.doi.org/10.2967/jnumed.111.096230.

97. Zerizer I, Al-Nahhas A, Towey D, et al. The role of early (1)(8)F-FDG PET/CT in prediction of progression-free survival after (9)(0)Y radioembolization: comparison with RECIST and tumour density criteria. Eur J Nucl Med Mol Imaging 2012;39(9):1391–9. http://dx.doi.org/10.1007/s00259-012-2149-1.

98. Zalom M, Yu R, Friedman M, et al. FDG PET/CT as a prognostic test after 90Y radioembolization in patients with metastatic hepatic disease. Clin Nucl Med 2012;37(9):862–5. http://dx.doi.org/10.1097/RLU.0b013e318262af7f.

99. Wong CY, Qing F, Savin M, et al. Reduction of metastatic load to liver after intraarterial hepatic yttrium-90 radioembolization as evaluated by [18F]fluorodeoxyglucose positron emission tomographic imaging. J Vasc Interv Radiol 2005;16(8):1101–6. http://dx.doi.org/10.1097/01.RVI.0000168104.32849.07.

100. Miller FH, Keppke AL, Reddy D, et al. Response of liver metastases after treatment with yttrium-90 microspheres: role of size, necrosis, and PET. AJR Am J Roentgenol 2007;188(3):776–83. http://dx.doi.org/10.2214/AJR.06.0707.

101. Szyszko T, Al-Nahhas A, Canelo R, et al. Assessment of response to treatment of unresectable liver tumours with 90Y microspheres: Value of FDG PET versus computed tomography. Nucl Med Commun 2007;28(1):15–20. http://dx.doi.org/10.1097/MNM.0b013e328011453b.

102. Tochetto SM, Rezai P, Rezvani M, et al. Does multidetector CT attenuation change in colon cancer liver metastases treated with 90Y help predict metabolic activity at FDG PET? Radiology 2010;255(1):164–72. http://dx.doi.org/10.1148/radiol.09091028.

103. Young H, Baum R, Cremerius U, et al. Measurement of clinical and subclinical tumour response using [18F]-fluorodeoxyglucose and positron emission tomography: review and 1999 EORTC recommendations. European Organization for Research and Treatment of Cancer (EORTC) PET study group. Eur J Cancer 1999;35(13):1773–82.

104. Zhao M, Wu PH, Zeng YX, et al. Evaluating efficacy of transcatheter arterial chemo-embolization combined with radiofrequency ablation on patients with hepatocellular carcinoma by ^{18}FDG-PET/CT. Ai Zheng 2005;24(9):1118–23.

105. Cascales Campos P, Ramirez P, Gonzalez R, et al. Value of 18-FDG-positron emission tomography/computed tomography before and after transarterial chemoembolization in patients with hepatocellular carcinoma undergoing liver transplantation: Initial results. Transplant Proc 2011;43(6):2213–5.

106. Vitola JV, Delbeke D, Meranze SG, et al. Positron emission tomography with F-18-fluorodeoxyglucose to evaluate the results of hepatic chemoembolization. Cancer 1996;78(10):2216–22.

107. Kim JW, Seong J, Yun M, et al. Usefulness of positron emission tomography with fluorine-18-fluorodeoxyglucose in predicting treatment response in unresectable hepatocellular carcinoma patients treated with external beam radiotherapy. Int J Radiat Oncol Biol Phys 2012;82(3):1172–8. http://dx.doi.org/10.1016/j.ijrobp.2010.11.076.

FDG-PET/CT in Infectious and Inflammatory Diseases

Søren Hess, MD[a],*, Susanne H. Hansson, MD[b],
Kasper T. Pedersen, MD[a], Sandip Basu, MD[c],
Poul Flemming Høilund-Carlsen, MD, DMSc[a]

KEYWORDS

- Positron emission tomography/computed tomography • PET/CT • Fluorodeoxyglucose • FDG
- Infection • Inflammation • Infectious disease • Inflammatory disease

KEY POINTS

- The advantages of fluorodeoxyglucose–positron emission tomography/computed tomography (FDG-PET/CT) over conventional radionuclide studies in infection and inflammation include high sensitivity, high-resolution images, high target-to-background ratio, and fast technique completed in one session.
- FDG-PET/CT is well established in several infectious and inflammatory diseases (eg, fever of unknown origin, spondylitis, and vasculitis).
- FDG-PET/CT is promising in several clinical settings of infection and inflammation (eg, bacteremia of unknown origin, prosthetic infections, and sarcoidosis).
- FDG-PET/CT is being investigated in several novel indications (eg, inflammatory bowel disease, rheumatoid arthritis, psoriasis, and venous thromboembolism).

INTRODUCTION

Nuclear medicine techniques have been an integral part of infection and inflammation imaging for decades. Conventional radionuclide imaging tests, such as bone scintigraphy, labeled white blood cell scintigraphy, and gallium scanning, have all been used; but the relatively low spatial resolution is a recognized shortcoming; they are technically demanding and time consuming (with requirement of 2 scans on 2 separate days) and lack sensitivity, specificity, or both. All of these have restricted their use in a busy department. Fluorodeoxyglucose–positron emission tomography/computed tomography (FDG-PET/CT) has several advantages over the conventional radionuclide imaging methodologies and morphologic imaging

alone (**Box 1**); in recent years, much of the indications for conventional radionuclide imaging have been taken over by FDG-PET/CT. This review provides a comprehensive overview of current and potential applications for FDG-PET/CT in infectious and inflammatory diseases.

SYSTEMIC INFECTIONS
Fever and Bacteremia of Unknown Origin

Fever of unknown origin (FUO) is a heterogeneous group of diseases with as many as 200 potential differential diagnoses. The causes of FUO may be divided into 4 major groups: infections, malignancies, noninfectious inflammation, and miscellaneous. However, establishing an etiologic diagnosis is challenging because many patients

[a] Department of Nuclear Medicine, Odense University Hospital, Soender Boulevard 29, 5000 Odense, Denmark; [b] Department of Nuclear Medicine, Næstved Hospital, Ringstedgade 61, Næstved 4700, Denmark; [c] Radiation Medicine Centre, Bhabha Atomic Research Centre, Tata Memorial Hospital Annexe, Jerbai Wadia Road, Parel, Mumbai 400012, India
* Corresponding author.
E-mail address: soeren.hess@rsyd.dk

PET Clin 9 (2014) 497–519
http://dx.doi.org/10.1016/j.cpet.2014.07.002

present with unspecific symptoms and few diagnostic clues.[1] Because many FUO cases have some element of hypermetabolism (**Figs. 1–3**), the sensitivity of whole-body FDG-PET/CT is used in guiding the clinician toward more specific investigations. FDG-PET has, in multiple studies, been reported to provide clinically important information with regard to the underlying pathologic condition in between 42% and 92% of cases (**Table 1**), which is substantially higher than with any other diagnostic procedure.[2] A recent meta-analysis has summed up the results from 15 available studies and found a pooled sensitivity of 85% for establishing the cause of FUO on a per-patient basis.[3]

In more specialized settings (eg, critically ill patients with severe sepsis/septic shock of unknown origin), FDG-PET/CT has had direct therapeutic consequences in one-third of patients[14]; a small case series also showed promise in a pediatric setting.[15] In bacteremia of unknown origin or with suspected metastatic spread, FDG-PET/CT finds clinically relevant foci in up to half of patients with high positive and negative predictive values.[16,17] One group found significantly more patients with metastatic infectious disease when applying FDG-PET/CT compared with a control group in which no PET scans were performed, and the relapse and mortality rates were significantly lower in the FDG-PET/CT group because of more timely and correct treatment regimens. These results proved cost-effective taking into account the number of prevented deaths.[18,19]

Immunocompromised Patients

FUO often develops in immunocompromised patients (eg, during the neutropenic stages of chemotherapy or in patients infected with human immunodeficiency virus (HIV), where conventional diagnostics often fail to identify the cause. The role of FDG-PET/CT in febrile neutropenia was corroborated in 2 recent studies. In one, FDG-PET/CT identified additional infection sites not seen by conventional imaging in half the patients and had

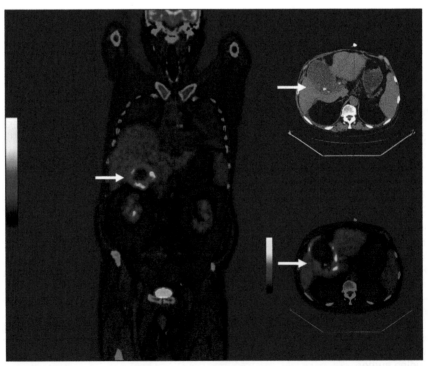

Fig. 1. FUO (infection). Coronal fused PET/CT image (*left*), axial CT image (*upper right*), and axial fused PET/CT image (*lower right*) show increased FDG uptake (*arrows*) in the circumference of the gall bladder. A previous CT and ultrasound were considered normal.

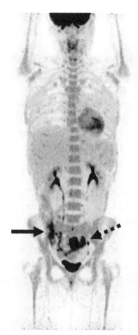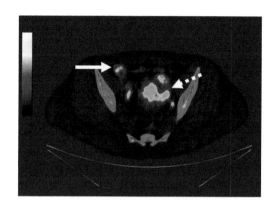

Fig. 2. FUO (inflammation). MIP PET image (*left*) and axial fused PET/CT image (*right*) show increased FDG uptake in the ileocecal area (*solid arrow*) with a fistula to an abscess in the pelvic region (*dotted arrow*). Surgery later confirmed Crohn disease. MIP, Maximum intensity projection. (*From* Hess S, Blomberg BA, Rakheja R, et al. A brief overview of novel approaches to FDG PET imaging and quantification. Clin Transl Imaging 2014;2:187–98. Reproduced with kind permission from Springer Science + Business Media.)

an overall clinical impact in 75% of cases,[20] and in another, FDG-PET/CT proved especially effective in detecting infection and thrombosis in central venous catheters and lung infections, while at the same time exhibiting a high negative predictive value of 94%.[21]

Immunosuppression in patients with HIV may result in fever caused by opportunistic infections or tumors, and locating the source is critical for reducing the time to initiating treatment. In their early landmark study of 80 patients who were HIV positive with fever, O'Doherty and colleagues[22] used FDG-PET/CT to locate sites of infections for sampling and the disease extent of lymphomas. Identification of focal pathology requiring treatment had a sensitivity and specificity of 92% and 94%, respectively. Furthermore, with PET they were able to distinguish between toxoplasmosis and central nervous system (CNS) lymphoma, which exhibits similar symptoms and similar features on morphologic imaging but needs different treatment and harbors very different prognoses. They reported the standard uptake value (SUV) in toxoplasmosis to be less than 3.7 in all cases and an SUV in CNS lymphoma greater than 3.9 in all respective cases. These data suggest that FDG-PET should be the modality of choice in patients with focal cerebral pathology. In a more recent study, Castaigne

and colleagues[23] similarly reported FDG-PET/CT to be helpful in locating disease and possible sampling sites in 9 out of 10 patients with HIV with FUO; the same group just published another report stating that FDG-PET/CT was helpful in diagnosing or excluding a focal cause for FUO in patients who are HIV positive, even in viremic stages.[24]

A novel entity within the realm of HIV/AIDS is tuberculosis (TB), which is also an increasing problem in developing countries in general. Early diagnosis of TB and especially differentiation from malignancies is of great importance, but FDG-PET/CT is not the modality of choice in this setting. Active granulomas are indeed highly FDG avid because the predominant cells are highly glucose-consuming lymphocytes and macrophages, but the lesions are indistinguishable from malignancies. As a consequence, dual-time-point imaging has been suggested, but the results have been disappointing because of comparable washout rates in TB and cancer. The most promising use for FDG-PET/CT seems to be staging or assessment of extrapulmonary disease activity and response evaluation.[25,26] The latter is important in both patients who are HIV positive and non-HIV patients, especially in developing countries because of the increasing incidence of multidrug-resistant and extensively drug resistant

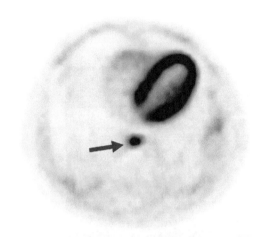

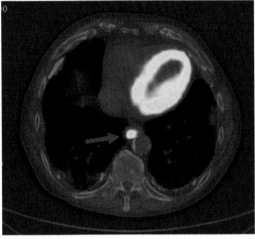

Fig. 3. FUO (cancer). Axial PET image (*top*) and fused axial PET/CT image (*bottom*) show focally increased FDG uptake in the distal esophagus (*arrows*). Endoscopy with biopsy confirmed adenocarcinoma.

TB. Two recent studies have assessed the treatment response in patients with TB who are HIV positive[27] and patients with TB who are HIV negative.[28] The former included 24 patients, and the investigators were able to differentiate responders from nonresponders with a sensitivity and specificity of 88% and 81%, respectively. The latter included 21 patients and found reduced FDG uptake in 19 patients, with a median decrease in maximum SUV (SUVmax) of 31% (range 2%–84%) after treatment was instituted.

Infectious Endocarditis

Infectious endocarditis (IE) is another clinical entity with the potential for metastatic infection, and early detection is very important for the successful management of this serious condition with high morbidity and mortality. The diagnosis is typically based on a synthesis of findings from the clinical presentation, blood cultures, echocardiography,[29,30] and the revised Duke criteria, which are considered the gold standard.[31] Transthoracic echocardiography and transesophageal echocardiography remain cornerstone modalities in the diagnostic workup. To be considered true positive, echocardiography should display vegetations on the valve, an abscess, or a new dehiscence of a prosthetic valve. It is important to remember that 30% of patients having IE have peripheral embolization at the time on diagnosis.[32]

So far, the literature regarding IE and FDG-PET and FDG-PET/CT consists mainly of numerous case studies; in 2013, Millar and colleagues[33] published a review of these. The PET findings were positive with evidence of IE in 86% of the cases, and 68% of them involved infection related to a prosthetic valve. Only 27% of the patients with IE on a prosthetic valve had vegetations on echocardiography, but all had a positive FDG PET; the investigators highlight this as a potential advantage of FDG-PET in such cases (**Fig. 4**).

Another potential advantage of FDG-PET/CT is the whole-body scan enabling findings of complications like peripheral embolization. In 2010, Van Riet and colleagues[34] published a study of 24 patients with IE examined with FDG-PET/CT and found peripheral embolization and/or metastatic infection in 44% of the patients; in 28%, there was no clinical suspicion of this. More recently, Ozcan and colleagues[35] published a retrospective study with 72 patients concluding that FDG-PET/CT may be an important diagnostic tool in detecting extracardiac infections in patients with IE, particularly in organs with low physiologic glucose uptake.

There are limitations to the use of FDG-PET/CT. There is normally variable focal or diffuse physiologic FDG uptake in the heart, and several factors may influence myocardial uptake (eg, fasting time, blood glucose level, and a low-carbohydrate diet). Thus, a low-carbohydrate diet and a high-fat, low--carbohydrate, protein-permitted meal followed by fasting in 6 hours before the injection might decrease the physiologic FDG uptake.[36] Also, FDG-PET/CT imaging is usually performed 1 hour after injection, but perhaps delayed imaging could provide a better target-to-background ratio because of the clearance of the background activity.[37] Furthermore, several diseases resemble IE on FDG-PET/CT (eg, soft arteriosclerotic plaques,[38] vasculitis,[39] primary cardiac tumors,[40] postsurgical inflammation,[41] and foreign body reactions).[42] There are also technical issues; the spatial resolution threshold of current PET/CT scanners is about 5 mm, but sites of peripheral

Table 1
Overview of studies on FUO

Author, Year	Design	Patients Included	PET/CT Helpful (%)	No Final Diagnosis (%)
Tokmak et al,[4] 2014	Prospective	25	60	—
Manohar et al,[5] 2013	Retrospective	103	60	40
Pedersen et al,[6] 2012	Retrospective	52	45	32
Pelosi et al,[7] 2011	Retrospective	24	46	29
Sheng et al,[8] 2011	Retrospective	48	67	12
Ferda et al,[9] 2010	Retrospective	48	92	8
Federici et al,[10] 2010	Retrospective	14	50	29
Kei et al,[11] 2010	Retrospective	12	42	42
Sheng et al,[8] 2011	Retrospective	48	67	12
Balink et al,[12] 2009	Retrospective	68	56	35
Keidar et al,[13] 2008	Prospective	48	46	40

Data from Refs.[4–13]

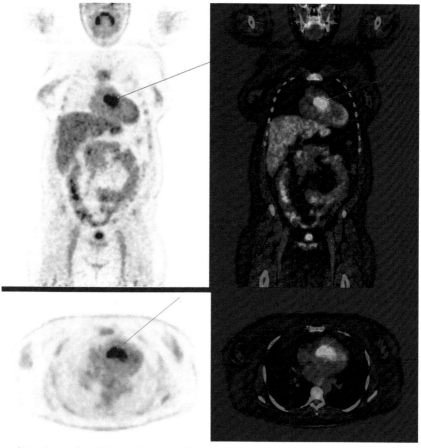

Fig. 4. Endocarditis. Coronal PET image (*upper left*), axial PET image (*lower left*), fused coronal PET/CT image (*upper right*), and fused axial PET/CT image show a focal area of increased FDG uptake in the heart at the position of the aortic valve (*arrows*). Echocardiographies were normal. (*From* Vind SH, Hess S. Possible role of PET/CT in infective endocarditis. J Nucl Cardiol 2010;17:516–9. Reproduced with kind permission from Springer Science + Business Media.)

embolization are often smaller, and there is a limit to finding peripheral embolization in the brain because of the high physiologic glucose consumption in the brain.

In summary, the data so far support the use of FDG-PET/CT to rule out or confirm IE in difficult cases; FDG-PET/CT has the advantage of showing concomitant extracardiac infection as a result of peripheral embolization. Furthermore, FDG-PET has shown potential in patients with IE related to prosthetic valve.

BONE INFECTIONS
Spinal Infection

Spinal infections account for 2% to 4 % of skeletal infections, and the diagnosis remains challenging but is facilitated by early and appropriate imaging together with histopathology or bacteriologic culture. Morphologic imaging modalities, such as conventional radiography, CT, and magnetic resonance (MR) imaging, are frequently used but are nonspecific. Moreover, CT and MR imaging are hampered by artifacts induced by spinal implants or hardware. MR imaging is the gold standard; but there are problems with differentiating spinal infection from neoplastic conditions, benign compression fractures, degenerative abnormalities, or postoperative changes.[43]

All of these issues may be alleviated by FDG-PET/CT (**Fig. 5**), and published data have indicated the potential for this imaging technique in diagnosing spinal infection.[44,45] In general, there is only faint FDG uptake in the spine; FDG uptake normalizes within 3 to 4 months following fracture or surgery. Furthermore, differentiation is possible because there tends to be less FDG uptake in benign fractures compared with malignant fractures or spinal infection; older fractures demonstrate from none to mildly or moderately increased FDG uptake.[46,47]

Many of the published studies are a mixture of patients with postoperative infection and hematogenous infection; many deal only with standalone FDG-PET and, thus, lack CT attenuation correction and proper anatomic localization.[48–53] A study by Schmitz and colleagues[54] concluded that, although limited experiences in diagnosing

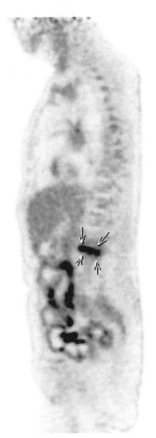 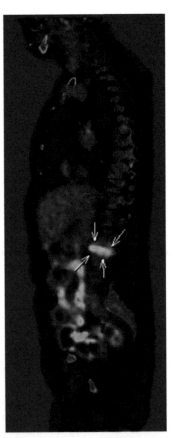

Fig. 5. Spondylodiscitis. Sagittal PET image (*left*) and sagittal fused PET/CT image (*right*) show intense FDG uptake in lumbar vertebras at L2/L3 consistent with spondylodiscitis (*arrows*). A subsequent MR imaging scan confirmed the diagnosis.

spinal infection are available, FDG-PET is a very sensitive imaging procedure for this purpose. Only very few studies include FDG-PET/CT. In 2007, Hartmann and colleagues[55] published a retrospective evaluation of 33 patients suspected of having chronic osteomyelitis in the axial and appendicular skeleton. In a subgroup analysis of 9 lumbar spinal regions, FDG-PET/CT was true positive in 7 patients with spinal infection and true negative in 2 patients without spinal infection (ie, sensitivity = specificity = 100%). In 2008, Kim and colleagues[56] performed FDG PET/CT in 22 patients with suspected spinal infection and concluded that FDG-PET/CT is a very sensitive method for the detection of spinal infection. More recently, Fuster and colleagues[57] and Seifen and colleagues[58] found sensitivities and specificities of 82% to 89% and 88% to 100%, respectively. In the latter article, the patients were complicated and with equivocal MR imaging findings. A recent meta-analysis[59] found pooled sensitivity, specificity, positive predictive value, and negative predictive value of 97%, 88%, 96%, and 85%, respectively; thus, results of FDG-PET and FDG-PET/CT for diagnosing spinal infections are very encouraging, although some issues remain. One problem could be FDG uptake in the degenerative spine as shown by Rosen and colleagues[60] in a retrospective study of 150 patients, but CT will be a powerful tool in this concern. Another problem could be the presence of a foreign body, which may give rise to a noninfectious immune response with increased FDG uptake. However, according to the abovementioned meta-analysis, this was not a consistent problem when PET/CT was used. Differentiating between spinal infection and tumor uptake may also be challenging, but dual-time-point FDG-PET/CT may mitigate this. A novel and very interesting potential indication is response evaluation as illustrated in a recent study by Nanni and colleagues[61] who used the change in SUVmax from baseline until 2 to 4 weeks of treatment to identify responders. In conclusion, although further data are desirable, the authors think that FDG-PET/CT should be the radionuclide examination of choice in spondylitis and spondylodiscitis in that a negative FDG-PET/CT excludes spinal infection with a good certainty, whereas increased FDG uptake contributes to the diagnosis in equivocal patients; response evaluation seems to be a promising option.

Periprosthetic Joint Infections

The numbers of prosthetic joints are increasing in the Western world. Hip and knee are the most commonly replaced joints; about 5% of the respective prostheses become infected, which is a serious complication with discomfort for patients; need of repeat surgery; potential loss of implant; and, in worst cases, invalidity or even death. A common differential diagnosis is prosthetic loosening presenting with much the same symptoms as infection, which makes discrimination difficult but imperative to ensure correct therapy.

An accurate noninvasive imaging modality is in high demand, and for many years In-111 labeled leukocyte scintigraphy in combination with sulfur colloid bone marrow scintigraphy has been considered the gold standard.[62] However, it is a time-consuming and expensive procedure that is inconvenient to patients and has awkward logistics, as it requires ex vivo labeling of patients' leukocytes and imaging after 4 and 24 hours. FDG-PET/CT is an attractive alternative (**Fig. 6**); several studies have shown its potential, especially in hip prostheses, with sensitivities and specificities around 90%. A meta-analysis from 2008 found pooled sensitivity and specificity of 86% and 82%, respectively.[63,64]

So far, there is no general consensus with regard to the interpretation of increased FDG uptake in relation to prostheses; but suggestions have been put forth with regard to hip prostheses (**Table 2**). Thus, uptake around the femoral neck may be regarded as nonspecific, whereas uptake in relation to the acetabular component or the parts of the femoral stem in direct contact with bone (except the tip of the implant) is considered consistent with infection.[65] Regarding knee prostheses, no specific pattern has gained general acceptance yet.

Diabetic Foot Infection and Charcot Foot

Diabetic foot infection is defined as an inframalleolar infection in diabetic patients, and the condition is associated with a high morbidity.[66] Ulcers are the major predisposing factors and result often from trauma or excessive pressure on a foot lacking protective sensation. Diabetic patients have a lifetime risk of 15% to 20% for a foot ulcer. The diagnosis is often overlooked because diabetic patients may not experience symptoms. Once there is infection, the risk of hospitalization and amputation increases dramatically. Diabetic foot infection can lead to lower extremity amputation and is the indication for about 60% of all amputations undertaken in developed countries. Thus, with the ongoing worldwide epidemic of diabetes, including third world countries, early detection of infection is essential.

The Charcot foot is a progressive, noninfectious, destructive disease of the bones and joints in the

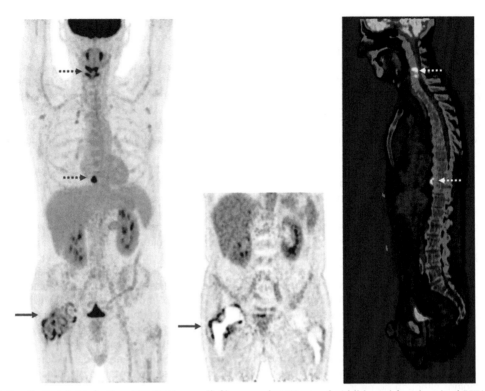

Fig. 6. Prosthetic joint infection. MIP PET image (*left*), coronal PET image (*middle*), and fused sagittal PET/CT image (*right*) show intense FDG uptake around the right hip prosthesis (*solid arrows*) and, furthermore, anteriorly in thoracic vertebras Th9/Th10 and cervical vertebras C3/C4 consistent with spondylodiscitis at 2 different levels (*dotted arrows*). MIP, Maximum intensity projection.

midfoot caused by neuropathy. The bones of the foot are weakened and may fracture. With continued walking, joints may collapse and the shape and function of the foot will change leading to deformity; disability; and, in serious cases, even amputation. With their tendency of peripheral neuropathy, diabetic patients are prone to develop Charcot feet and infection/inflammation may

superimpose and render diagnosis and differential diagnosis making, including osteomyelitis, extremely difficult. Reports on the use of FDG-PET and FDG-PET/CT in these settings exist (**Table 3**), but they are primarily from the era of stand-alone PET and quite heterogeneous with regard to material and image interpretation. Nonetheless, FDG-PET seems to be a very promising modality in patients with a diabetic foot infection and Charcot neuropathy, with accuracies near or more than 90%. This accuracy is at least comparable with MR imaging and, in some studies, associated with even better specificity.[67–74] Furthermore, in the study by Ruotolo and colleagues,[74] besides concluding that MR imaging and FDG PET/CT were comparable in Charcot neuropathy, they also found that FDG-PET/CT was useful for measuring the inflammatory response during treatment. Basu and colleagues[69] found the sensitivity of diagnosing neuropathy with FDG/PET and MR imaging to be 100% and 77%, respectively. Obviously, with patients being diabetic, blood glucose may be an issue. Some of the studies reported blood glucose levels and established the threshold for optimum-quality FDG-PET images for assessing infections to be less than 250 mg/dL ($\sim$14 mmol/L).

Table 2
Proposed interpretation points for FDG uptake pattern in suspected hip prosthesis infection

	Infection	Nonspecific Inflammation
Acetabular component	+	−
Femoral neck	−	+
Femur stem in contact with bone (− tip)	+	−
Tip of the femur stem	−	+

The + and − indicate presence and absence of abnormally high FDG uptake.

Table 3
Overview of studies on PET and PET/CT for diabetic complications

Author, Year	Modality	N	Population
Hopfner et al,[67] 2004	PET	16	Neuropathy
Keidar et al,[68] 2005	PET/CT	14	Clinically suspicious for infection
Basu et al,[69] 2007	PET	63	Neuropathy without infection
Schwegler et al,[70] 2008	PET	20	Ulcus without infection
Nawaz et al,[71] 2010	PET	110	Osteomyelitis
Familiari et al,[72] 2011	PET	13	High likelihood for infection
Kagna et al,[73] 2012	PET/CT	39	Possible infection
Ruotolo et al,[74] 2013	PET/CT	25	Charcot foot

Data from Refs.[67–74]

Therefore, although diabetic patients may have higher baseline blood glucose levels than nondiabetic patients, it is not a problem per se if only the diabetes is acceptably regulated. Further studies, especially addressing the usefulness of hybrid PET/CT, are desirable to confirm the potential of FDG-PET/CT in the management of the diabetic foot.

VASCULAR INFECTION AND INFLAMMATION
Vascular Graft Infection

Vascular graft infection is a rare complication with an incidence of 0.5% to 5.0% but a very serious one leading to amputation[75] and mortality rates of 25% up to 88%.[76] The diagnosis is not easily obtained; clinical symptoms and signs are variable and often nonspecific, especially depending on whether it is an early or late infection. Early and reliable diagnosis is important to institute adequate treatment as early as possible to ensure the best possible functional outcome for patients. Predominant current imaging modalities are ultrasound, CT, and MR imaging, although FDG-PET and FDG-PET/CT have shown great potential (**Fig. 7**). CT has a good diagnostic accuracy in patients with advanced infection but may fail in patients with a low-grade infection.[77]

To date, only a handful of smaller studies are available besides case reports, one on standalone PET and 3 on PET/CT.[78–81] In the first one, Fukuchi and colleagues[78] only looked at aortic graft infection (n = 33) but, nevertheless, found superior sensitivity of 91% compared with CT (64%). Specificity (64%) was lower than for CT (86%); but if focal uptake was chosen as a positive criterion, both specificity and positive predictive values increased to greater than 95%. The 3 evaluations of PET/CT (n = 25–76) all concluded that FDG-PET/CT is an excellent diagnostic modality in patients with

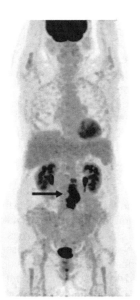
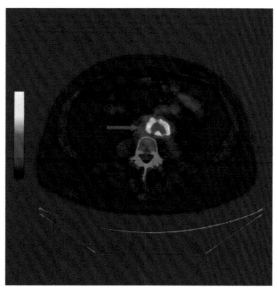

Fig. 7. Vascular graft infection. MIP PET image (*left*) and fused axial PET/CT image (*right*) show intense FDG uptake in connection with aortic vascular graft and adjacent soft tissue (*arrows*). MIP, Maximum intensity projection.

suspected vascular graft infection. The sensitivities, specificities, positive predictive values, and negative predictive values were 93%, 70% to 91%, 82% to 88%, and 88% to 96%, respectively, in papers by Keidar and colleagues[79] and Bruggink and colleagues[81] compared FDG-PET/CT to stand-alone CT and found corresponding values of 56%, 57%, 60%, and 58%. The third study by Spacek and colleagues[80] found an accuracy of greater than 95% in 75% of the cases and an accuracy of 70% to 75% in the remaining 25%. They also concluded that intense, focal FDG uptake and an irregular graft boundary were independent significant predictors for vascular graft infection. This finding underlines the importance of different FDG uptake patterns to govern the conclusions; a diffuse uptake has been described in nonspecific inflammation present postoperatively, whereas true infection was associated with focal FDG uptake.[78,80] FDG-PET has also been shown to be valuable for the assessment of vascular graft infection when CT results are negative.[82]

The results are promising, and further and larger prospective studies are needed; but FDG-PET/CT should be at the forefront in the diagnostic flow chart of patients with suspected vascular graft infections.

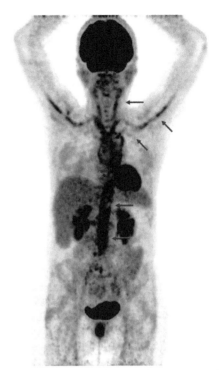

Fig. 8. Large vessel vasculitis. MIP PET image shows diffuse, intense FDG uptake in the central large arteries (ie, carotid arteries, subclavian artery, and the aorta [*arrows*]). MIP, Maximum intensity projection.

Vasculitis

Vasculitis is an inflammatory disease characterized by inflammation and necrosis in the vessel wall leading to reactive destruction of mural structures and surrounding tissues. Histopathologic analysis is considered the gold standard; but accurate imaging is obviously important because of the location of the disease, not only to confirm the diagnosis in case of inaccessibility to biopsy but also to find a suitable biopsy site, to evaluate the disease extent, and ideally to monitor the treatment response. Procedures include angiography, MR imaging, and ultrasound; but none of these are effective in early disease stages with subtle morphologic changes or for response assessment, as structural changes are slow. FDG-PET/CT, on the other hand, can detect metabolic activity with high sensitivity at a very early stage and monitor the response to treatment very promptly, at least in big- or medium-sized vessels,[83] whereas small vessel vasculitis is less than the detection limit of current PET scanners.

Polymyalgia rheumatica with giant cell arteritis is the most common vasculitis entity affecting medium and large vessels and, thus, the vasculitis type most frequently examined by FDG-PET (**Figs. 8** and **9**). A common location is the temporal artery; temporal biopsy is considered the gold standard, although it has a low sensitivity and a false-negative rate of 15% to 40%. A substantial part of patients have extracranial disease manifestations at the time of diagnosis, which underlines the importance of estimating correctly the disease extent. For instance, aortic involvement is a very serious implication with a need for specific treatment to prevent life-threatening complications, such as aortic dissection.

Since the first study more than a decade ago by Bleeker-Rovers and colleagues,[84] which showed FDG-PET to be a useful imaging technique in diagnosing and determining the extent of vasculitis, a great deal of studies has substantiated this; FDG-PET has been shown to have sensitivities of 77% to 92% and specificities of 89% to 100% in treatment-naïve patients.[85] Looking at separate studies, FDG-PET/CT locate more vascular sites involved than MR imaging; but the modalities were comparable with regard to making the initial diagnosis.[86] Steroid treatment has been shown to reduce the FDG uptake in vessels and may, thus, influence sensitivity. However, this aspect can be used to evaluate treatment response as FDG uptake normalizes with relevant treatment.[87] Compared with MR imaging, FDG-PET is probably better to predict an early response to therapy

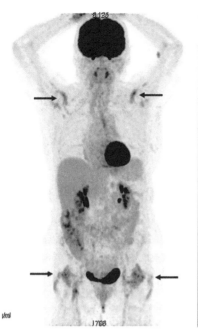 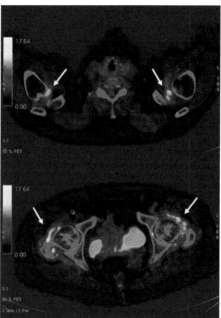

Fig. 9. Polymyalgia rheumatica. MIP PET image (*left*) and axial fused PET/CT images (*right*) show diffuse, intense FDG uptake in the muscles of the shoulders and hips (*arrows*). MIP, Maximum intensity projection.

because morphologic changes develop later than metabolic changes.

A recent systematic review by Treglia and colleagues[88] summed the results from 32 studies including more than 600 patients and concluded that FDG-PET and FDG-PET/CT are useful imaging methods in the initial diagnosis and extent of disease in patients with large vessel vasculitis while at the same time addressing some caveats (eg, assessing disease activity under immunosuppressive treatment). They suggested a much-needed standardization of the techniques used regarding PET analysis and diagnostic criteria for vasculitides.

There have been problems determining FDG uptake in the temporal artery because of the adjacent high brain uptake, but newer-generation high-resolution PET/CT scanners may alleviate these. Another problem is the possible false-positive finding from atherosclerotic plaques in, for instance, the aorta; but this problem might also be solved with fused PET/CT.

Takayasu arteritis is another group of large vessel vasculitis commonly that has been examined by FDG-PET/CT.[89] It is a rare disease predominantly affecting women, characteristically presenting with progressive inflammatory disease of the aorta and its branches. Angiography is considered the gold standard, but early disease may be missed because of late morphologic changes,[90] whereas FDG-PET/CT will reveal early changes in metabolism.

THORACIC AND ABDOMINAL INFLAMMATION
Sarcoidosis

The hallmark of sarcoidosis is the formation of noncaseating granulomas in one or more organ systems leading to a broad variety of symptoms, most often pulmonary ones, as the lungs and mediastinal lymph nodes are predominantly affected (**Fig. 10**). The prognosis ranges from spontaneous remission to severe debilitation and sudden cardiac death. Being caused by active immune cells, sarcoid lesions have been shown to display avid FDG uptake in countless reports; but the role of FDG-PET/CT has yet to be formally established in the diagnostic workup and monitoring of sarcoidosis.

So far, most studies on the properties of FDG in sarcoidosis have used strand-alone PET only. FDG-PET seems highly sensitive in detecting sarcoid lesions compared with traditional imaging modalities,[91–94] especially extrathoracic lesions. This point is particularly relevant if suitable biopsy sites are wanting[95] and in staging verified sarcoidosis, although in traditional staging of sarcoidosis, the focus is mainly on intrathoracic manifestations.[96] The distribution of FDG uptake may also be a predictor of prognosis and may help to identify patients with a need for treatment and to separate them from patients who may benefit more from a strategy of active surveillance.[94,97,98] Changes in FDG uptake in sarcoid lesions during

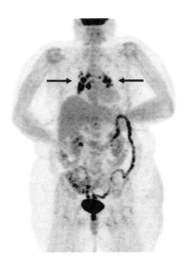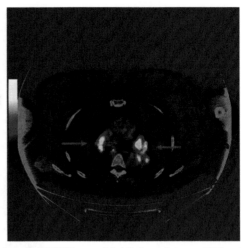

Fig. 10. Sarcoidosis. MIP PET image (*left*) and fused axial PET/CT image (*right*) show intense FDG uptake in mediastinal and hilar lymph nodes bilaterally (*arrows*). Subsequent biopsy confirmed granulomatous inflammation consistent with sarcoidosis, and the patient responded clinically to relevant treatment. MIP, Maximum intensity projection.

treatment have been shown to correlate to disease activity even when other markers of disease activity do not. Traditional markers of disease activity have been found within their normal ranges in up to 75% of patients (albeit in a strongly selected study population) even though active sarcoidosis was demonstrated by FDG-PET or PET/CT. These findings suggest that FDG-PET/CT may be suitable for monitoring disease activity and treatment response when traditional serologic markers are not elevated.[91,99–101] Ambrosini and colleagues[93] recently compared FDG-PET/CT and thoracic high-resolution CT, the usual modality of choice in sarcoidosis, in a prospective study of 28 patients with sarcoidosis. Concordance between these two modalities in assessing disease activity and extension was as low as 46%, mainly because of the ability of FDG-PET/CT to demonstrate extrathoracic granulomas. FDG-PET/CT results had a direct impact on the clinical management in 95% of cases of discordance.

Cardiac sarcoidosis (CS) is a manifestation responsible for a significant amount of disease-related deaths owing to severe arrhythmia caused by conduction abnormalities. It may be present in up to 25% of patients with sarcoidosis or even more frequently in certain subpopulations[102] that are often not diagnosed premortally. The guidelines of the Ministry of Health, Labor, and Welfare of Japan (MHLWJ) are often used as the gold standard for diagnosing CS. They recommend a composite of several clinical and paraclinical factors but not FDG-PET/CT. Studying FDG-PET/CT as a tool in assessing CS requires particular preparations to minimize FDG uptake in normal myocardium.[103] Sensitivity and specificity of FDG-PET is up to 89% and 78%, respectively, although with great variance; these figures can be further improved in combination with gadolinium-enhanced cardiac MR imaging.[102] FDG-PET/CT in combination with myocardial perfusion scintigraphy may predict the risk of major cardiac events.[104] If the MHLWJ criteria are tested with FDG-PET as the gold standard, the sensitivity of the MHLWJ criteria in diagnosing CS may be as low as 33% with a specificity of 97%, which suggests that the presence of CS may be underestimated by the traditional criteria, which is in line with the aforementioned large percentage of patients with undiagnosed CS.

Neurosarcoidosis (NS) is a rare manifestation of sarcoidosis, and studies of FDG-PET in NS are sparse.[105,106] However, when localized to the spinal cord, sarcoid granulomas can cause severe debilitation; the potential of FDG-PET to distinguish sarcoid lesions from noninflammatory myelopathies, thereby helping to direct treatment, has been suggested.[106]

The studies of FDG-PET and FDG-PET/CT in sarcoidosis are heterogeneous as are their results, partly because of the very diverse presentation and course of sarcoidosis. However, FDG-PET/CT seems to be potentially useful in many aspects of the diagnostic workup and in monitoring the course of sarcoidosis, especially given the reported high rate of undiagnosed cardiac or extrathoracic manifestations and the suboptimal sensitivity of the parameters that are traditionally used for assessing sarcoidosis activity and severity.

Inflammatory Bowel Diseases

Chronic inflammatory bowel disease (IBD) comprises Crohn disease (CD) (see **Fig. 2**) and ulcerative colitis (UC) (**Fig. 11**), which are similar in some respects but also very different with regard to other characteristics. They are both chronic with frequently relapsing inflammation but differ significantly in extent (ie, in being localized somewhere in the entire gastrointestinal tract [CD] or in the colon only [UC]). Nevertheless, the need to identify the disease activity and disease extent and to monitor the response to treatment is obvious for both diseases. Conventionally, these clinical issues rely on scoring systems requiring multiple invasive endoscopies (eg, gastroscopy, colonoscopy, capsule endoscopy) and imaging studies submitting the patients to rather high doses of radiation (eg, small bowel follow through CT enteroclysis); the results are often only indirect. Thus, an accurate and noninvasive method like FDG-PET/CT would be a significant improvement in the management of these patients.[107] The literature is sparse, but the potential is recognizable. Bicik and colleagues[108] published the first study with stand-alone PET in 1997. They studied 7 patients with suspected IBD and found a high FDG activity in areas of active inflammation on biopsy and a generally higher FDG uptake in patients with clinically active disease. Later, Neurath and colleagues[109] used FDG-PET in patients with known IBD to assess the disease extent and found PET to be much more sensitive (85%) than MR imaging (41%) at comparable specificity. A recent meta-analysis compiling the results of all FDG-PET and FDG-PET/CT studies to date found an overall pooled per-segment sensitivity and specificity of 85% and 87%, respectively.[110] Furthermore, the results also signify some potential for more specific indications (eg, in detecting and differentiating fibrostenosis [requiring surgery] vs inflammatory strictures requiring only conservative, medical treatment[111,112] and in assessing global, whole-body disease activity quantitatively,[113–119] including the response to treatment with implications for treatment strategy).[120]

IBD is also a diagnostic challenge in children and adolescents in the early stages or with episodes of flare-up. Contrary to adults, invasive endoscopies often require general anesthesia; noninvasive alternatives are in high demand. Despite the promising results in adults, only few original pediatric papers have been published. The authors recently published a review of the available literature.[121] During the period of 1999 to 2013, only 5 studies were published, 3 about

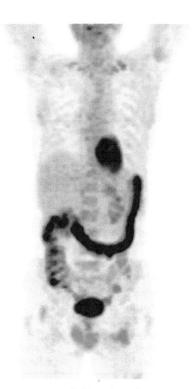

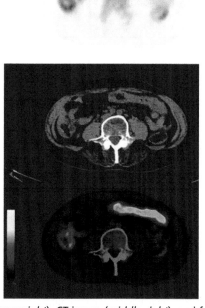

Fig. 11. IBD. MIP PET image (*left*) and axial PET image (*upper right*), CT image (*middle right*), and fused PET/CT image (*lower right*) show segmental, intense FDG uptake in the ascending and transverse colon. Subsequent colonoscopy confirmed ulcerative colitis. MIP, Maximum intensity projection.

stand-alone FDG-PET and 2 describing both FDG-PET and FDG-PET/CT (**Table 4**). The papers are heterogeneous, retrospective, and with different methodologies making comparisons difficult; but as for the adult population, results are encouraging by indicating a potential for detecting gastrointestinal inflammation by PET with high sensitivity and a reasonable specificity. Developments in instrumentation (ie, hybrid PET/CT) have greatly improved the sensitivity and specificity for uses in cancer[122–125] and are also expected to further enhance the diagnostic efficacy in inflammatory diseases. Thus, early reports based on stand-alone PET imaging can hardly be compared with novel studies using PET/CT; future studies with FDG-PET/CT in pediatric IBD will probably show even better overall results. Moreover, the ability of PET/CT to visualize the extraintestinal manifestations of IBD has proven valuable in the diagnostic workup of adults; the same may be expected to be the case in the pediatric setting.[116] Saboury and colleagues[126] recently published a paper emphasizing the use of a quantitative volume-based technique. In adult CD, they demonstrated the feasibility of calculating the global disease activity, in essence a single number summing up the inflammatory activity within the entire body, which seems to correlate to both clinical and endoscopic findings. Applying this technique in pediatric IBD would greatly improve noninvasive treatment monitoring particularly because it seems that as many as 44% of gold standard examinations in children suspected of having IBD may be incomplete.[121]

In conclusion, in both adults and children, FDG-PET/CT has a definite potential for noninvasive whole-body assessment of IBD adding accuracy to that of existing techniques in the preliminary assessment of disease extent, in the follow-up of indeterminate cases, for diagnosing flares or recurrence, for therapy planning in patients with stenosis, and for the assessment of the response to treatment. However, the scarcity of literature in both children and adults calls for prospective, randomized studies of well-characterized patient cohorts to firmly elucidate the impact of FDG-PET/CT in the management of patients with known or suspected IBD.

POTENTIAL NOVEL APPLICATIONS
Psoriasis and Rheumatoid Arthritis

Psoriasis is an inflammatory condition typically affecting the skin; but it is often associated with an inflammatory arthritis, psoriatic arthritis (PsA). In 2001, Yun and colleagues[127] described the first reported case of increased FDG uptake on a PET scan in joints with active PsA, demonstrating FDG-PET's potential ability to visualize the extent of PsA, an ability that subsequently has been confirmed by Takata and colleagues.[128] They showed that FDG-PET/CT can visualize arthritic joints and entheses in both patients with symptomatic and, jointwise, asymptomatic psoriasis. Moreover, it can be used to assess the efficacy of treatment with tumor necrosis factor-α (TNF-α) inhibitors of symptomatic and asymptomatic PsA.

Table 4
Overview of papers on PET/CT for pediatric IBD

Author, Year	n	Study Design	Modality Studied	Reference Examination	Sensitivity/Specificity (%)
Skehan et al,[155] 1999	25	Retrospective	FDG-PET	Colonoscopy and/or SBFT	81/85[a]
Lemberg et al,[156] 2005	65	Prospective	FDG-PET	Colonoscopy and SBFT	PET vs colonoscopy: 86/50 PET vs SBFT: 59/100[a]
Löffler et al,[157] 2006	23	Retrospective	FDG-PET	Colonoscopy and/or ultrasound	98/68[b]
Dabritz et al,[158] 2011	45	Retrospective	FDG-PET (±CT)	Colonoscopy, ultrasound, and gastroscopy	97/100[a] 82/97[b]
Berthold et al,[159] 2013	23	Retrospective	FDG-PET (±CT)	Colonoscopy, MR imaging, and gastroscopy	Stomach and duodenum: 25/100[b] Remaining bowel: 73/89[b]

Abbreviation: SBFT, small bowel follow-through.
[a] Per-patient sensitivity and specificity.
[b] Per-segment sensitivity and specificity.
Data from Refs.[155–159]

Rheumatoid arthritis (RA) is another notable inflammatory condition of unknown cause characterized by symmetric joint affection and the presence of various immunologic parameters. In the early symptomatic stages, RA joints are painful and swollen because of synovial inflammation, which in advances stages leads to joint irreversible destruction caused by the formation of pannus and cartilage erosion.[129] In 2011, Carey and colleagues[130] performed a systematic review of FDG-PET imaging in joint disorders comprising RA. The investigators highlighted the importance of detecting RA, specifically the synovial inflammation, as early as possible to arrest progression to advanced stages. FDG-PET seemed to be highly useful in asserting global disease activity and/or inflammation burden compared with the traditional methods of assessment. It has been discussed, if the degree of FDG uptake may be an indirect measure of neovascularization and consequently aggressive synovitis,[131] thereby possibly predicting the course of newly detected, early RA, but the investigators admitted that the supporting evidence was so far speculative. However, it was stated that high FDG uptake in large joints is correlated with the risk of developing atlantoaxial instability. Newer studies have shown that FDG-PET/CT may early on predict the outcome with

traditional treatment (steroids and disease-modifying antirheumatic drugs); some studies mention the assessment of lymph node activity as a special feature because it tends to decline earlier than joint activity and, thus, may represent a tool for early response assessment.[132–135] The response evaluation of biological treatment with, for instance, TNF-α inhibitors has shown promise[136]; but the sample sizes regarding the response assessment were small. In the first-mentioned study, all test subjects also improved clinically.

The inflammation in both psoriasis and RA is systemic in nature, and FDG-PET/CT has been used to illustrate that inflammation in these diseases may harbor not only in skin lesions and joints but also in the large blood vessels,[137,138] a finding which is thought to give rise to the increased cardiovascular risk in both psoriasis and RA.[129,139,140] A trial has been made to ascertain if treatment with TNF-α inhibitors given to patients with psoriasis and arterial inflammation can reduce this vascular inflammation as seen by FDG-PET/CT, but results are pending.[141] Nonetheless, treatment of psoriasis and RA could possibly benefit from focusing on the vascular component; FDG-PET/CT may prove useful to this end (**Fig. 12**).

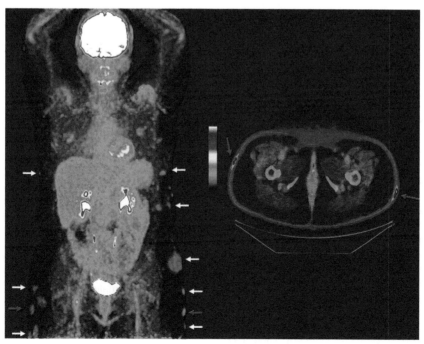

Fig. 12. Psoriasis. MIP PET image (*left*) and fused axial nonattenuation-corrected PET/CT image (*right*) show a patchy pattern of superficially increased FDG uptake in the skin (*arrows*) consistent with the patient's well-known psoriatic skin affections. MIP, Maximum intensity projection.

Chronic Obstructive Pulmonary Disease

Chronic obstructive pulmonary disease (COPD) covers a very broad disease spectrum from emphysema to bronchial inflammation and, in more advanced stages, cor pulmonale. It constitutes a major health care burden; but if correctly diagnosed, treatment options are available. Recently, the focus has been on systemic inflammation. Thus, patients with COPD have higher levels of systemic biomarkers of inflammation and probably have a worse cardiovascular risk profile and prognosis. Because of the heterogeneity of COPD, a more personalized treatment strategy could prove valuable; FDG-PET may offer several potential opportunities (ie, evaluating pulmonary and systemic inflammation and visualizing respiratory muscle activity and right heart function).[142]

Jones and colleagues[143] compared FDG-PET in 6 patients with COPD, 6 patients with chronic asthma, and 5 never-smoking controls and found significantly higher pulmonary FDG uptake in patients with COPD. Recently, another group demonstrated significant differences in pulmonary FDG uptake between patients with alpha-1-antitrypsin–deficient COPD and patients with COPD without alpha-1-antitrypsin deficiency.[144] As a surrogate measure for systemic inflammation, Coulson and colleagues[145] compared aortic FDG uptake in 7 ex-smokers with COPD and 7 ex-smokers without COPD and found significantly higher mean target-to-background ratio in COPD patients compared with ex-smoking patients without COPD (1.60 vs 1.34, $P = .001$). The investigators could offer no other potential explanation than COPD. Another study found prominent uptake in the right ventricle in 4 of 14 patients, and these 4 patients all had pulmonary hypertension confirmed by echocardiography.[146] Respiratory muscle uptake has also been studied as a marker of disease activity in several retrospective studies of patients scanned for other reasons than COPD (eg, malignant diseases). When comparing patients with and without COPD, these studies demonstrated significantly increased FDG uptake in respiratory muscles in all patients with COPD[147] and in the accessory respiration muscles in three-fourths of patients with COPD. Similar muscle uptake was only present in 4% of non-COPD patients.[148] FDG-PET is a quantitative modality, and all of the abovementioned studies use quantification to some extent. Other studies have clearly emphasized the importance of quantification as opposed to visual assessment. Thus, Torigian and colleagues[149] found the degree of pulmonary inflammation as visualized by FDG-PET to correlate with the severity of emphysema in 49 patients, much like the abovementioned study by Subramanian and colleagues,[144] but only when data were corrected for partial volume effect.

In conclusion, the current literature is sparse and heterogeneous with studies too small and exploratory to allow for general conclusions on the use of FDG-PET in COPD. However, it does indicate potential indications for FDG-PET in COPD: (1) for differentiating COPD from chronic asthma and alpha-1-antitrypsin deficiency, (2) to ascertain pulmonary and systemic inflammation for treatment guidance and prognosis estimates, (3) for quantifying respiratory muscle use, and perhaps also (4) for diagnosing cor pulmonale. Thus, clearly, the future role of FDG-PET in COPD deserves further studies.[142]

Venous Thromboembolic Disease

Venous thromboembolism (VTE) is a common and potentially fatal disease that comprises several different but interrelated clinical entities (eg, deep venous thrombosis [DVT] and pulmonary embolism [PE]), and the diagnosis of VTE remains challenging because of a vague and unspecific clinical presentation resembling other conditions. Standard imaging strategies are less than perfect; several issues remain, paving the way for novel modalities. Whole-body assessment with FDG-PET/CT shows promise for several reasons, first and foremost the intimate link between thrombosis and inflammation. DVT (**Fig. 13**) and PE are the most common manifestations; but VTE may occur globally in the venous vasculature, which promotes the whole-body approach of FDG-PET/CT.[150] Several studies have demonstrated DVT to be highly FDG avid, also in less accessible locations like sagittal sinuses, whereas PE tends to be less FDG avid.[150,151] FDG may also provide a means of quantifying global disease activity allowing for monitoring the disease course and response to treatment. In a recent study, Rondina and colleagues[152] addressed this and showed a decline in SUV over time with probable normalization after approximately 3 months.

Another advantage relates to the well-known association between VTE and malignancies; whole-body FDG-PET/CT provides a sensitive screening for underlying malignancies as cause of novel VTE.[153] Finally, patients with VTE are prone to relapse; but the morphologic changes that the current diagnostic methods base their diagnosis on may remain unchanged for years. Thus, FDG-avid VTE is metabolically active and more likely to be novel and treatment demanding, whereas

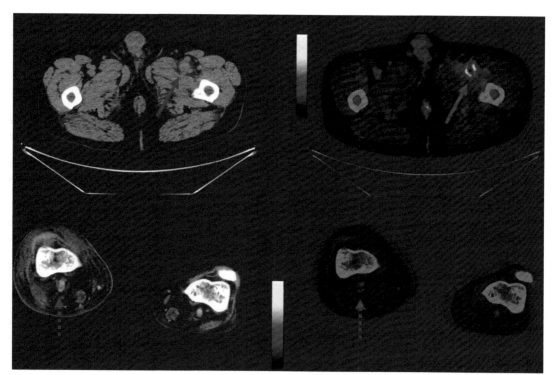

Fig. 13. VTE. Upper row shows axial CT image (*left*) and fused axial PET/CT image (*right*) in a patient with confirmed acute DVT with a short history. There is increased FDG uptake circumferentially in the dilated left femoral vein (*solid arrows*) consistent with acute, active inflammation. Lower row shows axial CT image (*left*) and fused axial PET/CT image (*right*) in a patient with a history of prior DVT but no current symptoms. There is no FDG uptake in the dilated right popliteal vein (*dotted arrows*) but stranding on CT consistent with prior (old) DVT without active inflammation.

nonavidity is more consistent with metabolically inactive chronic VTE better served by a conservative approach.[150]

In conclusion, further studies are needed; but evidence is emerging for VTE as a novel clinical application for FDG-PET/CT imaging. The authors think that the use of FDG as a marker of the inflammatory component of VTE may contribute substantially to patient management by providing whole-body assessment of both VTE and possible underlying malignancies, including a quantitative approach to characterize the disease course and assess the treatment response and to discriminate novel, metabolically active thrombi from older, inactive ones.

CONCLUDING REMARKS

One can envisage the potential role of FDG-PET/CT in several infectious and aseptic inflammatory processes. The list of applications is currently growing and will continue to do so in years to come. The assessment of disease extension and activity with functional FDG-PET/CT imaging as well as response evaluation by means of this method seem to have distinct advantages compared with the current conventional structural imaging. Their early and proper implementation in relevant patient courses may greatly improve patient management and contribute to more personalized strategies and potentially more effective therapies because early detection implies eo ipso "a perspective of cure instead of disease suppression."[154]

REFERENCES

1. Knockaert DC, Vanderschueren S, Blockmans D. Fever of unknown origin in adults: 40 years on. J Intern Med 2003;253(3):263–75.
2. Israel O, Keidar Z. PET/CT imaging in infectious conditions. Ann N Y Acad Sci 2011; 1228:150–66.
3. Hao R, Yuan L, Kan Y, et al. Diagnostic performance of 18F-FDG PET/CT in patients with fever of unknown origin: a meta-analysis. Nucl Med Commun 2013;34(7):682–8.
4. Tokmak H, Ergonul O, Demirkol O, et al. Diagnostic contribution of (18)F-FDG-PET/CT in fever of unknown origin. Int J Infect Dis 2014;19:53–8.
5. Manohar K, Mittal BR, Jain S, et al. F-18 FDG-PET/CT in evaluation of patients with fever of unknown origin. Jpn J Radiol 2013;31(5):320–7.

6. Pedersen TI, Roed C, Knudsen LS, et al. Fever of unknown origin: a retrospective study of 52 cases with evaluation of the diagnostic utility of FDG-PET/CT. Scand J Infect Dis 2012;44(1):18–23.

7. Pelosi E, Skanjeti A, Penna D, et al. Role of integrated PET/CT with [(1)(8)F]-FDG in the management of patients with fever of unknown origin: a single-centre experience. Radiol Med 2011; 116(5):809–20.

8. Sheng JF, Sheng ZK, Shen XM, et al. Diagnostic value of fluorine-18 fluorodeoxyglucose positron emission tomography/computed tomography in patients with fever of unknown origin. Eur J Intern Med 2011;22(1):112–6.

9. Ferda J, Ferdova E, Zahlava J, et al. Fever of unknown origin: a value of (18)F-FDG-PET/CT with integrated full diagnostic isotropic CT imaging. Eur J Radiol 2010;73(3):518–25.

10. Federici L, Blondet C, Imperiale A, et al. Value of (18)F-FDG-PET/CT in patients with fever of unknown origin and unexplained prolonged inflammatory syndrome: a single centre analysis experience. Int J Clin Pract 2010;64(1):55–60.

11. Kei PL, Kok TY, Padhy AK, et al. [18F] FDG PET/CT in patients with fever of unknown origin: a local experience. Nucl Med Commun 2010; 31(9):788–92.

12. Balink H, Collins J, Bruyn GA, et al. F-18 FDG PET/CT in the diagnosis of fever of unknown origin. Clin Nucl Med 2009;34(12):862–8.

13. Keidar Z, Gurman-Balbir A, Gaitini D, et al. Fever of unknown origin: the role of 18F-FDG PET/CT. J Nucl Med 2008;49(12):1980–5.

14. Kluge S, Braune S, Nierhaus A, et al. Diagnostic value of positron emission tomography combined with computed tomography for evaluating patients with septic shock of unknown origin. J Crit Care 2012;27(3):316.e1–7.

15. Del Rosal T, Goycochea WA, Mendez-Echevarria A, et al. F-FDG PET/CT in the diagnosis of occult bacterial infections in children. Eur J Pediatr 2013;172(8): 1111–5.

16. Bleeker-Rovers CP, Vos FJ, Wanten GJ, et al. 18F-FDG PET in detecting metastatic infectious disease. J Nucl Med 2005;46(12):2014–9.

17. Hess S, Vind SH, Skarphédinsson S, et al. Clinical value of PET/CT in bacteraemia of unknown origin. Results from an observational pilot study. Eur J Nucl Med Mol Imaging 2010;37(Suppl 2):1.

18. Vos FJ, Bleeker-Rovers CP, Kullberg BJ, et al. Cost-effectiveness of routine (18)F-FDG PET/CT in high-risk patients with gram-positive bacteremia. J Nucl Med 2011;52(11):1673–8.

19. Vos FJ, Bleeker-Rovers CP, Sturm PD, et al. 18F-FDG PET/CT for detection of metastatic infection in gram-positive bacteremia. J Nucl Med 2010;51(8): 1234–40.

20. Guy SD, Tramontana AR, Worth LJ, et al. Use of FDG PET/CT for investigation of febrile neutropenia: evaluation in high-risk cancer patients. Eur J Nucl Med Mol Imaging 2012;39(8):1348–55.

21. Vos FJ, Donnelly JP, Oyen WJ, et al. 18F-FDG PET/CT for diagnosing infectious complications in patients with severe neutropenia after intensive chemotherapy for haematological malignancy or stem cell transplantation. Eur J Nucl Med Mol Imaging 2012;39(1):120–8.

22. O'Doherty MJ, Barrington SF, Campbell M, et al. PET scanning and the human immunodeficiency virus-positive patient. J Nucl Med 1997;38(10): 1575–83.

23. Castaigne C, Tondeur M, de Wit S, et al. Clinical value of FDG-PET/CT for the diagnosis of human immunodeficiency virus-associated fever of unknown origin: a retrospective study. Nucl Med Commun 2009;30(1):41–7.

24. Martin C, Castaigne C, Tondeur M, et al. Role and interpretation of fluorodeoxyglucose-positron emission tomography/computed tomography in HIV-infected patients with fever of unknown origin: a prospective study. HIV Med 2013;14(8):455–62.

25. Sathekge M, Maes A, Van de Wiele C. FDG-PET imaging in HIV infection and tuberculosis. Semin Nucl Med 2013;43(5):349–66.

26. Ito K, Morooka M, Minamimoto R, et al. Imaging spectrum and pitfalls of 18F-fluorodeoxyglucose positron emission tomography/computed tomography in patients with tuberculosis. Jpn J Radiol 2013;31(8):511–20.

27. Sathekge M, Maes A, Kgomo M, et al. Use of 18F-FDG PET to predict response to first-line tuberculostatics in HIV-associated tuberculosis. J Nucl Med 2011;52(6):880–5.

28. Martinez V, Castilla-Lievre MA, Guillet-Caruba C, et al. (18)F-FDG PET/CT in tuberculosis: an early non-invasive marker of therapeutic response. Int J Tuberc Lung Dis 2012;16(9):1180–5.

29. Beynon RP, Bahl VK, Prendergast BD. Infective endocarditis. BMJ 2006;333(7563):334–9.

30. Evangelista A, Gonzalez-Alujas MT. Echocardiography in infective endocarditis. Heart 2004;90(6): 614–7.

31. Li JS, Sexton DJ, Mick N, et al. Proposed modifications to the Duke criteria for the diagnosis of infective endocarditis. Clin Infect Dis 2000;30(4):633–8.

32. Thuny F, Di Salvo G, Belliard O, et al. Risk of embolism and death in infective endocarditis: prognostic value of echocardiography: a prospective multicenter study. Circulation 2005;112(1):69–75.

33. Millar BC, Prendergast BD, Alavi A, et al. (18)FDG-positron emission tomography (PET) has a role to play in the diagnosis and therapy of infective endocarditis and cardiac device infection. Int J Cardiol 2013;167(5):1724–36.

34. Van Riet J, Hill EE, Gheysens O, et al. (18)F-FDG PET/CT for early detection of embolism and metastatic infection in patients with infective endocarditis. Eur J Nucl Med Mol Imaging 2010;37(6):1189–97.
35. Ozcan C, Asmar A, Gill S, et al. The value of FDG-PET/CT in the diagnostic work-up of extra cardiac infectious manifestations in infectious endocarditis. Int J Cardiovasc Imaging 2013;29(7):1629–37.
36. Williams G, Kolodny GM. Suppression of myocardial 18F-FDG uptake by preparing patients with a high-fat, low-carbohydrate diet. AJR Am J Roentgenol 2008;190(2):W151–6.
37. Treglia G, Bertagna F. Factors influencing the sensitivity of 18F-FDG PET/CT in the detection of infective endocarditis. Eur J Nucl Med Mol Imaging 2013;40(7):1112–3.
38. Williams G, Kolodny GM. Retrospective study of coronary uptake of 18F-fluorodeoxyglucose in association with calcification and coronary artery disease: a preliminary study. Nucl Med Commun 2009;30(4):287–91.
39. Kobayashi Y, Ishii K, Oda K, et al. Aortic wall inflammation due to Takayasu arteritis imaged with 18F-FDG PET coregistered with enhanced CT. J Nucl Med 2005;46(6):917–22.
40. Kaderli AA, Baran I, Aydin O, et al. Diffuse involvement of the heart and great vessels in primary cardiac lymphoma. Eur J Echocardiogr 2010;11(1):74–6.
41. Abidov A, D'Agnolo A, Hayes SW, et al. Uptake of FDG in the area of a recently implanted bioprosthetic mitral valve. Clin Nucl Med 2004;29(12):848.
42. Schouten LR, Verberne HJ, Bouma BJ, et al. Surgical glue for repair of the aortic root as a possible explanation for increased F-18 FDG uptake. J Nucl Cardiol 2008;15(1):146–7.
43. Hong SH, Choi JY, Lee JW, et al. MR imaging assessment of the spine: infection or an imitation? Radiographics 2009;29(2):599–612.
44. Gemmel F, Dumarey N, Palestro CJ. Radionuclide imaging of spinal infections. Eur J Nucl Med Mol Imaging 2006;33(10):1226–37.
45. Walker RC, Jones-Jackson LB, Martin W, et al. New imaging tools for the diagnosis of infection. Future Microbiol 2007;2(5):527–54.
46. Bredella MA, Essary B, Torriani M, et al. Use of FDG-PET in differentiating benign from malignant compression fractures. Skeletal Radiol 2008;37(5):405–13.
47. Schmitz A, Risse JH, Textor J, et al. FDG-PET findings of vertebral compression fractures in osteoporosis: preliminary results. Osteoporos Int 2002;13(9):755–61.
48. De Winter F, Gemmel F, Van De Wiele C, et al. 18-Fluorine fluorodeoxyglucose positron emission tomography for the diagnosis of infection in the postoperative spine. Spine 2003;28(12):1314–9.
49. Guhlmann A, Brecht-Krauss D, Suger G, et al. Chronic osteomyelitis: detection with FDG PET and correlation with histopathologic findings. Radiology 1998;206(3):749–54.
50. Zhuang H, Duarte PS, Pourdehand M, et al. Exclusion of chronic osteomyelitis with F-18 fluorodeoxyglucose positron emission tomographic imaging. Clin Nucl Med 2000;25(4):281–4.
51. Guhlmann A, Brecht-Krauss D, Suger G, et al. Fluorine-18-FDG PET and technetium-99m antigranulocyte antibody scintigraphy in chronic osteomyelitis. J Nucl Med 1998;39(12):2145–52.
52. Kalicke T, Schmitz A, Risse JH, et al. Fluorine-18 fluorodeoxyglucose PET in infectious bone diseases: results of histologically confirmed cases. Eur J Nucl Med 2000;27(5):524–8.
53. Schiesser M, Stumpe KD, Trentz O, et al. Detection of metallic implant-associated infections with FDG PET in patients with trauma: correlation with microbiologic results. Radiology 2003;226(2):391–8.
54. Schmitz A, Risse JH, Grunwald F, et al. Fluorine-18 fluorodeoxyglucose positron emission tomography findings in spondylodiscitis: preliminary results. Eur Spine J 2001;10(6):534–9.
55. Hartmann A, Eid K, Dora C, et al. Diagnostic value of 18F-FDG PET/CT in trauma patients with suspected chronic osteomyelitis. Eur J Nucl Med Mol Imaging 2007;34(5):704–14.
56. Kim SJ, Lee JS, Suh KT, et al. Differentiation of tuberculous and pyogenic spondylitis using double phase F-18 FDG PET. Open Med Imaging J 2008;2:6.
57. Fuster D, Sola O, Soriano A, et al. A prospective study comparing whole-body FDG PET/CT to combined planar bone scan with 67Ga SPECT/CT in the diagnosis of spondylodiskitis. Clin Nucl Med 2012;37(9):827–32.
58. Seifen T, Rettenbacher L, Thaler C, et al. Prolonged back pain attributed to suspected spondylodiscitis. The value of (1)(8)F-FDG PET/CT imaging in the diagnostic work-up of patients. Nuklearmedizin 2012;51(5):194–200.
59. Prodromou ML, Ziakas PD, Poulou LS, et al. FDG PET is a robust tool for the diagnosis of spondylodiscitis: a meta-analysis of diagnostic data. Clin Nucl Med 2014;39(4):330–5.
60. Rosen RS, Fayad L, Wahl RL. Increased 18F-FDG uptake in degenerative disease of the spine: characterization with 18F-FDG PET/CT. J Nucl Med 2006;47(8):1274–80.
61. Nanni C, Boriani L, Salvadori C, et al. FDG PET/CT is useful for the interim evaluation of response to therapy in patients affected by haematogenous spondylodiscitis. Eur J Nucl Med Mol Imaging 2012;39(10):1538–44.
62. Palestro CJ, Roumanas P, Swyer AJ, et al. Diagnosis of musculoskeletal infection using combined

In-111 labeled leukocyte and Tc-99m SC marrow imaging. Clin Nucl Med 1992;17(4):269–73.

63. Basu S, Chryssikos T, Moghadam-Kia S, et al. Positron emission tomography as a diagnostic tool in infection: present role and future possibilities. Semin Nucl Med 2009;39(1):36–51.

64. Kwee TC, Kwee RM, Alavi A. FDG-PET for diagnosing prosthetic joint infection: systematic review and metaanalysis. Eur J Nucl Med Mol Imaging 2008;35(11):2122–32.

65. Chacko TK, Zhuang H, Stevenson K, et al. The importance of the location of fluorodeoxyglucose uptake in periprosthetic infection in painful hip prostheses. Nucl Med Commun 2002;23(9):851–5.

66. Uckay I, Gariani K, Pataky Z, et al. Diabetic foot infections: state-of-the-art. Diabetes Obes Metab 2013;16(4):305–16.

67. Hopfner S, Krolak C, Kessler S, et al. Preoperative imaging of Charcot neuroarthropathy in diabetic patients: comparison of ring PET, hybrid PET, and magnetic resonance imaging. Foot Ankle Int 2004;25(12):890–5.

68. Keidar Z, Militianu D, Melamed E, et al. The diabetic foot: initial experience with 18F-FDG PET/CT. J Nucl Med 2005;46(3):444–9.

69. Basu S, Chryssikos T, Houseni M, et al. Potential role of FDG PET in the setting of diabetic neuro-osteoarthropathy: can it differentiate uncomplicated Charcot's neuroarthropathy from osteomyelitis and soft-tissue infection? Nucl Med Commun 2007;28(6):465–72.

70. Schwegler B, Stumpe KD, Weishaupt D, et al. Unsuspected osteomyelitis is frequent in persistent diabetic foot ulcer and better diagnosed by MRI than by 18F-FDG PET or 99mTc-MOAB. J Intern Med 2008;263(1):99–106.

71. Nawaz A, Torigian DA, Siegelman ES, et al. Diagnostic performance of FDG-PET, MRI, and plain film radiography (PFR) for the diagnosis of osteomyelitis in the diabetic foot. Mol Imaging Biol 2010;12(3):335–42.

72. Familiari D, Glaudemans AW, Vitale V, et al. Can sequential 18F-FDG PET/CT replace WBC imaging in the diabetic foot? J Nucl Med 2011;52(7):1012–9.

73. Kagna O, Srour S, Melamed E, et al. FDG PET/CT imaging in the diagnosis of osteomyelitis in the diabetic foot. Eur J Nucl Med Mol Imaging 2012;39(10):1545–50.

74. Ruotolo V, Di Pietro B, Giurato L, et al. A new natural history of Charcot foot: clinical evolution and final outcome of stage 0 Charcot neuroarthropathy in a tertiary referral diabetic foot clinic. Clin Nucl Med 2013;38(7):506–9.

75. Seeger JM. Management of patients with prosthetic vascular graft infection. Am Surg 2000;66(2):166–77.

76. Swain TW 3rd, Calligaro KD, Dougherty MD. Management of infected aortic prosthetic grafts. Vasc Endovascular Surg 2004;38(1):75–82.

77. Orton DF, LeVeen RF, Saigh JA, et al. Aortic prosthetic graft infections: radiologic manifestations and implications for management. Radiographics 2000;20(4):977–93.

78. Fukuchi K, Ishida Y, Higashi M, et al. Detection of aortic graft infection by fluorodeoxyglucose positron emission tomography: comparison with computed tomographic findings. J Vasc Surg 2005;42(5):919–25.

79. Keidar Z, Engel A, Hoffman A, et al. Prosthetic vascular graft infection: the role of 18F-FDG PET/CT. J Nucl Med 2007;48(8):1230–6.

80. Spacek M, Belohlavek O, Votrubova J, et al. Diagnostics of "on-acute" vascular prosthesis infection using 18F-FDG PET/CT: our experience with 96 prostheses. Eur J Nucl Med Mol Imaging 2009;36(5):850–8.

81. Bruggink JL, Glaudemans AW, Saleem BR, et al. Accuracy of FDG-PET-CT in the diagnostic work-up of vascular prosthetic graft infection. Eur J Vasc Endovasc Surg 2010;40(3):348–54.

82. Krupnick AS. 81-Fluorodeoxyglucose positron emission tomography as a novel imaging tool for the diagnosis of aortoenteric fistula and aortic graft infection: a case report. Vasc Endovascular Surg 2003;37(5):363–6.

83. Blockmans D, de Ceuninck L, Vanderschueren S, et al. Repetitive 18F-fluorodeoxyglucose positron emission tomography in giant cell arteritis: a prospective study of 35 patients. Arthritis Rheum 2006;55(1):131–7.

84. Bleeker-Rovers CP, Bredie SJ, van der Meer JW, et al. F-18-fluorodeoxyglucose positron emission tomography in diagnosis and follow-up of patients with different types of vasculitis. Neth J Med 2003;61(10):323–9.

85. Zerizer I, Tan K, Khan S, et al. Role of FDG-PET and PET/CT in the diagnosis and management of vasculitis. Eur J Radiol 2010;73(3):504–9.

86. Basu S, Zhuang H, Torigian DA, et al. Functional imaging of inflammatory diseases using nuclear medicine techniques. Semin Nucl Med 2009;39(2):124–45.

87. Walter MA, Melzer RA, Schindler C, et al. The value of [18F]FDG-PET in the diagnosis of large-vessel vasculitis and the assessment of activity and extent of disease. Eur J Nucl Med Mol Imaging 2005;32(6):674–81.

88. Treglia G, Mattoli MV, Leccisotti L, et al. Usefulness of whole-body fluorine-18-fluorodeoxyglucose positron emission tomography in patients with large-vessel vasculitis: a systematic review. Clin Rheumatol 2011;30(10):1265–75.

89. Lee KH, Cho A, Choi YJ, et al. The role of (18) F-fluorodeoxyglucose-positron emission tomography in

the assessment of disease activity in patients with Takayasu arteritis. Arthritis Rheum 2012;64(3): 866–75.

90. Webb M, Chambers A, AL-Nahhas A, et al. The role of 18F-FDG PET in characterising disease activity in Takayasu arteritis. Eur J Nucl Med Mol Imaging 2004;31(5):627–34.

91. Treglia G, Taralli S, Giordano A. Emerging role of whole-body 18F-fluorodeoxyglucose positron emission tomography as a marker of disease activity in patients with sarcoidosis: a systematic review. Sarcoidosis Vasc Diffuse Lung Dis 2011; 28(2):87–94.

92. Rubini G, Cappabianca S, Altini C, et al. Current clinical use of FDG-PET/CT in patients with thoracic and systemic sarcoidosis. Radiol Med 2014; 119(1):64–74.

93. Ambrosini V, Zompatori M, Fasano L, et al. (18) F-FDG PET/CT for the assessment of disease extension and activity in patients with sarcoidosis: results of a preliminary prospective study. Clin Nucl Med 2013;38(4):e171–7.

94. Keijsers RG, van den Heuvel DA, Grutters JC. Imaging the inflammatory activity of sarcoidosis. Eur Respir J 2013;41(3):743–51.

95. Teirstein AS, Machac J, Almeida O, et al. Results of 188 whole-body fluorodeoxyglucose positron emission tomography scans in 137 patients with sarcoidosis. Chest 2007;132(6):1949–53.

96. Valeyre D, Prasse A, Nunes H, et al. Sarcoidosis. Lancet 2014;383(9923):1155–67.

97. Glaudemans AW, de Vries EF, Galli F, et al. The use of (18)F-FDG-PET/CT for diagnosis and treatment monitoring of inflammatory and infectious diseases. Clin Dev Immunol 2013;2013:623036.

98. Keijsers RG, Verzijlbergen EJ, van den Bosch JM, et al. 18F-FDG PET as a predictor of pulmonary function in sarcoidosis. Sarcoidosis Vasc Diffuse Lung Dis 2011;28(2):123–9.

99. Sobic-Saranovic D, Grozdic I, Videnovic-Ivanov J, et al. The utility of 18F-FDG PET/CT for diagnosis and adjustment of therapy in patients with active chronic sarcoidosis. J Nucl Med 2012;53(10): 1543–9.

100. Sobic-Saranovic DP, Grozdic IT, Videnovic-Ivanov J, et al. Responsiveness of FDG PET/CT to treatment of patients with active chronic sarcoidosis. Clin Nucl Med 2013;38(7):516–21.

101. Mostard RL, Voo S, van Kroonenburgh MJ, et al. Inflammatory activity assessment by F18 FDG-PET/ CT in persistent symptomatic sarcoidosis. Respir Med 2011;105(12):1917–24.

102. Youssef G, Leung E, Mylonas I, et al. The use of 18F-FDG PET in the diagnosis of cardiac sarcoidosis: a systematic review and metaanalysis including the Ontario experience. J Nucl Med 2012;53(2):241–8.

103. Ohira H, Tsujino I, Yoshinaga K. (1)(8)F-Fluoro-2-deoxyglucose positron emission tomography in cardiac sarcoidosis. Eur J Nucl Med Mol Imaging 2011;38(9):1773–83.

104. Skali H, Schulman AR, Dorbala S. 18F-FDG PET/CT for the assessment of myocardial sarcoidosis. Curr Cardiol Rep 2013;15(4):352.

105. Segal BM. Neurosarcoidosis: diagnostic approaches and therapeutic strategies. Curr Opin Neurol 2013;26(3):307–13.

106. Sakushima K, Yabe I, Shiga T, et al. FDG-PET SUV can distinguish between spinal sarcoidosis and myelopathy with canal stenosis. J Neurol 2011; 258(2):227–30.

107. Perlman SB, Hall BS, Reichelderfer M. PET/CT imaging of inflammatory bowel disease. Semin Nucl Med 2013;43(6):420–6.

108. Bicik I, Bauerfeind P, Breitbach T, et al. Inflammatory bowel disease activity measured by positron-emission tomography. Lancet 1997;350(9073):262.

109. Neurath MF, Vehling D, Schunk K, et al. Noninvasive assessment of Crohn's disease activity: a comparison of 18F-fluorodeoxyglucose positron emission tomography, hydromagnetic resonance imaging, and granulocyte scintigraphy with labeled antibodies. Am J Gastroenterol 2002;97(8):1978–85.

110. Treglia G, Quartuccio N, Sadeghi R, et al. Diagnostic performance of fluorine-18-fluorodeoxyglucose positron emission tomography in patients with chronic inflammatory bowel disease: a systematic review and a meta-analysis. J Crohns Colitis 2013; 7(5):345–54.

111. Lenze F, Wessling J, Bremer J, et al. Detection and differentiation of inflammatory versus fibromatous Crohn's disease strictures: prospective comparison of 18F-FDG-PET/CT, MR-enteroclysis, and transabdominal ultrasound versus endoscopic/histologic evaluation. Inflamm Bowel Dis 2012;18(12): 2252–60.

112. Jacene HA, Ginsburg P, Kwon J, et al. Prediction of the need for surgical intervention in obstructive Crohn's disease by 18F-FDG PET/CT. J Nucl Med 2009;50(11):1751–9.

113. Lapp RT, Spier BJ, Perlman SB, et al. Clinical utility of positron emission tomography/computed tomography in inflammatory bowel disease. Mol Imaging Biol 2011;13(3):573–6.

114. Groshar D, Bernstine H, Stern D, et al. PET/CT enterography in Crohn disease: correlation of disease activity on CT enterography with 18F-FDG uptake. J Nucl Med 2010;51(7):1009–14.

115. Das CJ, Makharia G, Kumar R, et al. PET-CT enteroclysis: a new technique for evaluation of inflammatory diseases of the intestine. Eur J Nucl Med Mol Imaging 2007;34(12):2106–14.

116. Das CJ, Makharia GK, Kumar R, et al. PET/CT colonography: a novel non-invasive technique for

assessment of extent and activity of ulcerative colitis. Eur J Nucl Med Mol Imaging 2010;37(4):714–21.

117. Bettenworth D, Reuter S, Hermann S, et al. Translational 18F-FDG PET/CT imaging to monitor lesion activity in intestinal inflammation. J Nucl Med 2013;54(5):748–55.

118. Meisner RS, Spier BJ, Einarsson S, et al. Pilot study using PET/CT as a novel, noninvasive assessment of disease activity in inflammatory bowel disease. Inflamm Bowel Dis 2007;13(8):993–1000.

119. Louis E, Ancion G, Colard A, et al. Noninvasive assessment of Crohn's disease intestinal lesions with (18)F-FDG PET/CT. J Nucl Med 2007;48(7):1053–9.

120. Spier BJ, Perlman SB, Jaskowiak CJ, et al. PET/CT in the evaluation of inflammatory bowel disease: studies in patients before and after treatment. Mol Imaging Biol 2010;12(1):85–8.

121. Malham MH, Nielse RG, Husby S, et al. PET/CT in the diagnosis of inflammatory bowel disease in pediatric patients: a review. Am J Nucl Med Mol Imaging 2014;4(3):225–30.

122. Bockisch A, Freudenberg LS, Schmidt D, et al. Hybrid imaging by SPECT/CT and PET/CT: proven outcomes in cancer imaging. Semin Nucl Med 2009;39(4):276–89.

123. Czernin J, Allen-Auerbach M, Schelbert HR. Improvements in cancer staging with PET/CT: literature-based evidence as of 2006. J Nucl Med 2007;48(Suppl 1):78S–88S.

124. Facey K, Bradbury I, Laking G, et al. Overview of the clinical effectiveness of positron emission tomography imaging in selected cancers. Health Technol Assess 2007;11(44):iii–iv. xi-267.

125. Histed SN, Lindenberg ML, Mena E, et al. Review of functional/anatomical imaging in oncology. Nucl Med Commun 2012;33(4):349–61.

126. Saboury B, Salavati A, Brothers A, et al. FDG PET/CT in Crohn's disease: correlation of quantitative FDG PET/CT parameters with clinical and endoscopic surrogate markers of disease activity. Eur J Nucl Med Mol Imaging 2014;41(4):605–14.

127. Yun M, Kim W, Adam LE, et al. F-18 FDG uptake in a patient with psoriatic arthritis: imaging correlation with patient symptoms. Clin Nucl Med 2001;26(8):692–3.

128. Takata T, Taniguchi Y, Ohnishi T, et al. (18)FDG PET/CT is a powerful tool for detecting subclinical arthritis in patients with psoriatic arthritis and/or psoriasis vulgaris. J Dermatol Sci 2011;64(2):144–7.

129. Harris ED Jr. Rheumatoid arthritis. Pathophysiology and implications for therapy. N Engl J Med 1990;322(18):1277–89.

130. Carey K, Saboury B, Basu S, et al. Evolving role of FDG PET imaging in assessing joint disorders: a systematic review. Eur J Nucl Med Mol Imaging 2011;38(10):1939–55.

131. Beckers C, Ribbens C, Andre B, et al. Assessment of disease activity in rheumatoid arthritis with (18)F-FDG PET. J Nucl Med 2004;45(6):956–64.

132. Sarma M, Vijayant V, Basu S. (18)F-FDG-PET assessment of early treatment response of articular and extra-articular foci in newly diagnosed rheumatoid arthritis. Hell J Nucl Med 2012;15(1):70–1.

133. Vijayant V, Sarma M, Aurangabadkar H, et al. Potential of (18)F-FDG-PET as a valuable adjunct to clinical and response assessment in rheumatoid arthritis and seronegative spondyloarthropathies. World J Radiol 2012;4(12):462–8.

134. Basu S, Shejul Y. Regional lymph node hypermetabolism corresponding to the involved joints on FDG-PET in newly diagnosed patients of rheumatoid arthritis: observation and illustration in symmetrical and asymmetric joint involvement. Rheumatol Int 2014;34(3):413–5.

135. Roivainen A, Hautaniemi S, Mottonen T, et al. Correlation of 18F-FDG PET/CT assessments with disease activity and markers of inflammation in patients with early rheumatoid arthritis following the initiation of combination therapy with triple oral antirheumatic drugs. Eur J Nucl Med Mol Imaging 2013;40(3):403–10.

136. Okamura K, Yonemoto Y, Arisaka Y, et al. The assessment of biologic treatment in patients with rheumatoid arthritis using FDG-PET/CT. Rheumatology 2012;51(8):1484–91.

137. Mehta NN, Yu Y, Saboury B, et al. Systemic and vascular inflammation in patients with moderate to severe psoriasis as measured by [18F]-fluorodeoxyglucose positron emission tomography-computed tomography (FDG-PET/CT): a pilot study. Arch Dermatol 2011;147(9):1031–9.

138. Rose S, Sheth NH, Baker JF, et al. A comparison of vascular inflammation in psoriasis, rheumatoid arthritis, and healthy subjects by FDG-PET/CT: a pilot study. Am J Cardiovasc Dis 2013;3(4):273–8.

139. Gelfand JM, Neimann AL, Shin DB, et al. Risk of myocardial infarction in patients with psoriasis. JAMA 2006;296(14):1735–41.

140. Roman MJ, Salmon JE. Cardiovascular manifestations of rheumatologic diseases. Circulation 2007;116(20):2346–55.

141. Bissonnette R, Tardif JC, Harel F, et al. Effects of the tumor necrosis factor-alpha antagonist adalimumab on arterial inflammation assessed by positron emission tomography in patients with psoriasis: results of a randomized controlled trial. Circ Cardiovasc Imaging 2013;6(1):83–90.

142. Madsen PH, Hess S, Hoilund-Carlsen PF, et al. Positron emission tomography in chronic obstructive pulmonary disease. Hell J Nucl Med 2013;16(2):121–4.

143. Jones HA, Marino PS, Shakur BH, et al. In vivo assessment of lung inflammatory cell activity in

patients with COPD and asthma. Eur Respir J 2003;21(4):567–73.

144. Subramanian DR, Jenkins L, Edgar R, et al. Assessment of pulmonary neutrophilic inflammation in emphysema by quantitative positron emission tomography. Am J Respir Crit Care Med 2012;186(11):1125–32.

145. Coulson JM, Rudd JH, Duckers JM, et al. Excessive aortic inflammation in chronic obstructive pulmonary disease: an 18F-FDG PET pilot study. J Nucl Med 2010;51(9):1357–60.

146. Basu S, Alzeair S, Li G, et al. Etiopathologies associated with intercostal muscle hypermetabolism and prominent right ventricle visualization on 2-deoxy-2[F-18]fluoro-D-glucose-positron emission tomography: significance of an incidental finding and in the setting of a known pulmonary disease. Mol Imaging Biol 2007;9(6):333–9.

147. Aydin A, Hickeson M, Yu JQ, et al. Demonstration of excessive metabolic activity of thoracic and abdominal muscles on FDG-PET in patients with chronic obstructive pulmonary disease. Clin Nucl Med 2005;30(3):159–64.

148. Osman MM, Tran IT, Muzaffar R, et al. Does ^{18}F-FDG uptake by respiratory muscles on PET/CT correlate with chronic obstructive pulmonary disease? J Nucl Med Technol 2011;39(4):252–7.

149. Torigian DA, Dam V, Chen X, et al. In vivo quantification of pulmonary inflammation in relation to emphysema severity via partial volume corrected (18)F-FDG-PET using computer-assisted analysis of diagnostic chest CT. Hell J Nucl Med 2013;16(1):12–8.

150. Hess S, Madsen PH, Basu S, et al. Potential role of FDG PET/CT imaging for assessing venous thromboembolic disorders. Clin Nucl Med 2012;37(12):1170–2.

151. Hess S, Madsen PH, Iversen ED, et al. Efficacy of FDG-PET/CT imaging for venous thromboembolic disorders: preliminary results from a prospective, observational pilot study. Clin Nucl Med 2014. [Epub ahead of print].

152. Rondina MT, Lam UT, Pendleton RC, et al. (18)F-FDG PET in the evaluation of acuity of deep vein thrombosis. Clin Nucl Med 2012;37(12):1139–45.

153. Rondina MT, Wanner N, Pendleton RC, et al. A pilot study utilizing whole body 18 F-FDG-PET/CT as a comprehensive screening strategy for occult malignancy in patients with unprovoked venous thromboembolism. Thromb Res 2012;129(1):22–7.

154. Hunziker P. "Knowledge-based (personalized) medicine" instead of "evidence-based (cohort) medicine". Eur J Nanomed 2012;4(1):5–6.

155. Skehan SJ, Issenman R, Mernagh J, et al. 18F-fluorodeoxyglucose positron tomography in diagnosis of paediatric inflammatory bowel disease. Lancet 1999;354:836–7.

156. Lemberg DA, Issenman RM, Cawdron R, et al. Positron emission tomography in the investigation of pediatric inflammatory bowel disease. Inflamm Bowel Dis 2005;11:733–8.

157. Loffler M, Weckesser M, Franzius C, et al. High diagnostic value of 18F-FDG-PET in pediatric patients with chronic inflammatory bowel disease. Ann N Y Acad Sci 2006;1072:379–85.

158. Dabritz J, Jasper N, Loeffler M, et al. Noninvasive assessment of pediatric inflammatory bowel disease with 18-F-fluorodeoxyglucose-positron emission tomography and computed tomography. Eur J Gastroenterol Hepatol 2011;23(1):81–9.

159. Berthold LD, Steiner D, Scholz D, et al. Imaging of chronic inflammatory bowel disease with 18F-FDG PET in children and adolescents. Klin Padiatr 2013;225:212–7.

Index

Note: Page numbers of article titles are in **boldface** type.

PET Clin 9 (2014) 521–524
http://dx.doi.org/10.1016/S1556-8598(14)00084-4
1556-8598/14/$ – see front matter © 2014 Elsevier Inc. All rights reserved.

pet.theclinics.com

Printed and bound by CPI Group (UK) Ltd, Croydon, CR0 4YY

03/10/2024

01040379-0016